T0390951

I TATTI STUDIES IN
ITALIAN RENAISSANCE HISTORY

Published in collaboration with I Tatti
The Harvard University Center for Italian Renaissance Studies
Florence, Italy

GENERAL EDITOR
Nicholas Terpstra

ADVISORY COMMITTEE
Nicholas Scott Baker
Giorgio Caravale
Eric Dursteler
Paula Findlen
Cécile Fromont
Tamar Herzig
Mary Laven
Katherine Park
Sarah Gwyneth Ross
Kaya Şahin
Francesca Trivellato

THE STATE DRUG

*Theriac, Pharmacy, and Politics
in Early Modern Italy*

BARBARA DI GENNARO SPLENDORE

Harvard University Press

Cambridge, Massachusetts
London, England
2025

Copyright © 2025 by the President and Fellows of Harvard College
All rights reserved
Printed in the United States of America

First printing

Library of Congress Cataloging-in-Publication Data

Names: Di Gennaro Splendore, Barbara, 1971– author.
Title: The state drug : theriac, pharmacy, and politics in early modern
   Italy / Barbara Di Gennaro Splendore.
Other titles: I Tatti studies in Italian Renaissance history.
Description: Cambridge, Massachusetts : Harvard University Press, 2025. |
   Series: I Tatti studies in Italian Renaissance history | Includes bibliographical
   references and index.
Identifiers: LCCN 2024049803 | ISBN 9780674299788 (cloth)
Subjects: LCSH: Public health—Italy—History. | Pharmaceutical policy—Italy—History. |
   Antidotes—History. | Materia medica—Italy—History. | Medicine—Formulae, receipts,
   prescriptions—History.
Classification: LCC RS67.I8 D5 2025 | DDC 362.10945/0903—dc23/eng/20250218
LC record available at https://lccn.loc.gov/2024049803

*To Antonio, Neri, and Mira,
with love and gratitude*

CONTENTS

NOTE ON CONVENTIONS *ix*

Introduction *1*

I EARLY HISTORY AND SENSORY EXPERIENCE OF THERIAC

1 The Reinvention of Theriac *19*

2 The Experience of Theriac *50*

II PHARMACY AND STATECRAFT

3 Imperial Antidotes for Renaissance Rulers *87*

4 A Public Health Measure against Poison and Plague *112*

5 Theriaca Magna on the Marketplace *145*

6 A Preservative of the Social Order *175*

III PARADOXES OF SUCCESS

7 From "Antidote of All Antidotes" to Pharmaceutical Monster *201*

Conclusion *231*

ABBREVIATIONS *245*

NOTES *247*

BIBLIOGRAPHY *283*

ACKNOWLEDGMENTS *321*

INDEX *325*

NOTE ON CONVENTIONS

Weights and measures differed greatly from city to city in early modern Europe. At least nominally, *apothecary* measures for medicaments were similar:

1 pound = 12 ounces
1 ounce = 8 drachms
1 drachm = 3 scruples
1 scruple = 24 grains

However, the value of these measures changed from place to place, for example, 1 medicinal pound in Venice (*libra sottile*) = 302.229 grams, while in Bologna 1 medicinal pound = 325.665 grams. The fundamental reference for measures and currencies in early modern Italy is still Angelo Martini, *Manuale di metrologia ossia Misure pesi e monete in uso attualmente e presso tutti i popoli* (Turin: Loescher, 1883), to which I also refer the reader.

For *dates* I consulted Adriano Cappelli, *Cronologia e calendario perpetuo: Tavole chronografiche e quadri sinottici* (Milan: Ulrico Hoepli, 1930). In Italy, the beginning of the new year also differed greatly from city to city. For example, in Venice until 1797 the year began on March 1 (*more Veneto*). In Rome, while private citizens started the year on December 25, each pope adopted a different solution for official documents. In Florence until 1751, the new year began on March 25, the feast of the Annunciation. I chose to leave dates as indicated in the original documents, except when this led to confusion, in which case this is made clear to the reader in the endnotes.

The majority of Latin and non-English names of plants and animals given in the texts and notes are those used by Renaissance naturalists and in pharmacopoeias. It is not always possible to determine the Linnean equivalent of any given sixteenth-century name, but I did so when useful (or indeed possible).

Historical names and titles of books are given in their original language. The translation has been added to clarify meaning when necessary.

THE STATE DRUG

But I don't understand. Where did they draw the treacle from?
Lewis Carroll, *Alice in Wonderland*

Introduction

*A*NTOINE THOMAS (1644–1709) was a Jesuit mathematician who spent more than twenty years at the imperial court of China, where he was known as An Duo. In a memorial, a Chinese official informed the emperor Kangxi (r. 1662–1722) that in 1709 Thomas had become very sick. He was visited by court physician Ru Huang, who reported: "[Because] An Duo's illness is very serious, I now wish to request for deliyage [theriac] and to use it with a variable quantity of Lizhong tang for medical treatment."[1] Lizhong tang was a Chinese medicament, which Huang combined with non-Chinese theriac, a compound remedy containing about seventy plant, mineral, and animal-derived ingredients, including viper flesh and opium. Theriac was one of the most famous medicines of the Galenic tradition, the most widely adopted medical framework in Europe and the Middle East.

Emperor Kangxi and his court used theriac alongside Chinese medicines. The emperor even funded an ultimately unsuccessful expedition of Chinese and Western botanists, asking them to make theriac using ingredients sourced from the "nearby mountains."[2] The imperial court's adoption of theriac highlights the extent of the remedy's worldwide success in the early modern period. This episode also points to two essential characteristics of early modern theriac: its proximity to the state, and its use as a status symbol.

Theriac was in use since the first century CE, and over the course of two millennia it spread across four continents.[3] Its material constitution, as well as its long and complex textual transmission across languages and cultures, make for a history that is at helped local, regional, and global. According to tradition, theriac was an improvement on mithridate, an earlier antidote. These two medicines' histories are inextricably intertwined; throughout the centuries, though, physicians discussed theriac more often and generally considered it more effective than mithridate.[4] A dark and sticky substance usually taken dissolved in a liquid, theriac was primarily an antidote against venoms and poisons, although it was also prescribed to treat a wide variety of ailments, including the plague. Theriac comprised a fluid cornucopia of ingredients, elaborate but also unusually universal in an era when medicines were supposed to be specific to individual patients and not to diseases. Nevertheless, theriac was an emblem of Galenic pharmacy, a rich and long-lasting pharmaceutical tradition. Eighteenth-century physician William Heberden (1710–1801), author of *Antitheriaka: An Essay on Mithridatium and Theriaca* (1745), admitted against his better judgment that this now-forgotten remedy had enjoyed a "tryal of near two thousand years with a constant prepossession in its favor."[5]

Often referred to as an improbable "universal panacea," theriac and its history in the early modern period raise several questions.[6] Why did it last so long? What did people hope it would do for them? Why did theriac become especially relevant in the sixteenth to eighteenth centuries, and to whom was it important? How vast was its reach, both socially and geographically? When did its use decline, and why? In this book I trace the history of theriac from the 1490s to the end of the eighteenth century, with a focus on Italy. Although theriac had been known and revered for many centuries prior to the early modern period, it was during this era that theriac reached its maximum diffusion and relevance worldwide. Although theriac was never an exclusively Italian drug, I argue that the Italian Renaissance was a hinge moment in its history, leading to the pinnacle of theriac use and production in the seventeenth and eighteenth centuries, as well as to its global spread.

I make three interconnected arguments. First, I argue that the early modern Italian states were directly concerned with pharmacy as a fundamental part of their well-documented preoccupation with public health. Compared to other drugs, theriac offers an exceptional instance of how this concern developed through the early modern period. Because governments used both provisions of theriac in public health and public performances of its preparation to assert their legitimacy, theriac was a *state drug* during this time. Second, I argue that theriac was *socially effective*. Beyond and regardless of its biological effects, real or supposed, theriac affected the *social* body by helping to preserve the social order. Third, because of theriac's social effectiveness and political currency, its history in early modern Italy epitomizes the official role played by Galenic pharmacy during that era, which accounted for the persistence of this pharmaceutical tradition. The reputation theriac acquired in Italy advanced its spread and use, first across Europe, and subsequently in colonial settings, at the very time the medicament was being challenged in Europe as part of the reevaluation of all Galenic medicine during the late seventeenth and eighteenth centuries.

A State Drug

In the past, as today, medicines have embodied fluid meanings that patients, healers, producers, and legislators have both shared and contested. Drugs are powerful objects of inquiry, not only for historians but also, for anthropologists, sociologists, and philosophers.[7] Focusing on the eighteenth century, for example, Zachary Dorner has shown that English chemical medicines aided the expansion of the British Empire.[8] For the early modern world, Benjamin Breen has argued that drugs were a "key component of economic and social modernization," affirming that the "age of reason" was, in fact, an "age of intoxication." Breen has linked cultural histories of empire, the process of commodification, and the biological bases of drugs.[9] I follow this line of inquiry while drawing on the medieval, ancient, and Mediterranean roots of the interplay among drugs, economy, politics and medicine, demonstrating that theriac and mithridate were especially well connected to the early modern state.

In the early modern period, medical and political authorities needed to respond to widespread demand for both reliable cures and reliable defenses against enemies and myriad other threats—internal or external, real or imagined. Amid these calls, theriac transcended its pharmaceutical origins. While the term *theriac* had long connoted an antidote to anything threatening one's spiritual or physical health, the metaphor came to the fore during the early modern period: "theriac" now denoted anything that protected society not only from medical threats, such as plague, but also from nonmedical threats, such as war and heresy. The title of a political pamphlet published in 1590 unmistakably exemplifies the metaphor's reach: *Theriaque et anthidot prepare, pour chasser le venin, poison, ou peste, des Heretiques, Navaroois, et Athees Politiques de la France* (Theriac and antidote prepared to cast out the venom, poison, or plague of heretics, Navarres and political atheists of France).[10] Moreover, as we shall see, theriac now symbolized opposing forces: it was new, yet rooted in ancient texts; it revived tradition while incorporating the exotic; and it simultaneously offered hope and containment.

In the early modern states of Italy, medical theories, public health policies, and economic and social interests converged around theriac. By a "state drug" I mean a drug that the state leverages to realize its objectives and preserve the social order and hierarchy. However, theriac was not a state drug only in early modern Italy, nor was it the only state drug in history. This book illustrates that theriac's origin story—tied to King Mithradates, General Pompey, and Emperor Nero—inextricably tied the drug to state figures, and therefore was a perfect candidate to become a state drug during the early modern period. In other historical contexts, state drugs may assume different characteristics. For example, when vaccines are mandated for the population and those who refuse them are barred from accessing activities such as travel, education, and socializing, those vaccines may fairly be described as state drugs, too. Moreover, while theriac was arguably one of the most long-lived state drugs, it was not the most impactful in either biological or economic terms. That being said, I propose that theriac was a successful instance of symbiosis between drug and state, and served as a blueprint for state drugs to come.

Social order and *state* are terms fraught with both historical and philosophical meaning. By *social order* I refer to "a relatively persistent system of institutional regulations, hierarchical structures and beliefs, and patterns of conduct which guide both individual and group behavior and interactions and thereby support the reproduction of a social system."[11] By *state* I refer primarily to the structures of government. The historical definition of what constituted an early modern state is subject to much historical debate, and the Italian peninsula itself comprised a mosaic of states under a variety of systems of government. However, I imbue *state* with a comprehensive meaning, referring not only to governments but also to rulers, such as the pope and the Medicis; governing institutions, such as the Senate in Bologna and the Signoria and Collegio dei Savij in Venice; offices and administrations that directly reported to the highest political authorities, such as health boards; and institutions that came to act in lieu of the state in specific areas of intervention, such as medical colleges.

When addressing how the state was involved in medical practices and how it approached public health, historians have typically focused on control of the medical professions; the standardization of remedies through pharmacopoeias; preventive measures against the plague such as *cordons sanitaires*, quarantines, pest houses, and health passports; and the evolution of temporary health offices into permanent institutions.[12] These state interventions in the sphere of public health aimed to exert control, whether directly or indirectly, over bodies, objects, spaces, and practices. Conversely, theriac worked mainly through *hope*, not control. While other public measures closed borders to contain epidemics, theriac symbolically "opened" them by incorporating exotic ingredients. Moreover, theriac brought people together in a shared and reassuring ritual, the theriac-making public ceremony, a display of medical knowledge and apothecary craft. By ingesting theriac, patients incorporated what was necessary to keep poisons away, which was indeed a form of protection against (and closure to) danger coming from "outside." However, as we shall see, because theriac integrated both divine and earthly healing powers and resonated with people across the social spectrum, it instilled hope in large civic populations—which political and medical authorities then exploited to soothe anxieties. Drugs can acquire political and economic currency, even when they are unavailable on the market or their effects are subjected to scrutiny, simply by virtue of the hopes placed on resolutive therapies.

Venice and Bologna appear more than other Italian cities throughout this book because they offer two opposing but complementary declinations of the possible social meanings embodied by theriac. Furthermore, both cities offer rich documentary materials. Theriac's huge commercial success in Venice swayed state decisions on the composition of the drug, whereas decisions about theriac in Bologna were derived almost exclusively from medical determinations. Of course, divergent outcomes stem from distinct contexts: Venice was the center of a commercial empire, whereas Bologna was a rich university town and part of the Papal States. The cities' political structures were different, yet what made the difference in how the two handled theriac was not only their respective political setups but also their unique social, cultural, and economic organizations. I employ plenty of examples from other cities, including Rome, Florence, Naples, and Mantua, to show similarities and differences. Most importantly, although Venetian theriac was especially well known all over Europe, Venice itself played little part in shaping other cities' theriac cultures, even those cities under its political dominion such as Padua and Vicenza. In each of these cities, theriac followed a peculiar path. Theriac was a distinctly urban drug—but documenting its history in every one of Italy's early modern cities would have gone beyond my purposes in this work.

Social Effectiveness: Beyond Pharmaceutical Determinism

The efficacy of medicines is commonly defined in biological terms: Do they cure the diseases they are supposed to cure? However, if we understand medicines not just as medicines but also as symbols, commodities, and cultural artifacts, their biological effects are only one side of the story. I argue that theriac held transformative powers over the *social body,* and so in this book I explore its effectiveness in social, economic, and political terms, as well as biological.

This book contends that early modern theriac primarily acted as a preservative of the social order. A preservative is a transformative substance that prevents the spoilage and extends the life of organic matter. I also contend that theriac was neither a revolutionary nor a subversive drug. If theriac had narcotic power, it would have been incorporated into what Breen calls the "normative model of intoxication."[13] Nonetheless, during the sixteenth century theriac could influence social dynamics, as well as spur scientific research by renovating scholars' interest in *materia medica,* natural matter with medical properties.[14] Thus, in this case theriac also served as an agent of change and innovation, albeit for restricted groups and a limited time span.

Despite this, theriac mainly preserved the early modern hierarchy in the service of political authority. Such service was exemplified throughout this period by theriac's consistent association with men, and possibly high-ranking men. Kings, emperors, and prominent physicians are portrayed with theriac in images and stories. In fact, its intimate association with political authority and medical hierarchy is so consistent that, despite theriac's having acquired the moniker "queen of all medicaments," I could identify only one woman during this period who was linked to theriac: Camilla Erculiani, an ambitious apothecary from Padua.[15] It was only as theriac's prestige started to diminish toward the end of the eighteenth century that prints and journal articles began linking theriac to women, as well as to men from the lower classes and other continents. By the mid-eighteenth century, medical and political elites had slowly begun abandoning theriac as other medicaments came into vogue. Yet political and medical authorities ensured that its production continued to satiate the public's strong and unwavering appetite for the drug's "wonderous" quality, and they leveraged this appeasement to shore up their power during the nineteenth century. In 1803 the Austrian governor of Venice kept theriac alongside other traditional medicaments in the new pharmacopoeia to maintain social order. He suggested the guidelines to make a new pharmacopoeia: follow the example of notable pharmacopoeias—and "avoid the scandals deriving from ignorance and imposture, but one should not grieve men of good faith by putting out of use some medicaments protected by the blind faith of the plebs."[16] Thus, "ignorance and imposture" still had their place in official policies, including pharmacopoeias, provided they served to keep the population at bay. In this case and others, theriac's social effectiveness as a state drug outlived its perceived biological effectiveness.

This book is the next piece of research initiated by Erwin Ackerknecht's call for a history of therapeutics, and by the necessity of situating pharmacy in a broad context.[17] In the late 1970s, Charles Rosenberg argued that patients and physicians share a common framework, which involves a cognitive system of explanation, as well as social rituals.[18] The biological effects of drugs are not without consequence, as John Warner has shown, but they also do not necessarily "work" in the way we think they do.[19] Substances' biological and physical properties constitute part of the material world and historians must take them into account, while cautiously not using such properties as the sole *explanans*.[20]

Theriac's supposedly boundless capacity to treat a plethora of ailments, even the plague and venomous bites, is blatantly untenable by today's standards. To explain the durable popularity of this medicament, several historians have presupposed that theriac must have had therapeutic benefits, pointing to the opium it contained.[21] Michael Stein has argued that "from today's point of view, we attribute the effects of theriac primarily to opium."[22] Similarly, Christiane Nockels Fabbri has maintained that, above all, "the therapeutic effects of theriac . . . are explained by the pharmacokinetics of opium."[23] Indeed, I have found references to the narcotic effects of opium in theriac. Physician Bartolomeo Maranta (1500–1571), one of the highest early modern authorities on theriac, wrote that fresh theriac (no more than four years old) had narcotic powers because of the opium therein.[24] Nineteenth-century physicians complained that mothers employed in factories were adding theriac to their babies' polenta to keep them quiet at night.[25] It is important to note, though, that other sources do not mention any narcotic effect of theriac at all.

Meanwhile, for decades other historians have neglected the material and biological qualities of substances, contrary to biological explanations, to avoid anachronism (How can we actually know how substances affected bodies in the past?). While I share these historians' propensity for cultural explanations, the constraints and possibilities that materials present have an undeniable impact on historical events and processes. Nobody would go as far as to postulate that substances we consider biologically active today, such as opium, had no effect on early modern bodies. Therefore, the question of the biological effectiveness of theriac derived from opium requires careful examination.

Overall, I agree with those who believe that *if* theriac had significant physiological effects, they likely helped its persistence. However, I have two objections to the opium hypothesis. First, theriac was only one of several compound remedies used at the time that contained opium. Why then was theriac more popular than other drugs? Second, medicaments sold under the name *theriac* varied tremendously, and some "theriacs" were likely more "effective" than others, making it impossible to state the biological effects of "theriac."²⁶ When apothecaries followed an official recipe—official formulas used in different cities were remarkably similar—the final product was identifiable.²⁷ However, apothecaries in Venice let theriac age for three months; those in Bologna left it for twelve; and still others let it age for only one month. Early modern physicians believed fermentation neutralized the effects of opium. Accordingly, early modern legislation prohibited the sale or gifting of theriac that had not been fermented.²⁸ Of course, the necessity of these provisions implies that at least some producers sold theriac without fermenting it. As Jean-Pierre Bénézet and Jean Flahaut have noted, not all the theriac on the market was produced legally or according to set standards.²⁹ Moreover, theriac's shelf life spanned several decades, meaning the same theriac might have been more or less "active" depending on when it was ingested.

To understand the biological effects of theriac (or at least of official theriacs), we would need to reconstruct it and run the appropriate experiments in vitro and in vivo, which would be an expensive endeavor. Maranta held that the most important effects of theriac and mithridate developed after fermentation, when the powers of opium had been "weakened" and "broken."³⁰ Did fermentation create a new substance with different "powers" (virtues), as maintained by the preeminent philosopher Ibn Sīnā (latinized as Avicenna, 980–1037)? Biologists today cannot predict what molecules a fermented mixture may create, nor even say which among conflicting bonds will prevail. The possible biomedical effects of ancient remedies could be tested only through experimentation. We will never know the biomedical effects of early modern theriac on early modern patients. Substances affect different bodies in different ways, as early modern physicians and indeed patients well understood. Even if it were possible to prove the biomedical effects of a freshly prepared theriac, the ingredients used today would be different. Nonetheless, I hope such trials will take place in the near future, as there is much historians and biologists can learn through historical reconstructions.³¹

The Persistence of Galenic Pharmacy

Theriac's trajectory shows that the Galenic pharmaceutical tradition acquired the status of official pharmacy in many European states during the early modern period. I suggest that such status helps explain the longevity of Galenic pharmacy. In this sense, the history of theriac serves as a synecdoche, a part that represents the whole of Galenic pharmacy.

Within Galenic pharmacy, theriac and mithridate were universally recognized as the most powerful antidotes, glorified by generations of physicians and scholars. Ironically, neither was representative of the broad range of Galenic remedies, compounds made to respond to specific humoral imbalances. Galenic remedies helped reestablish the balance among the four humors (blood, phlegm, yellow bile, and black bile), curing the individual and not targeting a disease. In contrast with the general tenets of Galenic pharmacy, theriac and mithridate were ready-made medicines, similar for all patients, and contained ingredients with opposing qualities. But by virtue of their extraordinariness, and because of the status they enjoyed, they reveal more about Galenic pharmacy in early modern society than any other remedy.

From the first century CE to the nineteenth century, Galenic pharmacy dominated pharmaceutical theory and practice across most of Europe and the Middle East. Derived from the writings of Galen of Pergamon (ca. 130–210 CE), Galenic pharmacy was an integral part of Galenic medicine, one of the most durable and widespread medical systems in history.[32] Pagan, Christian, Jewish, and Muslim authors kept alive and contributed to this veritable multicultural tradition, which is sometimes wrongly defined as "Western."[33] In early modern Italy and in many European regions, pharmacy was primarily practiced domestically, especially by women. Local pharmaceutical lore was often strongly rooted, yet the influence of Galenic pharmacy was paramount. But Galenic pharmacy faced fundamental challenges, especially during the early modern period, such as internal revision, the arrival of new materia medica, and the rising popularity of alchemical pharmacy.

New trade routes opening across the globe led to previously unknown plants, animals, and diseases arriving in Eurasia. This raised questions about the natural world and the possibility of novel cures and economic prospects, generating excitement among scholars and physicians as well as merchants and trading companies.[34] In most of Europe, demand for *exotica* grew consistently, triggering debates about remedies specific to one disease, such as guaiacum wood for syphilis.[35] In parallel, humanists put ancient texts under philological scrutiny in an attempt to retrieve knowledge lost during what they called the "Dark Ages." At a time when the word *reform* was applied to many fields of life and learning, several scholars advocated for "reforming" materia medica.[36] Such revision had profound consequences on the methods of producing natural knowledge, as well as on pharmacy.

While apothecaries and physicians researched materia medica from other continents, alchemical procedures were rising in popularity. Like Galenic pharmacy, alchemy was a tradition shared across Europe and the Mediterranean. Historians long attributed the introduction of alchemical pharmacy into Europe to the theories of the Swiss physician Paracelsus (1493–1541), but Galenic and alchemic pharmacy had actually already existed in tandem for several centuries.[37] Numerous alchemical preparations, such as distilled waters, entered common apothecary use in the late Middle Ages. In the early modern period, the growth of alchemical pharmacy was accompanied by bitter controversies between Paracelsians and their detractors. The weight of such controversies should not be exaggerated, however. Even in Germany, the homeland of alchemical medicine, physicians scrutinized Paracelsian texts to extract what was compatible with Galenic pharmacy.[38] Remedy sellers, charlatans, and healers inundated the market with secrets and patent medicines. But charlatans usually collaborated with apothecaries, and alchemical secret remedies were often indistinguishable from Galenic remedies.[39] The two pharmaceutical traditions eventually merged, but historians have yet to consider how Galenic pharmacy was affected by the rise of alchemy.[40] Regardless, Galenic pharmacy survived internal revision, incorporated foreign materia medica, blended with alchemy, and prospered throughout the early modern period.

The longevity of Galenic pharmacy is puzzling and yet underexplored. Historian Owsei Temkin dedicated only a few pages to Galenic pharmacy in his pathbreaking book on Galenism, which for decades remained the most comprehensive account on the topic. According to Temkin, Galenic pharmacology "offered a blend of the rational and experiential," a mixture that "gave the appearance of reliable knowledge." However, he continued, "judged by our standards, the majority of drugs in Galen's materia medica did not have the curative effects ascribed to them." To explain why Galenic pharmacology persisted so much longer than Galenic anatomy despite its lack of curative abilities, Temkin argued that a "different sense of reality" led people to believe in "revealed authority" over "empirical verification."[41] Temkin's cultural explanation is no longer tenable today.

Interdisciplinary teams of scholars and scientists have proven that researching traditional pharmaceutical practices can shed light on efficacious cures.[42] According to present standards, even some unexpected remedies in these traditions have been proven biologically effective. Although research on ancient remedies is not yet fully developed, it is attracting increasing attention. On their part, historians lack a full explanation of why Galenic pharmacy persisted for so many centuries. Paula De Vos has argued that "malleability" and "flexibility" were defining characteristics of Galenic pharmacy because of its multicultural history.[43] Others have argued that the Galenic system was able to incorporate novelties intrinsic to its theoretical framework, and in particular to "substitution," which posited that different medical materials (matters) could possess qualities in similar degrees (hot, humid, dry, and cold), and were therefore interchangeable. Through substitution, practitioners of pharmacy could incorporate fresh materia medica from their own region, instead of using the Mediterranean plants mostly listed in classical texts. Furthermore, once they were outside Europe, they could adapt the recipes using different ingredients.[44]

Inclusiveness, flexibility, and substitution were crucial factors contributing to the persistence of Galenic pharmacy, but they do not fully account for the resilience of this tradition in Europe and its global success. By considering the official status of Galenic pharmacy—that is, its direct connection to the political and medical structures of the ancien régime—we gain a more complete understanding of why this pharmaceutical tradition endured for so long. The main tradition of pharmacy since antiquity, Galenic pharmacy became the official pharmacy in the Italian states, and a similar process happened in other European polities. For example, physicians in sixteenth-century Nuremberg were able to establish a new order of medicine based squarely on Galenic pharmacy.[45] The history of theriac in early modern Italy exemplifies the process through which Galenic pharmacy became a fundamental reference point for rulers and political and medical authorities. In the early modern global age, Galenic pharmacy was the pharmacy of conquerors and missionaries; it was therefore associated with political, economic, and cultural authority, and thus gained an edge over other medical systems. Exporting Galenic phar-

·

macy constituted part of European colonization.⁴⁶ Once abroad, Galenic pharmacy was challenged and transformed as it encountered different cultures and environments, and so was theriac. However, the adoption of theriac at the Chinese imperial court shows that the ability of Galenic pharmacy to enter other cultures and medical systems rested, at least in part, on its prestige, not just on colonial domination or violence.

Organization of the Book

Like any other drug, theriac was at once a commodity, a medicinal substance, and an object of scientific inquiry. Previous literature on theriac often shifted from one aspect of the drug to another without a robust analytical structure. Only by first isolating each different perspective and then recombining them has it been possible to reconstruct a comprehensive understanding of its history. This multifaceted approach, which required me to blend a variety of disparate sources—quantitative and qualitative, as well as micro and macro scales of analysis—has illuminated and enriched the subject. Integrating these varied materials and analyses was not without its challenges, particularly in terms of organization and narrative cohesion. Nonetheless, these obstacles presented me with opportunities for creative structuring. While the chapters follow a broadly chronological order, there are exceptions. Chapter 2 has a distinct focus on the materiality of theriac, privileging a thematic approach; Chapter 5 delves into theriac's economic history. Chapter 6 is structured around two case studies, adopting a microhistorical analysis in one section for a more specific exploration of Venetian political economy.

The book is divided into three parts. Part I presents an overview of what theriac was, and how it emerged and developed. Chapter 1 revises the refashioning of theriac into "true theriac" during the sixteenth century. This process, initiated by a dispute in Venice in the 1490s and concluded in the 1570s, involved a community of physicians, collectors, and apothecaries reviving a tradition of prestigious pedigree that had fallen into disrepute. Unlike previous analyses, in this chapter I examine the reformation of theriac within the context of its medical, economic, institutional, and commercial frameworks. I explore physicians' understanding of the functioning of theriac; the *types* of theriac actually accessible to patients on the market; the legal procedures governing their distribution; and the key institutions pivotal to theriac's history during the early modern period, such as medical colleges and apothecary guilds. The export of Venetian theriac all across Europe earned it the status of a renowned brand. This recognition necessitated early involvement from the Venetian state in theriac-related affairs. Against this backdrop, the evolution of theriac science unfolded as a continual negotiation between the realms of scholarship and production, carrying significant social, institutional, and intellectual implications. During the reformation of theriac, a select group of apothecaries notably transformed themselves into an elite of "learned apothecaries."

Chapter 2 departs from the chronological narrative to explore the sensory qualities of theriac: its taste, aroma, and texture, and even its auditory qualities, along with its intricate production process. Theriac existed not just as a medicinal substance but also as a tangible object, experienced both by patients when taking it and by apothecaries during its meticulous preparation. Through a rare trial assessing the quality of theriac available on the market, I gained precious insights into the sensory knowledge possessed by apothecaries, which further contextualized the language used by physicians and apothecaries to describe their products. Moreover, the chapter delves into the composition of the theriac recipe, which was one of history's most debated formulations despite never having actually been kept secret. The final sections of the chapter examine two significant aspects of theriac's most iconic ingredient—viper—whose incorporation imbued the medicine with religious symbolism. Early modern patients revered this spiritual dimension of theriac's medicinal efficacy, whose endorsement by the state only elevated its stature further. Lastly, the chapter investigates the environmental ramifications of large-scale theriac production, shedding light on the broader impacts of its manufacture.

Part II expands on what it means to describe theriac as a state drug in the early modern period. Chapter 3 builds on the discussion introduced in Chapter 1, shifting the focus from Venice to other Italian cities to investigate the allure that the concept of "true theriac" held for rulers and court physicians. The chapter first analyzes the origin tale of theriac, involving kings, generals, and emperors, which positioned the remedy as aspirational and deepened the lore surrounding it. This narrative propelled theriac to new prominence among rulers and the medical elite. In numerous Renaissance courts, rulers displayed an interest in pharmaceutical experimentation, as they understood that pharmacy was part of state building. This explains why they were inclined to accept and follow physicians' assertions in this domain. The last sections of the chapter examine treatises on theriac, elucidating how authors utilized theriac to promote a comprehensive overhaul of pharmacy and advocate for increased regulation by state authorities. However, these treatises also reveal the different relations of power between apothecaries and physicians across various Italian cities.

Italian magistrates commonly believed that the state had to offer some level of health care. Chapter 4 considers how distributing "true theriac" came to be seen as an effective response to crises, as the state made provisions of theriac, forbade exports, and asked physicians to assess its usefulness in case of epidemics. By the time of the plague of 1630, theriac was widely used in hospitals. To ensure recognition and appreciation of their commitment to public health, magistrates and medical professionals launched elaborate public ceremonies for the production of theriac. By describing the history of and analyzing theriac celebrations, I investigate the different meanings acquired by these public performances across several contexts. In the final part of the chapter, I explore the pamphlets printed by apothecaries to accompany these celebrations, and how they served to promote apothecaries' status and activities.

Chapter 5 examines the history of theriac as a commodity, and highlights the role of apothecaries in spreading medical knowledge. Tariffs and other sources enable quantitative analyses of prices and production. During the seventeenth century, the reinvention of theriac as "true theriac" led to an increase in theriac production, which in turn bolstered its economy. As a point of comparison to Italy, I describe the business of theriac in England. I devote the central part of the chapter to a controversial question, that of the price and affordability of theriac. I challenge the widely held historiographical notion that theriac was always expensive, arguing that in early modern Italy it was in fact transformed from an elite drug into one accessible to a sizable proportion of the public, at least in times of need. Alongside theriac, apothecaries and other pharmaceutical operators inundated the market with various theriacal by-products. An analysis of the printed material that accompanied theriac, leaflets called *virtues,* suggests that theriac constituted apothecaries' official response to both exotica and charlatans' wares. *Virtues* also show what kind of medical information apothecaries disseminated, and how such information changed over time.

While public ceremonies of theriac production projected the vision of a harmonious medical establishment, medical colleges and apothecary guilds were fighting to control the pharmaceutical field. In Chapter 6, I draw on legal, medical, and literary sources to highlight these social dynamics by comparing developments in seventeenth-century Venice and Bologna and the bitter battles around theriac production. The scale of this analysis in the first part of the chapter is microhistorical, focusing on a controversy in 1620s Venice: a dispute over the quantity of honey in the theriac recipe. Through the lens of theriac, the chapter investigates different local political economies, and how they shaped states' interventions in local feuds such as those in Venice and Bologna. The chapter underscores the fact that theriac increasingly proved a conservative agent insofar as it enabled established elites to maintain power.

Part III highlights the peak of theriac's global success in the late-seventeenth and eighteenth centuries, and introduces the beginning of its demise. Chapter 7 follows multiple versions of theriac as they mushroom across four continents, illuminating Galenic pharmacy's flexibility to thrive in markedly different environments, and demonstrating how the commercial potential and political significance of theriac transcended latitude and longitude. An assessment of evolving medical theories in eighteenth-century Italy shows how its prestige waned despite production increased over the course of the century. The fall of the ancien régime heralded the end of the ceremonial productions of theriac, although its consumption continued well into the nineteenth century.

I

Early History and Sensory Experience of Theriac

CHAPTER 1

The Reinvention of Theriac

*G*IROLAMO CALESTANI (1510–1582?) was a well-traveled apothecary from Parma and the author of a successful manual for apothecaries. In the 1560s he noted: "As one might expect, vendible theriac (as we call the theriac that merchants bring to the most important markets and fairs and sell in big quantities, labeling it as exquisite [*finissima*]), has neither the qualities nor the properties that truest theriac should have."[1] Calestani contrasted the commercial theriac sold across Europe, which he called "vendible" (*vendereccia*), with an ideal antidote (*verissima*) made with the "truest" ingredients: those described in the recipe handed down over the centuries from Andromachus the Elder (fl. first cent. CE) through Galen.

The Great Theriac of Andromachus the Elder (*Theriaca magna Andromachi senioris*) was a celebrated medical preparation believed to have exceptional healing properties. Naturalist Ulisse Aldrovandi (1522–1605), an unwavering researcher of theriac for more than forty years, proclaimed the drug the "antidote of antidotes," deserving the title "hand of God, for the immediate health that it brings to infinite ailments and above all to pestilential diseases and the plague itself."[2] Theriac derived from the tradition of antivenoms—antidotes counteracting the bites of venomous creatures—associated with physicians active in Egypt in the third century BCE.[3] The name itself, *theriac*, is a generic noun derived from the Greek *thēriakē*, which in turn comes from *thēríon*, "wild and venomous animal."[4] The name *theriac* was synonymous with *antidote*, and was also used generically for numerous medical preparations. When Andromachus the Elder served as the chief physician (archiater) to Emperor Nero during the first century CE, he revised the recipe for an existing compound remedy called *mithridate*. Andromachus made several changes, including adding such components as viper flesh and increasing the quantity of opium, all of which resulted in a new antidote comprising over sixty ingredients.[5] This was Andromachus's theriac, the theriac referred to by Calestani as the "truest."

During the Renaissance, various scholars took on the challenge of identifying the ingredients of Andromachus's theriac. Physicians and apothecaries alike hoped to recreate the formidable antidote that would ostensibly enable them to cure innumerable diseases. Many naturalists believed the gradual loss of reliable knowledge about materia medica compromised the possibility of making theriac as potent as Andromachus's, and that any such production would lead to ineffective or even deleterious drugs. The term *materia medica* encompassed any plant, animal, or mineral matters (called "simples") with medicinal properties that were used to make medicaments. Materia medica was at the heart of natural history, a field in which questions of observation, description, representation, and experimentation played crucial roles in fresh understandings of natural knowledge.[6] Richard Palmer, Paula Findlen, and Giuseppe Olmi have shown the centrality of the early modern pursuit of "true theriac" to the renewed interest in materia medica.[7] Apothecary and collector Francesco Calzolari (1522–1609) visually emphasized this importance in his museum, placing at the center of the last room the quasi-altar of "legitimate theriac and mithridate ingredients," which from the visitor's perspective appeared as a vanishing point (Figures 1.1, 1.2). Findlen has also demonstrated that theriac helped several collectors advance their careers.[8] Other scholars have highlighted the fact that Italian apothecaries attached their reputations to theriac and mithridate, and have acknowledged the institutional and economic significance of theriac, despite having limited their investigations to specific times and places.[9]

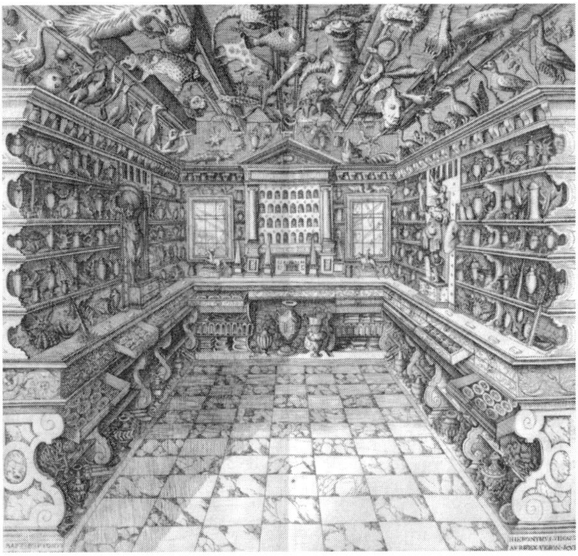

Fig. 1.1. (a.) Francesco Calzolari's natural collection and museum featured the tabernacle of theriac's ingredients at its very center. Folded engraving from Ceruti, *Musaeum Francisci Calceolari,* 53–54. (b.) Detail of Francesco Calzolari's tabernacle of theriac.
Zentralbibliothek, Zürich, NM 53 | G.

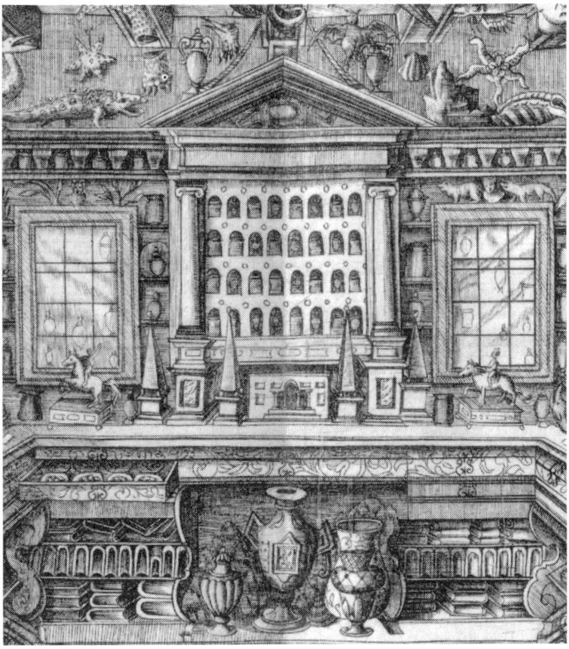

```
        "Legitimate" Theriac
        and Mithridatum
           Ingredients
                │
                ▼
        ┌───────────────┐
        │    Natural    │
        │    objects    │
        ├───────────────┤
        │ Books, mss. & │
        │  distillation │
        │   equipment   │
        ├───────────────┤
        │  Portraits of │
        │    famous     │
        │  naturalists  │
        └───────────────┘
```

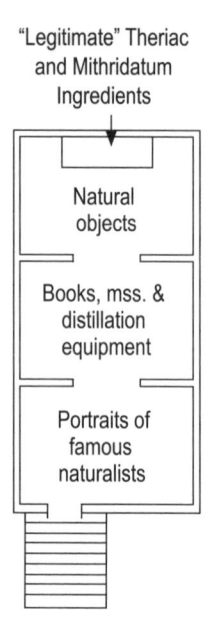

Fig. 1.2. The plan of Calzolari's museum in the reconstruction shows the rooms on the second floor of his home in the order in which the visitor would encounter them when entering by the stairway.

In this chapter I present a revised account of the context underpinning the quest for "true theriac." I argue this was a process of reinvention that took place between the 1490s and 1570s, mainly in Italy but also involving several scholars and apothecaries from elsewhere in Europe.[10] I emphasize that, although refashioning theriac into "true theriac" was a scientific and intellectual endeavor, it was also a legal, social, economic, and institutional process. Such complexity is revealed by the case study of Venice, a city that takes center stage in the following pages for three reasons. First, Venice holds a special place in the history of medieval and early modern theriac for its long and steady association with the remedy. Second, in the fifteenth century theriac was already a brand linked to the "honor" of Venice, an early instance of a state drug. Officials believed its quality reflected the city's commercial reputation, so they kept its production and sale under careful control. Finally, the reformulation of the recipe of theriac shows that stable pharmacological knowledge was already a matter of state interest in fifteenth- and sixteenth-century Venice.

Among apothecaries—a multifaceted group of artisans associated in guilds and by the nature of their activities—a number of especially learned individuals emerged in the quest for "true" theriac. This elite group created an internal hierarchy based on prestige, and received recognition from scholars and physicians by virtue of their theriac. This new hierarchy was one of the many ways theriac affected society. The "learned apothecaries" distinguished themselves by asserting that they had superior knowledge, claiming exclusive expertise in producing "true theriac," and declaring moral superiority over their rank-and-file contemporaries who could make only "vendible" theriac. Learned apothecaries eventually gained a commercial advantage, too, when the price of theriac increased considerably in the wake of its refashioning.

This chapter begins by examining vendible theriacs and their cost, regulation, and reputation. Some, such as Egyptian theriac, enjoyed great prestige; others lacked recognition and were metaphorically associated with treachery. A brief overview of theriac's medical history illuminates its centuries-long prominence in medical literature, and is also essential for understanding the shift in early modern debates about the drug. The refashioning of theriac started in Venice in the 1490s, with a physician arguing that local viper was the correct snake for the recipe. The emergence of learned apothecaries and the enthusiastic quest for theriac's "true" ingredients developed in parallel, from the years of initial disbelief and setbacks in the 1530s to the 1560s, when some claimed to have finally created "true theriac."

Material Theriacs

Vendible Theriac and Its Low Prestige

During the fifteenth century, theriac was widely accessible to patients in Italy and across Europe, vended by apothecary shops in large cities and provincial towns, as well as by peddlers in rural areas alongside other goods.[11] Apothecary inventories from diverse locations confirm theriac's availability in provincial settings, such as a Jewish community in Sicily and the small town of Gandino in the Venetian state.[12] Its widespread accessibility reflects the fifteenth-century expansion of the apothecary trade. Apothecaries' productions grew in the main Italian cities, such as Venice and Rome. Apothecaries distributed their compounds through established networks of peddlers, retailers, and hospitals, cultivating these networks through guilds, trade partners, and other enduring associations, such as relatives or compatriots.[13] In Genoa and Venice, apothecaries produced theriac in bulk, exporting it as far afield as France, England, and Germany.[14] Jean-Pierre Bénézet and Jean Flahaut have estimated that approximately 2,200 pounds (1.1 tons) were sold at the annual Beaucaire fair, which attracted up to 300,000 visitors.[15] This was precisely the type of theriac Calestani referred to as "vendible."

Not just anyone could manufacture theriac. Apothecaries held the exclusive legal right to its production, along with that of other medicines. To become a master apothecary, one had to secure approval from the local guild after having served as an apprentice for several years. The craft of the apothecary was considered a mechanical art, requiring manual skills and knowledge but lacking the prestige of liberal professions. However, apothecaries were some of the most literate artisans, often proficient in writing and at least somewhat conversant with Latin. The apothecary functioned not only as an artisan but also as a healer and a merchant, contributing to the wealth of his guild. In fact, apothecary guilds were usually among the most affluent in town.[16] Not every apothecary could produce theriac, given its costly ingredients and complex manufacturing procedure. Unlike most remedies, produced on site for individual patients following a physician's prescription, theriac was produced in bulk, stored, and sold ready for use.

Our knowledge of the production of theriac for fifteenth-century Venice is limited to one apothecary involved in the theriac trade: Agostino Altucci, a merchant from Arezzo who became one of the city's major producers of theriac. Connected to suppliers in the Levant, between 1465 and 1475 Altucci imported simples (plant, animal, and mineral matter) and other goods from Cyprus and Syria, as well as from Egypt. He enjoyed substantial sales, despite his records revealing that his theriac lacked some essential ingredients, such as snake flesh and maritime squill (*Drimia maritima*). Over ten years Altucci sold approximately 1,540 pounds (about 0.8 tons) of theriac, mostly in wholesale quantities to local clients, both in Arezzo and in Venice, but he also exported it to other locations in Italy, such as Rome, as well as to cities farther afield, such as Cologne.[17]

In the fifteenth and early-sixteenth centuries, the price of theriac was kept reasonable by demand, bulk production, and the components used. Furthermore, other drugs were more fashionable. For example, in 1493–1494 theriac ranked only tenth among the best-selling drugs at the Florentine apothecary Al Giglio's, which had only thirty-nine sales of it that year, enjoying moderate popularity. Purveyed at 40 soldi per pound, theriac was not expensive, considering that an unskilled laborer earned 7–8 soldi per day and an average dose was just a few grams.[18] When bought in bulk, theriac was even cheaper; in Venice throughout the 1460s and 1470s, it cost about 22 soldi per pound.[19] The low cost of theriac in the fifteenth century reflected the widespread awareness that its availability at fairs and in apothecary shops meant it may have been counterfeit or otherwise of poor quality. However, the drug's price increased significantly after its refashioning into "true theriac." In Venice in 1636, for example, theriac was retailing at 576 soldi per pound—a twenty-six-fold increase.[20]

There had been misgivings about theriac's quality for centuries. Even medical texts such as Michele Savonarola's *Practica Major*, written in Ferrara and Padua in the 1440s, denounced the low quality of "our" theriac, which he attributed to apothecaries not adhering to proper production methods.[21] What was questioned was not the effectiveness of medical theriac as Galen and other authors described it, but instead the quality of the actual compound, which would be inefficacious if it had been made following an improper procedure or recipe.

Doubts surrounding the quality of theriac were so common that the term often served as a metaphor for quackery in literary texts, symbolizing deceit and treachery. Theriac abounded in the paraphernalia of charlatans and rogues. In his 1481 knightly burlesque poem, Luigi Pulci—a favorite of Lord Byron—included a case of theriac among the possessions of Gano the traitor: "Imagine, reader, that the betrayer tides up all his lies and knickknacks . . . and opens the tin of theriac."[22] Similarly, François Rabelais's *Gargantua et Pantagruel* described one of the main characters, Panurge, as "a quack touting theriac," equipped with "a dentist's pincers, a hooked prod, a pelican, and certain other implements."[23] These authors portrayed theriac as representing a deceptive promise of recovery. Its poor reputation preoccupied many, albeit for different reasons. Patients and physicians wanted a powerful remedy; apothecaries and state officials were concerned about their revenues and commercial reputation.

Egyptian Theriac

When high-ranking patients such as princes and diplomats were worried for their health, they could draw on their illustrious connections to source Egyptian theriac. In 1429, for example, Pope Martin V (r. 1417–1431) requested the theriac he needed for various ailments from the sultan of Egypt.[24] Egyptian theriac was a sought-after gift. After completing a diplomatic mission to Egypt in 1443, Andrea Donato returned to Venice with gifts from the sultan, including musk, porcelain, and theriac.[25] In 1575, when Sultana Nūr Bānū (Cecilia Baffo, 1525–1583) sent precious gifts to Venice from Istanbul, theriac figured among them once again.[26] Egyptian theriac was so renowned in Italy that a 1549 map of Cairo printed in Venice marked a square with the caption "Theriac is made here."[27]

Egyptian and Syrian theriacs were highly prized because those countries were closer to the point of origin of several ingredients, especially the Syrian tyrus, the snake that was traditionally a key component of the compound. Because the genesis of the production of theriac in Venice remains elusive, it is also possible that Venetian apothecaries adopted production practices from the Eastern Mediterranean and considered this region its place of origin.[28] Moreover, in Cairo and Baghdad the production of theriac had been conducted publicly since the Middle Ages.[29] Christian travelers bought Egyptian theriac during their pilgrimages to Egypt and the Holy Land. Egyptians profited from selling theriac to "Italians, Poles, English, French, Flemish, and other nations."[30] Egyptians refused to disclose the remedy's composition to Christians, probably to maintain their commercial advantage, or possibly because "it was prohibited by their laws."[31] However, I have found no mention of consistent imports of Egyptian or Syrian theriac into Europe.

By the mid-sixteenth century, Egyptian theriac's stellar reputation in Europe started to falter. In a 1559 letter to Aldrovandi, Melchiorre Guilandino (Melchior Weiland, ca. 1520–1589) stated with disenchantment: "The pyramids of Cairo that we see today are not those that the ancients count among the seven marvels of the world . . . , Cairo is not Memphis, balsam is not from Egypt, tyrus of these lands is not viper, and finally theriac of Cairo is the saddest of any theriac made in Europe."[32] After then becoming a professor at the University of Padua and prefect of its Botanical Garden, Guilandino traveled extensively across Egypt and Asia, amassing a natural collection that was later lost in an assault by corsairs.[33] Regardless of Guilandino's perplexities about Egyptian theriac, the Venetian physician Prospero Alpini (1553–1616), while generally unimpressed by Egyptian medicines, demonstrated that Egyptian theriac was still worth his efforts. During his journey to Egypt in the 1580s, Alpini outsmarted a local scholar to obtain the Egyptian recipe for theriac, and had a Jewish acquaintance translate the Arabic text for him.[34] By gathering firsthand experience of Egyptian pharmacy, Guilandino and Alpini initiated a new season of materia medica and pharmaceutical product exchanges across the Mediterranean. Such new knowledge, together with substantial economic and political changes, would alter a centuries-long-held balance. As we will have explored by the end of this book, in the eighteenth century Venetian theriac became more prestigious than Egyptian theriac in Europe and the Ottoman Empire.

The First Certified Drug, and an Early Instance of Branding

Only a handful of wealthy patients with international connections could fetch theriac from Egypt; everyone else had to rely on local production. From the twelfth century, various institutions guaranteed customers medicaments of a certain quality. The problem of counterfeit electuaries was as old as theriac and mithridate themselves, and it is no exaggeration to argue that theriac triggered all subsequent pharmaceutical regulation in Europe.[35] Governance of medicines began with artisanal guilds, which emphasized trade over medical concerns. Such emphasis may have played a role in theriac's early association with Venice, which resulted in what can be considered an early instance of branding.

Apothecary guilds were associations of apothecaries that self-regulated via statute. Since the inception of the apothecary as a profession in the twelfth century, statutes in Pisa, Bologna, Verona, and Venice explicitly mentioned theriac,—but not wax and sugar, which actually accounted for the majority of apothecary sales.[36] Guild officials examined and approved the ingredients of theriac and mithridate in apothecary shops before their compounding. In Bologna, such approval had to be notarized, indicating a high degree of bureaucratization.[37] Medieval norms about theriac centered around two objectives: safeguarding the interests of the guild and its members, and ensuring quality control and consumer safety. Some regulations prohibited the sale of foreign theriac to protect guild members from external competition. For instance, the apothecary statute of Venice of the year 1258 obligated apothecaries to swear an oath not to buy or sell foreign theriac unless it had been inspected by appointed apothecaries.[38] Similarly, in 1496 apothecaries in Pisa introduced a ban on imported theriac, particularly from Genoa.[39] Other norms were aimed at protecting consumers by forbidding adulterations or the addition of dangerous herbs, such as caper spurge (*Euphorbia lathyris*) and hellebore.[40]

Alongside the guilds, state offices in medieval Italy oversaw the production of goods such as textiles, flours, glass, and theriac. As a significant commercial and productive hub, Venice presents a comprehensive example of the institutional actors involved in the theriac trade. As early as the thirteenth century, theriac was a lucrative product for Venetian apothecaries, and its production was officially sanctioned and regulated by state authorities. A twelfth-century government office known as the Giustizia Vecchia oversaw the production and regulation of large consumer goods and the prevention of consumer fraud. This magistrate supervised artisan guilds, including those of apothecaries, and had jurisdiction over weights and measures, prices, sales and exports, manual labor, and exemptions. A tribunal protected the interests of both state and consumer.[41]

During the first half of the fifteenth century, the Giustizia Vecchia issued several provisions on theriac.[42] The recurring reissuance of these regulations suggests a fast-growing production that state officials had difficulty controlling. In 1432 and 1437, the Giustizia Vecchia outlined the procedures apothecaries had to follow when making electuaries.[43] In 1441 the office decreed that "very fake" (*falsissime*) theriac and mithridate should be burned in Rialto, a meeting place for physicians. In 1442 it reiterated producers' obligation to publicly display the certified ingredients of their theriacs for three days after their approval by superintendents.[44] In 1480 a new regulation mandated that a small quantity from each batch be sealed in a lead case (*bossolo*) marked with the sign of the apothecary and the production date. The Giustizia Vecchia kept this sample in a locked cupboard and documented it in the Book of Theriacs (*Libro delle Triache*) with the intended date of sale. This record served as a point of comparison in case of suspicion.[45]

Alongside the apothecary guild and state magistrates such as the Giustizia Vecchia, another institution supervising theriac production was the Collegio Medico.[46] Collegiate physicians determined the recipe of theriac, inspected the ingredients, monitored apothecary procedures during production, and from 1507 accorded permission to apothecaries to compose theriac.[47] At the most fundamental level, medical colleges conferred medical degrees, organized scientific disputes and public dissections, and oversaw the composition of theriac. The influence of medical colleges increased in the sixteenth century, in Venice as well as other cities. The expansion of medical colleges during the early modern period, along with the growing reliance of states and rulers on these institutions, led to their commanding increasing authority over theriac and mithridate. Richard Palmer has argued that, since their inception in the thirteenth century, throughout Italy medical colleges "took on the character of organs of the state."[48] Palmer might have overstated the relationship between states and medical colleges somewhat; the nature of each college should be examined in its specific local context.[49] Nonetheless, in Venice the Collegio Medico did indeed function as part of the state. Besides granting access to the medical profession, collegiate physicians performed state duties, including service during times of plague. They also enjoyed privileges that conferred status, such as tax exemption and permission to dress as aristocrats.[50]

Such deployment of offices, attention, and regulation shows that the Venetian state considered theriac no ordinary good. In 1480 a Giustizia Vecchia state official acknowledged this explicitly: "Large quantities [of theriac] are taken from this land [Venice] to different places, and if theriac is good, it goes to the honor of our city; otherwise, it brings great disrepute."[51] Controlling the quality of theriac meant protecting the name of the city. The term *Venetian treacle* (as theriac was known in England) was like a brand. Since the state gained revenues from taxing apothecaries and exports, counterfeiting theriac was considered a crime against the "honor, and the reputation of this city."[52] Well before mercantilism and the Industrial Revolution, states and producers alike considered quality relevant for exports.[53] The branding of theriac endured for centuries. For example, when a French traveler in eighteenth-century Rome visited the apothecary shop at the Collegio Romano, the chief Jesuit school, he noted that "all sorts of medicines and drugs are prepared and sold.... *Venetian treacle* is likewise made here in the greatest perfection and in vast quantity." Jesuits in Rome could certainly not make "Venetian treacle" but, as far as patients were concerned, *any* theriac was a "Venetian treacle."[54]

By the end of the fifteenth century, some theriacs, such as the elusive Egyptian theriac and the more available Venetian theriac, were considered better than others simply by virtue of their origin. Overall, the reputation of material theriacs was at a low; the very word *theriac* was synonymous with *deceit*. However, if physicians held doubts, these only concerned theriacs that were actually produced, not the concept of the drug itself.

A Short History of Medical Theriac up to the Fifteenth Century

A history of medical theriac and the textual transmission of its recipe in antiquity and the Middle Ages is beyond the scope of this book, but a swift overview of some fundamental points regarding theriac and mithridate is in order.

Since antiquity, a long line of medical authors transmitted medical information about theriac.[55] Four works in the Galenic corpus directly discussed *Theriaca magna* (*De theriaca ad Pisonem, De theriaca ad Pamphilianum*, and *De Antidotis lib. I* and *lib. II*), although only the last two were definitively penned by Galen.[56] Roman authors such as Celsius (Aulus Cornelius, 25 BCE–50 CE) and Scribonius Largus (10 BCE–54 CE) also discussed theriac and mithridate. Indeed, the latter was possibly the first to use the word *theriaca* in Latin.

Theriac and mithridate posed an unsolvable conundrum within Galen's pharmacological theory because their complex composition made their workings inexplicable in terms of humoral theory.[57] Galen's reformulation of humoral theory described how each individual had a peculiar mixture of humors (blood, phlegm, yellow bile, and black bile). Illness derived from humoral imbalance was created either within the body or by external conditions. According to Galen, single substances (or simples) had properties (or powers) called *dunameis*. Each simple could be a mix of one active quality (hot or cold) and one passive quality (dry or humid) in four different degrees of intensity, depending on their effects on the body.

The extent of the humoral imbalance, together with the patient's individual constitution, dictated the remedy required by each patient. Therefore, different patients might require different remedies for similar symptoms.[58]

There are numerous discrepancies between Galen's pharmacological theory and his suggestions regarding remedies in medical practice. For example, he never explained how the qualities of simples interacted and how they affected bodies once mixed in large numbers, as in theriac and mithridate. Furthermore, the author of *De theriaca ad Pisonem* presented theriac as a preventive medicine, informing readers that Emperor Marcus Aurelius took it every day, while elsewhere Galen stated that antidotes (*alexipharmacons*) should not be taken as prophylactics.[59] Later physicians knew about these discrepancies and tried to make sense of them to establish a definitive interpretation.

What did not cause any confusion among physicians was the remarkable array of ailments supposedly cured by theriac and mithridate, possibly explained by the fact that humoral imbalances could generate different symptoms. First and foremost, theriac and mithridate were antidotes against venoms and poisons, such as the bites of snakes, spiders, toads, scorpions, and rabid dogs. Additionally, both were supposed to cure headaches and migraines, sore throats, fevers, constriction of the chest, epilepsy, asthma, heart problems, palsy, arthritis, swelling, kidney stones, and blockages—to name only a few more eligible ailments. This list may seem ridiculously long to our modern sensibility, but importantly it was not endless. For certain diseases such as pestilential fevers, physicians actually discouraged the use of theriac.

Nowhere did Galen fully explain theriac's mechanism of action, although he did comment on each ingredient individually. As Sabine Vogt has noted, this is surprising because at least one reason for theriac's efficacy could have been derived implicitly from his texts. Most of the ingredients were hot and dry to some degree; and because most venoms and poisons were considered cold, it made sense that antidotes had heating qualities to counteract them directly.[60] Patients taking theriac might feel such heating qualities. The presence of viper's flesh also suggested the Hippocratic principle of curing like with like, which Galen dismissed. Moreover, since viper's flesh itself was considered akin to poison, once ingested it would accustom the patient's body to poison. However, several

Renaissance authors believed that viper's flesh would exert by sympathy an attraction on the poison in the body and drive it toward the heart. Only once all the nefarious substances had entered the heart would the other ingredients neutralize them.[61]

Instead of offering any of these answers to explain the workings of theriac, *De theriaca ad Pisonem* resorted to both authority and experience: "I think the best of the old doctors ... developed the best combination of drugs, developing the art of blending from the nature of each drug, rectifying the drugs which are most intense in their own nature by blending with others, and in the same way blunting those which are sharp and in general for the rest skillfully using drugs with an eye to the different ailments and the composition of human beings."[62] Thus, the efficacy of the compound depended on the experience of the most learned physicians ("the best of the old doctors"), who created theriac carefully through progressive tweaking. Overall, theriac's strength and virtues were believed to lie in both its history and its creators' expertise. Theriac was designed and tested by a succession of exceptional creators: Mithradates, Andromachus, and Galen himself. Competing understandings of medicine, empirical and rational, converged in this one compound remedy.

The uncertainties around theriac's workings fueled centuries of medical debate. During late antiquity, knowledge about theriac spread unevenly to Europe and Asia from the Mediterranean, its origin point. Authors offered contradictory information while several Galenic texts became unavailable in Latin. In the Middle Ages, theriac was discussed by Arab scholars active in not only the Middle East but also Europe, such as Ibn Juljul (ca. 944–ca. 994) and al-Zahrawi (latinized as Abulcasis, 936-1013).

Probably none of these Arab scholars was more influential than Ibn Sīnā. In the fifth book of his *Qanūn*, Ibn Sīnā affirmed that theriac should not be considered a sum of its ingredients, and instead proposed an elegant solution to the question of its workings: that theriac's medical properties derived from fermentation.[63] Indeed, he argued that theriac should rest for several months after a laborious preparation. According to Ibn Sīnā, fermentation changed the virtues and qualities of the ingredients, causing them to lose their peculiarities and acquire new ones.[64] Ibn Sīnā also elaborated on Galen's notion of "total substance" (*ex tota sui substantia*), and on Arab philosophers' concept of the "specific form," which ascribed particular characteristics to a substance or class of objects when it could not be explained by its simple qualities. For example, the specific form *poisonousness* was attributed to poison.[65] Medieval authors used this concept to discuss the power of magnets, a paramount example of natural wonder.[66] Ibn Sīnā remained an influential medical author throughout the sixteenth century, and Renaissance scholars and apothecaries continually referred to his notions regarding theriac.[67]

Medical and philosophical debates over theriac continued in medieval Europe. The first Latin translation of the influential treatise *Tractatus de tyriaca* by Ibn Rushd (latinized as Averroes, 1126–1198) appeared in Montpellier in the 1280s. This translation ignited an intellectual debate that contributed to shaping key medical figures, such as Arnald of Villanova (ca. 1240–ca. 1312).[68] In Arnald's works, the ontological nature of theriac had repercussions on aspects of its practical use, such as dosage.[69] After the Black Death, mithridate and especially theriac figured as consistent favorites among antipestilential compound remedies. Directed to a general public, plague tracts rarely mentioned ingredients, the recipe, or indeed ontological questions, focusing instead on how and when to use the compound. For instance, they recommended theriac be mostly taken by ingestion, but noted it could also be applied to buboes and near the heart.[70]

Throughout the early modern period, the term *poison* designated a variety of not only substances—venoms and plant-related poisons both natural and artificial—but also illnesses, which could be caused by external or internal poison, including the plague.[71] According to historian Melissa Chase, authors affiliated with the school of medicine in Montpellier associated the category "poisonous" with plague in the wake of the Black Death.[72] Most Montpellier authors in the fifteenth century claimed that pestilence was different from other diseases specifically because it was poisonous. Traditional medical explanations could not account for the devastating experience of the plague, and poison offered a convincing cause for a disease that hit with unprecedented ferocity without regard for individual differences.[73] This partially accounts for the reliance on theriac and other antidotes.

Also in the fifteenth century, many physicians still claimed that theriac was the most potent antidote. For example, in his influential book *Opus de venenis*, written between 1424 and 1426, the physician and philosopher Sante Ardoini (fl. fourteenth–fifteenth cent.) dedicated several pages to theriac and mithridate: their uses, composition, and preservation, as well as common mistakes surrounding their application.[74] Similarly, the prominent philosopher and humanist Marsilio Ficino (1433–1499), son of a physician and brother of two apothecaries, wrote: "All doctors unanimously agree that nothing is more beneficial than theriac for supporting and strengthening both particular parts and powers and also the spirits and the intelligence... If we have no theriac, we will use mithridate."[75] His endorsement of theriac in *De vita libri tres* has been rightly interpreted as a "simple acknowledgement" of the status of the compound at the time.[76] Then in *Consiglio contro la pestilenza*, Ficino restated the relation between poison, the plague, and theriac: "Plague is a poisonous vapor created in the air enemy of the vital spirit. I say enemy not for its elementary quality, but for a specific property, like theriac is an ally [to the vital spirit]."[77] According to Ficino, as an external poison the plague had to meet favorable conditions in the internal humoral imbalance to cause illness. *Consiglio* was a popular text, written during the epidemic of 1478 for physicians and lay readers alike. Theriac was a necessary preventive according to *Consiglio:* "Without theriac... one cannot well preserve oneself."[78]

In the fifteenth and early-sixteenth centuries, theriac and mithridate were considered medical staples, even by critics of Galenic pharmacy. For example, the medical iconoclast Paracelsus, well-known detractor of not only Galenic pharmacy but also apothecaries in general, spared theriac and mithridate from his cutting remarks. In fact, he listed them as two of only three apothecary preparations with any value: "What would you do if I were to exclude three of the recipes, *theriaca, triferae, mithridati;* the other ones, of which there must be a hundred, cannot amount to anything then."[79] The alleged low quality of the theriac in circulation had not remotely damaged the remedy's reputation among physicians, who mostly discussed its properties in principle, not those of the theriac actually available to patients.

I shall end this short overview by clarifying what theriac was *not*. Theriac was considered neither magic nor an artificial wonder, unlike automata and ever-burning lamps; nor was it related to alchemy—at least not until the seventeenth century. Physicians might have argued over its properties, but again these were considered neither magical nor preternatural. As we shall see in later chapters, theriac shared with artificial wonders a courtly character and a "civilizing intent"; that is, its healing properties endowed its owners and makers with prestige and authority.[80]

Physicians, apothecaries, and alchemists shared much knowledge in the Middle Ages. Historian Antoine Calvet has scoured medieval literature for a direct link between theriac and alchemy. His starting point was the hypothesis that the concept of "universal remedy" established a connection between theriac and alchemical products, such as elixirs. Calvet has convincingly demonstrated that analogies between theriac and the alchemical universal remedies were only episodic. While it is possible that literature about theriac influenced alchemists, there is no trace of the opposite being true.[81] Similarly, alchemists in the seventeenth century drew inspiration from Theriaca magna to create alchemical theriacs and products, such as *Theriaca coelestis*. Theriac would attract the interest of physicians at various junctures for several centuries, raising medical questions and prompting sharp speculations. While this preeminence did not falter in the early modern period, the sixteenth century marked an especially high tide of scholarly interest in theriac.

Refashioning Theriac into "True Theriac"

From the beginning, the process of researching ingredients and procedures for recreating Andromachus's theriac involved numerous individuals, overwhelmingly men, in several capacities. Many scholars, physicians, and collectors held institutional positions in universities, medical colleges, and state offices, and many apothecaries were officials in apothecary guilds. The proximity and interconnectedness of natural history, pharmacy, the state, and commercial institutions were pivotal to the process of reforming materia medica, which shaped institutions and was in turn shaped by the social dynamics of these institutions, as well as by their language. The process of transforming theriac into "true theriac" created friction, whose consequences will become especially evident in Part II of this book.

Lost objects such as theriac and its ingredients served as intellectual benchmarks for scholars studying the past while calling themselves "modern." In his treatise on lost things (*deperdida*) from antiquity, Guido Panciroli (1523–1599) listed several of theriac's lost ingredients, including costus, amomum, malabathrum, opobalsamum, storax, and cassia.[82] Attempting to make a theriac worthy of Andromachus meant striving to reestablish "lost knowledge," realizing an ancient ideal—and eventually superseding it. Naturalists engaged with the complex culture they had inherited from the ancients, a relationship that would take centuries to untangle.[83]

Naturalists striving to make "true theriac" engaged in an intellectual as well as a material dialogue with ancient authors. Scholars spent long hours on manuscript parchments, compiling revised editions of foundational medical texts, such as those of Galen, Theofrastus, and Dioscorides. They also engaged in a material relationship with the ancients, collecting stones, exchanging specimens, drawing plants and animals, and herborizing in the fields. One of the earliest mentions of a scholar directly involved in making theriac dates to 1533, when Girolamo Fracastoro (ca. 1478–1553), a physician from Verona, thanked his correspondent Giovan Battista Ramusio (1485–1557) for having sent him a translation of Nicander's and Andromachus's poems about antidotes and poisons. Fracastoro had longed to read Nicander, whom he regarded as a "splendid poet." He added: "If your lordship would like to help us with his means and favors, we would willingly make theriac here, ready to all necessary expenses; and it would be a useful thing, which I desire very much. Think about it, and let us know how you could help us. I fancy it, I think about it every day, but I need help. I have the viper ready."[84] Fracastoro read Nicander and was ready to cut up vipers. His enthusiasm for the possibility of remaking "true theriac" was tangible.

The ambition of scholars such as Fracastoro represented a reinvigorated aspiration to achieve reciprocity between words and objects. Many of those involved in the quest for "true theriac" built their authority within institutions—such as universities, medical colleges, and apothecary guilds—whose denizens spoke the language of law and legitimacy. Thus, this reciprocity between words and objects was not just a philosophical or philological enterprise, but also one with practical applications. The word *true* marked an important shift in the identities of Renaissance naturalists. According to the ancients, *true* meant *philologically accurate*; according to the law it meant both *legitimate* and *trustworthy*.[85] The use of the terms *true* and *fake* became a feature of Renaissance natural history, although such usage was hardly novel. For example, in the early fifteenth century, physician Sante Ardoini wrote about "vera [true] theriaca Andromachi" to distinguish it from other medical recipes called *theriac*. He also mentioned "vera Mithridatis," "vera ruta agrestis," and "vera terra sigillata."[86] In 1442 the Giustizia Vecchia used the term *fake* to refer to those medicinal compounds made "against the medical authors."[87] *True* also often appeared in relation to apothecaries and their practices and products—for example, "true preparation," "untrue apothecaries."[88] Those attempting to refashion theriac fulfilled or at least aspired to fulfill the social role of provider of reliable knowledge. They claimed such a role precisely by demonstrating the necessity of their pharmaceutical knowledge—such as understanding materia medica—to society. They distinguished what was "true" from what was not, and made only the former "legal."

The Beginnings of "True" Theriac: "Tyrus Is Viper"

The fact that snake flesh was considered the most important ingredient of theriac was widely known both within the medical world and among laypeople. Moreover, most people, not just physicians and apothecaries, understood the vital importance of using the right snake in theriac. From the Middle Ages, metaphors of snake and theriac abounded in nonmedical texts such as religious sermons, philosophical treatises, and even love poems. "Where does the physician more likely look for the antidote if not from poison? Who offers better theriac than the viper? In the best poison is the most excellent antidote," wrote philosopher Giordano Bruno (1548–1600), arguing that there was only one universal principle: generation is corruption, as corruption is generation.[89] Although the Catholic Church did not much appreciate Bruno's philosophy, the metaphor of viper and theriac had currency among Catholic preachers as well as Calvinists and Anglicans. One Anglican preacher used the metaphor to recall how ingenuity could overcome misfortune: "The art of the Apothecary doth make a poisonfull Viper into a wholesome Triacle."[90]

In 1565 the apothecary Francesco Calzolari located the start of new hopes for theriac in a specific moment in time: "More than anything, [what made the remaking of "true" theriac possible was] finding that the true vipers were among us, and that we did not need to go to the Levant to find the fake ones."[91] Calzolari believed that making "true" theriac became possible when the snake used in the recipe was identified as the local viper. Many scholars agreed, including physician Bartolomeo Maranta, who noted that "until recently" the viper "was not known."[92] In asserting "that the true vipers were among us," Calzolari was referring to a specific dispute in the 1490s, when Alessandro Agathimero, a physician active in Venice, claimed that local vipers were the equivalent of the tyrus snake, which sparked fiery debates (*acerrima disputationes*).[93]

At the end of the fifteenth century, most physicians maintained the traditional understanding that the tyrus and the viper were different types of snake, and that only tyrus was right for theriac. This belief derived from eleventh-century medical texts, in which the viper in Andromachus's recipe had become the tyrus snake. *Tyrus* is neither an Arab nor a Greek term. Medieval Latin authors later identified "tyrus" as a specific snake living in the Jericho region of Syria. The word *tyrus* was probably an unintentional neologism, the outcome of mistranslation because of the assonance of the terms *tyriaca* and *thérion* (venomous animal).[94] Ibn Sīnā's Latin translators used both *tyrus* and *viper* interchangeably for the Arabic word for serpent, *af'an*.[95] In subsequent literature, both medical and nonmedical, tyrus became the poisonous snake for compounding theriac. The serpent tyrus continued to figure in sixteenth-century treatises, such as Giovan Battista Ramusio's *Navigazioni e Viaggi*, as well as in many medical and apothecary books.[96]

Sometime in the 1490s Alessandro Agathimero claimed that the local viper was equivalent to tyrus for the purpose of making theriac.[97] At the time, apothecaries were obligated (at least in theory) to use *only* tyrus to make theriac, according to the Collegio Medico, the college of physicians of Venice that held authority over the recipes of theriac and mithridate. But importing tyrus from the Levant was both costly and risky: one snake could cost up to 200 ducats, and the sultan had banned exports.[98] Since tyrus was expensive and hard to acquire, the Collegio Medico allowed Venetian apothecaries to make theriac without tyrus—or indeed without any snake at all—although this practice would cast doubt on the quality of the product.

Agathimero had derived his opinion from a controversial work of his former professor Niccolò Leoniceno (1428–1524), famous for his critique of the errors of Pliny. Leoniceno was one of the most prestigious professors at the University of Ferrara, and is considered one of the initiators of Renaissance natural history.[99] In light of the dispute, Leoniceno wrote a brief treatise, *De tiro seu vipera*, supporting his former student. According to Leoniceno, the dispute stemmed from the new philological interpretation of medical texts. He proclaimed that "tyrus is viper" (*tirus vipera est*), and attributed the confusion between *viper* and *tyrus* to the imprecise pharmacological terminology of Ibn Sīnā.[100] Leoniceno also criticized Bartolomeo Montagnana, author of a popular medical compendium for students and physicians, for following Ibn Sīnā on this point.[101] Furthermore, he chastised the popular apothecary manual *Luminare Maior* for stating that apothecaries should use tyrus instead of local vipers. He even castigated the Collegio Medico for allowing apothecaries to make *trocisci* (dry round preparations) without tyrus. In typically aggravating Renaissance prose, he mocked the college's authority: "men of such high doctrine that one would suppose no knowledge remained unknown to them."[102]

Leoniceno must have been aware that his claim went beyond academic trivia. His treatise not only accused the Collegio Medico and other authors of incompetence, but also implied that actual practices were contravening patients' best interests. Furthermore, Leoniceno's position might have had an impact on the reputation of theriac, and implicitly freed apothecaries from having to import expensive tyrus from Syria, since local vipers were both cheaper and more available. Yet at the same time it forced them to actually make theriac with vipers, which were expensive and required intensive preparation. Unfortunately we do not know whether the Collegio Medico accepted Leoniceno's suggestion, because the papers of the Collegio predating 1545 burned in a fire.[103]

Pharmaceutical Recipes as a Matter of State

Another controversy in Venice, this time in 1531, shows that conflict was rife in the establishment of new pharmaceutical knowledge, and highlights how this process sowed division both within and between local professional groups. That year, prominent apothecary Cechino Martinelli (d. 1535) sought to update the recipe for mithridate. His attempt instigated a dispute involving apothecaries, collegiate physicians, and officers of the Giustizia Vecchia; eventually it escalated to the highest organ of the Venetian state.

Apothecaries in Venice had an edge over their counterparts in other Italian cities. In the sixteenth century, Venice was a unique emporium in both Italy and the wider European context, as well as an important publishing center. Thanks to the Republic's commercial networks, for centuries Venetian apothecaries enjoyed privileged access to spices and materia medica from the Middle East. Two of Venice's possessions, Cyprus and Crete, were considered the greenhouses of the Roman Empire, and were the origin of many theriac ingredients. Apothecaries such as Giovanni Battista Fulcheri from Lucca and Domenico Caravallo from Piedmont came to Venice to perfect their education in its famous Venetian apothecary shops, such as that of Galeazzo Corniani "at the sign of the Coral." (Each apothecary and their shop were identified by a specific sign.) Cechino Martinelli was the apothecary at the sign of the Angel, and himself the progenitor of a distinguished family of apothecaries. He had also served as the superintendent of the apothecary guild.[104]

In 1531 Martinelli asked the Giustizia Vecchia for permission to make mithridate according to Galen's instructions instead of the recipe approved by the Collegio Medico. He wanted to include in his mithridate "all the spices that should go in it, and not make it as it was actually done [*che non se fa cussi*], putting too much honey in it."[105] The recipe for mithridate from Servilius Damocrates (first cent. CE), as transmitted by Galen, was to become the remedy's most popular recipe in the early modern period. Unfortunately we never directly hear Martinelli's voice in the sources, and it is not clear how he articulated his request or what motivated him. Most likely he was influenced by the latest trends in medical scholarship, inspired by the rediscovery of Galen in the sixteenth century. He may have hoped that mithridate made according to Galen would favor his production or prestige over other apothecaries. Whatever Martinelli's reasons, his request was initially opposed by both the Giustizia Vecchia and the Collegio Medico.

In an unusual turn of events, the question reached the Collegio dei Savj, an executive organ of the Venetian government.[106] Since both the Giustizia Vecchia and the Collegio Medico agreed to use the old recipe, it is not clear why this uniquely apothecary matter reached such a high institution as the Collegio dei Savj. Three physicians from the Collegio Medico were received by Giovan Battista Ramusio, who was secretary of the Collegio dei Savj as well as a refined humanist and famous geographer. Against Martinelli's proposal, these collegiate physicians maintained that apothecaries should compound mithridate according to tradition, following "the mind of Avicenna" (Ibn Sīnā). According to Venetian diarist Marin Sanudo, Ramusio's response was unambiguous. He showed "that he knew medicine better than them, in spite of the fact that they were doctors. He took from the shelf a Greek version of Galen, and on the spot read the recipe to compose mithridate."[107] The book Ramusio cited was almost certainly the first Greek edition of Galen, the 1525–1526 Aldine edition.[108] Ramusio drew on his humanism to support Martinelli in exposing these physicians' backwardness. However, the Giustizia Vecchia continued to back the Collegio Medico. Caught in the crossfire, the Collegio dei Savj respected the institutional hierarchy; the final jurisdiction over a recipe belonged to the Collegio Medico. Ramusio referred the question back to the Collegio, "where they discuss men's lives."[109]

The college was unable to reach a decision. Some doctors followed Galen; others were inclined to use Ibn Sīnā's recipe. Pitting Galen against Ibn Sīnā raised a broader question surrounding competing medical references. Criticism against Arab authors such as Ibn Sīnā dated back a few centuries and gained momentum in light of the philological work of such scholars as Leoniceno. By the 1520s, academic criticisms of Arab authors intensified beyond scholarly circles. Many physicians kept referring to these authors as "barbarians," but several editions and commentaries of Ibn Sīnā's *Qanūn* continued to be published in the sixteenth century. As Nancy Siraisi has shown, at the time when Galen was "rediscovered," Ibn Sīnā was still a highly respected medical author both in universities and among practitioners, and remained so for many years to come.[110]

The Collegio dei Savj appointed a political committee to decide on the matter on the basis of the two factions' written medical reports.[111] State officials had to engage with pharmaceutical problems, despite not necessarily being knowledgeable about medicine and materia medica. In the end, the Collegio Medico diplomatically approved both Damocrates's and Ibn Sīnā's recipes for mithridate, allowing the "new" while maintaining the old custom.[112] But the question was settled only temporarily, and the regulation of recipes for mithridate and theriac was contested over the following years. In 1548 the Collegio Medico reaffirmed that apothecaries had to follow Ibn Sīnā "until true simples are found." The Collegio split again in 1559, and Damocrates's version of mithridate prevailed. Then in 1561 and again in 1572, Zuan Alberto Martinelli, son of Cechino, engaged in a new debate over the recipe of theriac.[113] In Venice pharmaceutical matters often became political questions requiring political answers.

The Race for "the Most Perfect Theriac"

The debate ignited by Agathimero in the 1490s over the recipe and ingredients of theriac took decades to gain momentum—but when it had, the search for "the most perfect theriac" thrilled the entire peninsula for more than half a century.[114] This process gained traction in the 1530s and went through an experimental phase during the 1540s to 1560s. By the late 1570s the Italian medical elite were convinced that "true theriac" had been achieved. From a practical standpoint, making "true theriac" first entailed establishing a definitive recipe by comparing recipes handed down over the centuries, such as those of Ibn Sīnā and Galen. Second, it required determination of the ingredients whose identity was uncertain, such as costus and amomum (two of the most elusive of all the missing ingredients) and supplying those whose commerce had been interrupted because of their costliness or shortage. For some ingredients, such as opobalsamum, these two problems coincided. Third, one had to perfect a number of discontinued apothecary procedures, such as making *trocisci hedicroi*, a compound that was an ingredient of theriac. Finally, it was necessary to overcome the skepticism of those scholars who believed that "true theriac" was simply impossible to achieve.

In the 1530s one such skeptical scholar was Symphorien Champier (ca. 1472–ca. 1540), who affirmed, "We want to demonstrate that, in our own times, we cannot have true theriac, because neither in France, nor in Italy nor Spain, and even less in Germany, do we have any knowledge of many simples that enter in the theriac of Andromachus and Galen."[115] Bolognese physician Giovanni Battista Teodosio (1475–1538) was also pessimistic. In a letter published posthumously in 1553, he confirmed he had tested theriac on doves—a trial described by Galen—with negative results because it was made with the wrong ingredients. He would later refuse to use theriac during an epidemic of plague, and he discouraged other doctors from doing so.[116] Teodosio concluded it was unlikely that anyone would have been able to make a good theriac, as so many ingredients were missing.[117] In Germany, Euricius Cordus (1486–1535), a Saxon physician who studied in Ferrara, published a treatise lamenting the low quality of German theriac, with a focus on the compound's production.

He affirmed that apothecaries produced bad theriac just like charlatans and "untrue apothecaries."[118] Skepticism abounded in the 1530s, dampening the enthusiasm of all but a few determined researchers.

The editions of *Discorsi* by Pier Andrea Mattioli (1501-1578) serve as a useful sociocultural barometer for gauging changing attitudes to "true theriac." In 1544 his Italian translation of and commentary on the five books of Dioscorides's *Materia Medica* gripped the attention of a public interested in plants. The work had thirteen editions during Mattioli's lifetime and was translated into Latin and several vernacular languages. As physician Bartolomeo Maranta put it, in the sixteenth century *Discorsi* went "through everybody's hands."[119] Such success testifies to Mattioli's outstanding sensitivity to the public's taste for changing trends and fashions. In fact, I assume the stances he took on theriac in *Discorsi* reflected, not necessarily his own views, but instead what he thought his readers would find both acceptable and convenient.

Mattioli did not even mention theriac in the first edition of *Discorsi* (1544).[120] Its success led to the second edition in 1548, published by Vincenzo Valgrisi; in this edition Mattioli added the sixth book on antidotes of Dioscorides. This book comprised two treatises on antidotes and venoms, that had been transmitted through the centuries in various versions and today are considered spurious.[121] In a world where every planet, plant, and mineral was placed in a precise hierarchy, antidotes were the most valued of all medicaments, and theriac and mithridate the most glorious of antidotes—and yet they were lost. Mattioli expressed his regret for this "truly damaging loss, greater than human life," explaining the problem thus: "Even if it is possible to find antidotes by these names compounded and everything, we cannot take advantage of Mithridatium and Theriaca of Andromachus..., in truth we completely lack them because they do not have the glorious and miraculous effects Galen and all his successors describe."[122] In line with Champier, Cordus, and Teodosio, Mattioli's baseline in 1548 was that the theriac available on the market was ineffective. So he publicized an alternative antidote of his own formulation: scorpion oil.[123]

The intellectual climate changed in the 1550s, by which point both classical texts on theriac and new works on pharmacy and materia medica had been available to scholars for several years.[124] The first published translation of *De theriaca ad Pisonem* appeared both in Paris and Basel in

1531, with a commentary by Johann Guenther.[125] A new translation of *De theriaca ad Pamphilianum* by Joachim Camerarius (1500–1574) was published in Nuremberg in 1533.[126] Nicander's *Theriaca* and *Alexipharmaca* were republished numerous times.[127] In 1561 Aldrovandi read Galen's *De theriaca ad Pisonem* to inaugurate a series of lectures at the University of Bologna.[128] By the 1550s scholars and medical students had become more familiar with classical texts.

Together with physicians' philological studies and fundamental research into materia medica, early modern natural history also benefited greatly from the engagement of members of the lower classes, such as apothecaries, surgeons, assayers, healers, and artisans.[129] Venetian apothecaries were especially well placed to contribute to the identification of materia medica, but those in other cities were just as active. Attempts to make "true theriac" took place in Rome, Perugia, Cortona, Padua, Bologna, Verona, Naples, Urbino, and Florence.[130] In Rome, for example, during the papacy of Pope Paul III (r. 1534–1549), Pellegrino Fulginate and Bartolomeo of Orvieto concocted theriac twice in the convent of Aracoeli, in an effort to make their compound "as legitimately as possible."[131] The convent was renowned for its apothecary shop, where Franciscan Angelo Paglia from Giovinazzo and Bartolomeo of Orvieto carried out their botanical research. Their work culminated in the 1543 publication of a commentary on Mesue, one of the authors most consulted by apothecaries.[132]

While the enthusiasm for simples was widespread, as evidenced by the wild success of Mattioli's *Dioscorides,* practical research into theriac itself was restricted to a relatively tight network of apothecaries and physicians. Making theriac was as expensive as it was complex, and therefore only those with means, connections, and large workshops could attempt it. Within this collaborative network, naturalists shared information, recipes, specimens, and apothecary procedures. Sharing was as much a practical necessity as a social practice. Maranta, a physician from Naples, wrote in 1558 to naturalist Aldrovandi in Bologna: "I prayed you let me know the way in which mithridate is made in Bologna and which substitutes you used . . . we wrote to all famous cities with the same request. Then we will choose the one that we will deem best."[133] A few months later he added: "I am only going to say that I am thankful for the two compositions of theriac and mithridate I received, and I am waiting for the one Falloppia is making in Padua."[134] Apothecaries often joined forces to organize theriac production, as was the case with Giulio Affaruosi from Reggio Emilia and Francesco Lauro de' Lavoranti from Pavia.[135] Sometimes, however, colleagues showed reluctance: in 1554 and 1555, and then again in 1558, apothecary Calzolari asked Aldrovandi for the substitutes used in Bologna. All three requests went unanswered.[136] Competition was as much a part of the game as cooperation.

In the late 1550s apothecaries started seeing exciting results. In Naples in 1557 the apothecary Ferrante Imperato (ca. 1525–ca. 1615) made theriac after having spent three years gathering all the necessary ingredients.[137] In 1561 Francesco Calzolari compounded theriac twice with only six substitutes.[138] In 1566 he did his best with only three substitutes. In 1563, sensible of the changing winds, a still reluctant Mattioli felt it was "troublesome to find theriac duly composed," but wrote that "if theriac must be used" then doctors should at least make sure it had been made with the authorities' approval. He also warned his readers against theriac sold in the public squares by charlatans who "eat poison as it if were bread" in front of a public ignorant of their tricks.[139] To help consumers avoid being misled or confused, Mattioli disclosed the nature of some of these deceptions. For example, he highlighted how charlatans would eat poison on a full stomach, but only after having first stuffed themselves with plentiful tripes in the winter or salads copiously dressed in oil in the summer, thus rendering the poison ineffective and allowing them to give credit to the low-quality theriac they had ingested.[140] In this edition of *Discorsi*, Mattioli still emphasized the untrustworthiness of theriac. But in the 1573 edition he finally had to yield and endorse at least one exception: "If in Italy can be found any theriac that I could myself declare the best according to my taste, it is the one made in Verona at the apothecary at the Golden Bell of the most virtuous M. Francesco Calceolario, rare simplicist of our own times." To endorse Calzolari's theriac, Mattioli claimed to have witnessed (*che n'ho vedute io*) several successful trials in "dangerous, almost desperate cases." He provided a few accounts of saved patients, including that of the seven-year-old son of Vespasiano Gonzaga, who had ingested sublimate having mistaken it for sugar.[141] Unable to outdo his rivals, Mattioli thought it wiser to side with them.

Refashioning Apothecaries While Refashioning Theriac

In his *Discorsi,* Mattioli distinguished between two types of apothecary. The first included apothecaries who made theriac in famous cities, "who desire universal health [*salute universale*], are very knowledgeable herbalists, and spend all their money and time fetching the right ingredients." The second type sold theriac "vulgarly" in great quantities, and would "dabble themselves in deceiving the world, in order to fill their purse with gold and silver."[142] These latter apothecaries were willing to make any compound remedy "as long as they can call it theriac and profit from it."[143] Even though all apothecaries had to belong to the local guild to practice, some were richer or more knowledgeable than others, and there could be subtle hierarchies and competition within a guild as much as anywhere else.

While researching theriac, a restricted number of apothecaries refashioned themselves as "learned apothecaries." As Mattioli noted, many attempted to profit from the refashioning of theriac into "true theriac," despite not having necessarily given equal contribution to the process. A few especially erudite and ambitious apothecaries secured a place for themselves among the learned elite. They advanced their careers by corresponding and collaborating with well-known physicians, building collections of *naturalia,* penning successful publications, and of course making "true theriac." These learned few included court apothecaries such as Evangelista Quattrami (1527–1608), herbalist of the Este family, and Antonio Bertioli (?–post-1608), apothecary of the Duke of Mantua. They took important positions in the local guilds, as did Ferrante Imperato in Naples; became successful authors, such as Georg Melich (fl. 1545–1590) in Venice; and became renowned collectors, such as Francesco Calzolari.[144] In the ancien régime, social mobility was modest. By fashioning themselves as learned apothecaries, artisans could achieve elevated status within their guilds, cities, and in the network of scholars studying materia medica.

Learned apothecaries emphasized what they considered to be the three characteristics that gave them authority over their rank-and-file counterparts. The first was their knowledge, both scholarly and practical, which they were proactive in demonstrating and sharing. They claimed to have researched, worked, and sometimes traveled more than other apothecaries. Key practices included studying texts, publishing, collecting simples, learning from other experienced apothecaries, and experimenting to reconstruct the right procedures. Camilla Erculiani, an apothecary in sixteenth-century Padua and the only learned apothecary woman we know of, wrote in one of her letters, "Now I struggle on our Galen, because I write about the nature, properties, and qualities of the ingredients of theriac, and which of these properties are beneficial against poisons."[145] Girolamo Calestani traveled extensively to master the art of apothecary, and bore witness to Roman apothecaries' first attempt to make theriac.[146] The compound would not stick together, and became so dry as to fall apart. Calestani affirmed that attending the two productions in Aracoeli removed any doubt he had had about performing the procedure.[147] More than anything, publishing helped learned apothecaries establish their authority.[148] Erculiani, Imperato, Melich, Calzolari, Bertioli, and Quattrami all published their works to prove their worth and knowledge. At times these works were institutionalized, such as when Calestani's *Delle osservationi nel comporre gli antidoti* (1564) became the official pharmacopoeia of Parma and Piacenza in 1667.[149]

The second way learned apothecaries asserted their difference was to proclaim their theriac to be "true," thereby all but disqualifying tons of vendible theriac on the market, and by extension discrediting the apothecaries producing it. In 1548 Galeazzo Corniani, apothecary at the sign of the Coral, informed the authorities he wanted to make theriac, which had not been made "for many years."[150] "Until recently," echoed Calzolari, the production of theriac "was left aside, and many reckoned it was impossible to compound it."[151] When affirming that theriac had not been made for years, learned apothecaries referred to "true theriac," which they considered the only acceptable theriac. Nonlearned apothecaries and even some physicians were put in a different category: those who did not know "true theriac." Calestani reported the story of a physician from Rome "who had never seen a production of theriac in his days (as many others), but following only the lesson of the books went in apothecary shops asking for *hedicroi*, believing it was a herb, a simple, or another medicine."[152] *Hedicroi* was solidified batter made of eighteen expensive ingredients, and was itself one of the ingredients of theriac.[153] Calestani was also skeptical of the Bolognese apothecaries who attempted to make theriac using an "extravagant" recipe in 1554—by simply omitting all the ingredients they lacked.[154] Knowing and making "true theriac" was a mark of distinction.

The third and final way learned apothecaries distinguished themselves from their more ordinary counterparts was to cast severe moral judgment on other producers of theriac. Author and well-traveled apothecary Georg Melich wrote: "Because in the composition of such a precious antidote I took great care and effort, I cannot but rest admired seeing that many sell these antidotes at a [low] price. I cannot but judge that together with the antidote they sell their soul to Satan."[155] According to learned apothecaries, those selling ordinary theriac not only had less knowledge, but were also of lesser morality—or were even diabolical. Complaints related to the risks of bad medicaments were as old as pharmacy, and popular healers and apothecaries alike sowed anxieties across all social levels.[156] Apothecaries occupied a liminal position, their interests split between profit and healing.[157] They were just as much in the public eye as charlatans. Popular writers such as Tommaso Garzoni, in his compilation about "all the professions of the world," described apothecaries as shrewd traders.[158] Some were honest enough to admit that their art was not beyond reproach: "In such an important Art, many errors are to be found, and . . . there are great flaws among the apothecaries who, because of greed, ignorance, or clumsiness, do not accurately follow the doctors' prescriptions."[159] By making "true theriac," learned apothecaries created a hierarchy within their profession based on morals as well as knowledge and practice.

Authoritative physicians such as Aldrovandi and Mattioli explicitly recognized this occupational distinction. As we saw in the passages at the beginning of this section, Mattioli endorsed the learned apothecaries as being both more knowledgeable and more honest than their counterparts.[160] Even Aldrovandi, who generally held a low opinion of apothecaries, admitted, "It is true that today we find some [apothecaries] who are very experienced [*molto bene essercitati*] and experts [*periti*] in their profession, they understand very well Latin authors who have written about this subject, and I know some of them in Rome, Bologna, Venice, Padua, Naples, Lucca, Florence, Mantua, Verona, Trento. God grant that all would imitate these few for the universal good."[161] Even though the endorsement of Mattioli, Aldrovandi, and other physicians could not grant learned apothecaries universal acceptance in the academic world, it nonetheless helped create a new community of scholars and researchers of natural history.

This chapter has offered a revision of the historical quest for "true theriac" by introducing different theriacs with parallel histories. More than a topic of scientific inquiry debated in erudite Latin medical books, theriac was a commodity sold by peddlers and apothecaries, controlled by officials, and consumed by patients. In the pursuit of recreating Theriaca magna as potent as that of Andromachus, a select group of physicians and apothecaries disrupted a network of well-established economic interests and legal traditions. This assessment has shown that the endeavor of recreating "true theriac" entailed intellectual, institutional, and social processes, spanning the whole of Renaissance Italy between the 1490s and 1570s.

The emergence of the concept of "true theriac" rested on the implication that vendible theriac was of bad quality, where quality was assessed according to both the recipe and the procedures employed in production. In their quest for "true" theriac, physicians, naturalists, and apothecaries reconceptualized and appropriated theriac. During this process, "learned apothecaries" conceived a new hierarchy based on their superior knowledge and expertise, the quality of their theriac, and their greater morality. Physicians explicitly recognized this new hierarchy by accepting learned apothecaries into their own circle of scholars involved in renovating knowledge on materia medica.

The case study of Venice exemplifies the interconnection between the intellectual and institutional spheres. Early on, the Venetian state itself was interested in defining the recipe of theriac, not only because of the revenues its commerce brought to state coffers, but also because of the city's deeply embedded association with theriac. Meanwhile in other Italian cities, whose theriac trade was less developed than Venice's, the reinvention of theriac from vendible to *verissima* (very true) took on a courtly character, as discussed in Chapter 3. The next chapter investigates patients' and apothecaries' experience of material theriac.

CHAPTER 2

The Experience of Theriac

"*O*FTEN I receive letters from our friend Salvuccio; sometimes he asks me for theriac and other times for mithridate, and he berates me for not providing them quickly enough, although I do my best to serve him swiftly and well."[1] Florentine linguist Giorgio Bartoli (1534–1583) playfully teased his friend Salvuccio, who would ask for theriac and mithridate so frequently that Bartoli was sometimes unable to fulfill his whimsical requests. Salvuccio likely hoped theriac would better his health. From an anthropological perspective, all medicines are "tokens of hope." So theriac and mithridate were not merely physical substances, but also catalysts for both physical and emotional experiences.[2] Early modern accounts of patients' experiences of illness, healing practices, and their relationship with drugs are scarcer than historians of medicine desire, and reports on theriac are no exception. Nonetheless, we have gained significant insights into how, when, and why patients employed theriac.

Theriac's potency resulted from the convergence of biological, cultural, and psychological processes. It was a physically recognizable substance that induced specific and distinctive sensory experiences, surpassing just its biomedical effects. Culturally theriac was infused with symbolism drawn from its history, recipe, production, ingredients, and popularity. Finally, theriac raised feelings of pride, hope, and security (or despair in its absence), all of which were integral to the acts of taking it and making it.

In the first section of this chapter I analyze theriac as an object by detailing its sensory qualities. What did it taste, look, smell, and even sound like? What did it mean to consume theriac? Both early modern patients and physicians relied heavily on their senses and own bodily experiences, ascribing great importance to the sensory characteristics of substances, even apart from those substances' medical qualities.[3] Early modern patients cherished theriac; like Salvuccio they would anxiously request it from friends and patrons; travelers carried it as protection from "bad airs." Those with means used theriac as a preservative to maintain good health. Patients of all social levels employed theriac and mithridate in cases of poisoning or acute conditions.

In the second, third, and fourth sections I explore the perspective of apothecaries. What did it mean to make theriac? What were the specificities of theriac recipe? How did they conceptualize their artisanal work when crafting theriac? Often produced simultaneously, theriac and mithridate were representative of Galenic pharmacy, yet were unique compared to other compound remedies. Making theriac presented numerous practical questions, such as how to grind its solid ingredients, melt gums, and ferment the compound. Crafting theriac demanded significant artisanal skills and knowledge, as well as a substantial economic investment. Producers sourced their ingredients from their business networks, which involved complex organization but afforded immense prestige. In the fourth section, an unusual trial in 1609 provides insight into how physicians and apothecaries perceived the materiality of pharmaceutical compounds.

Discussing all sixty-three ingredients of theriac one by one would result in a detailed list more akin to a Renaissance *herbarium* than a chapter in a contemporary monograph. Instead the fifth section of this chapter delves into one of the ingredients most laden with meaning: viper. A medieval legacy linked the snake in theriac to Christ, thus symbolically correlating the salvation of the soul with the recovery of the body. I suggest that the memory of this religious significance embedded in theriac was still alive in the early modern period, further intensifying the emotional power of the drug. In an intricate twist, however, the production of such spiritual and physical "salvation" posed a burden on the environment: the increased production of Theriaca magna in Venice led to the extinction of vipers in an area where they were exhaustively harvested for several centuries. The intensive early modern pharmacological production of theriac was not a sustainable practice.

What Was It Like Taking Theriac?

There was no standardization of goods in the early modern period, yet theriac possessed specific characteristics and a well-recognized taste. The compound varied from city to city according to recipe variations, and the quality of supplies could cause theriac to change from one year to the next. Nevertheless, theriac and mithridate had distinct flavors. Apothecaries and physicians claimed that a trained tongue could distinguish between high-quality and poor-quality theriac and mithridate.[4]

The chief rule of the art of producing these two compounds mandated that all ingredients be blended properly. To taste or smell an individual ingredient was considered a sign of incompetence. In his pamphlet "compiled rather for those which are to use it, [than] for the learned," physician Walter Baley taught patients "how to know good Mithridatium" by its taste:

> In like sort, the taste must not expresse any one simple, but be as a common sapore [taste] resulting of all the simples: so that if in tasting of Mithridatium you may manifestly discerne or discry any one simple in it, surely that Mithridatium is not well confected. Therefore it may not ha[v]e in it any excesse of [u]ngratefull bitternes, which doth sometimes happen, when the confectioner doth either take hony ouerold, or boyle ye same o[v]ermuch. So it may not shew to the taste any sowrenes, which happeneth if the wyne [u]sed be not well chosen, or not well handled in the compounding.[5]

In both manuals for apothecaries and pamphlets for patients, taste was the baseline for recognizing a good theriac.

What did theriac taste like? In a good theriac, the honey appeased the flavor of several bitter ingredients, and the taste lingered. According to physicians in seventeenth-century Bologna, the taste of a good theriac was "sweet at first, then rather bitter, and finally aromatic and sharp [*acuto*]."⁶ Humanist Marsilio Ficino, a firm supporter of theriac, conceded that "the taste of true theriac lasts in the mouth and gives thirst, and it constipates the bowels."⁷ Both theriac and mithridate contained several markedly bitter ingredients: opium, bdellium resin (possibly *Commiphora wightii*), opopanax (gummi-resina of *Opopanax chironium*), and thlaspi seed (possibly field pennycress or *Thlaspi arvense*). So the main function of honey was "to water down with its sweetness the bitterness of the simples with which theriac is made."⁸ Three scholars in the 1960s, unaware of the description of the Bolognese physicians, analyzed a sample of eighteenth-century theriac, concluding with a strikingly similar description: "at first fully sweet, then pungent, almost astringent."⁹

More recently, several groups have reconstructed theriac following different recipes and procedures. A panel of food experts evaluated a theriac made according to an eighteenth-century Swedish recipe, concurring that theriac had a specific aromatic and flavor profile, with sweetness and bitterness the most profound tastes.¹⁰ They concluded that "the flavour and odour of theriac were part of a sensory regime which is now lost to us, but which was once culturally shared and agreed."¹¹ After tasting a sample of theriac reconstructed in Wrocław, historian Larry Principe confirmed it provided a warming sensation, "a spreading out of warmth into the chest." This could corroborate the perceived heating qualities patients might anticipate from what was deemed a "hot medicament."¹²

The smell of theriac was just as distinctive as its taste: "heavy [*grave*], then acute, then penetrating and it fills the brain." It was also "somewhat ungrateful [*ingrato*]."¹³ Indeed, the smell was strong enough—albeit less ungrateful than other bad odors—that in his poem *Parvizal* Wolfram von Eschenbach (ca. 1170–1219/1225) described theriac being used to mitigate foul odors on the deathbed of the knight Amfortas:

And, to purify, they had theriac,
And costly ambergris, to attack
Foul odours with their wholesomeness.¹⁴

The early modern belief that smells carried the materials from which they emanated is maintained by scientific theories today. Odors were considered real substances that penetrated the brain and could affect the body.¹⁵

Thus, even the smell of theriac conveyed a little of the remedy's healing properties.

Alongside taste and smell, packaging and consistency were essential aspects of patients' experience with theriac. Apothecaries stored theriac in large or medium-sized jars in their shops, and sold it in small cylindrical containers. In 1962 researchers opened a typical eighteenth-century pewter container kept in the Museum of the Pharmacology Institute of Florence. The little box was 4.5 cm in length and sealed with a pewter lid, and contained 4 drachms (about half an ounce) of dehydrated matter. It was wrapped in a label with the engraving of the producer, secured with a twine sealed with red wax. Below the label was another protective wrapping, this time paper, folded four times. Upon opening, researchers found a dry black substance with an aroma like that of dry figs. Its core was still relatively soft.[16] A batch of theriac could supposedly last several decades, and depending on its age had the consistency of thick molasses or a soft paste. According to physicians, a four-year-old theriac "should stay together, not be runny, and when picked up remain attached to the spatula . . . when touched with a finger it should leave an odor and its coloring [dark brown]."[17]

Having opened the container, patients would dissolve a small dose of paste into a liquid for ingestion. According to sixteenth-century empiric Mario di Marino Galasso (fl. sixteenth cent.), rich men preferred taking their theriac in white wine: "Also a drachm of good theriac with or without white wine as rich men like it best. We heard from a trustworthy man who got the plague that someone gave him a drachm of theriac diluted in two fingers of water and two of oil and two of little child's urine on an empty stomach and he recovered, while everyone else in his household died of plague."[18] As this passage suggests, aside from wine, various liquids were considered suitable for dissolving theriac: juice, broth, water, oil, vinegar, tea, rum—even child's urine.

Patients used theriac not just for ingestion. It was often mixed with other medicines or used as an ingredient in more complex preparations. During the plague of 1624–1625 in Leiden, naturalist Jacobus Bontius (1592–1631) used human bladder stone mixed with theriac, mithridate, and drops of amber and juniper.[19] Similarly, in 1797 George Washington paid 25 dollars to Dr. Henry William Stoy in Lebanon, Pennsylvania, who cured "persons bit by wild animals" with a remedy made with red chickweed, theriac, and beer.[20] Theriac was also used as a cataplasm, a poultice applied to some parts of the body or to buboes. "Professor of secrets" Leonardo Fioravanti (1517–1588) advised applying a cataplasm to the region of the heart around the nipple to fend off the plague.[21] To protect themselves from miasmas, physicians and priests placed theriac soaked in wine or vinegar in the nostrils when visiting lazarettos or other potentially dangerous places.[22]

Apothecaries and physicians promoted theriac as a ready-made remedy for use by both sick and healthy individuals. Patients primarily trusted theriac for acute conditions or poisoning. For either purpose, a single dose varied from a scruple (1/24 of an ounce; 1–1.3 grams, depending on the system) to a drachm (3.9–4 grams), to be taken once or a few times if needed. After having been poisoned in China, Jesuit missionary Father Jean de Fontaney (1643–1710) reported a day of intense pain and two nights of distress, after which he vomited copiously, and then, he stated, "I took a good bit of theriac, and I felt better right away."[23] From his account, it seems Fontaney got rid of the poison *before* taking theriac, but nevertheless evidently attributed his immediate improvement to the remedy. Trust in theriac's efficacy was deeply rooted, and persisted despite the arrival of exotic remedies. Writing from India in 1586, merchant and humanist Filippo Sassetti (1540–1588) declared: "To be honest, I believe in these marvels [bezoar stone] only up to a certain point. I took it a few times and I felt neither better nor worse. I prefer to stick to theriac, mithridate, aloe, agaric, and rhubarb, whose effects are also known here."[24] Like Fontaney, most patients took theriac only occasionally, such as when they felt sick, had received a venomous bite, feared poisoning, or hoped to alleviate pain. The use of fresh theriac after a purge brought "substantial benefit" to Eleonora de' Medici-Gonzaga (1567–1611), who had been fatigued from "atrocious pains."[25] The apothecary shop at the monastery of Nunziatina in Florence purchased theriac in bulk for internal use from a single apothecary.[26] The monastery apothecary recorded the quantity, cost, and timing of theriac taken by the nuns. The monastery budgeted up to 8 soldi per year per nun for medicines, and also paid for physicians' visits. After that, nuns had to pay for medicines themselves. Nuns at Nunziatina usually took one ounce of theriac over the course of several days, together with other remedies.[27] In 1762 nun Margherita Masini took theriac for several days in August and September, at a total cost of 17soldi soldi. In the same year, nun Teresa Mannini took theriac in June and August for a total of 12 soldi. Many of the Nunziatina nuns came from families that were comfortably well off, and were willing to pay for theriac out of pocket if they needed it.

Only wealthy patients could afford to use theriac as a preventative. Physicians such as Oratio Guarguanti (1554–1611), author of a short treatise on the advantages of theriac, promoted its regular use: "I confess to taking [theriac] at least once a month during autumn and winter, as I deem it highly beneficial for preserving my health."[28] Patients followed this advice. For instance, in a eulogy for Antonio Magliabecchi (1633–1714), who died at eighty-one, the librarian of Cosimo III de' Medici attributed his longevity to four habits: never leaving the house in the morning except to attend disputes or declamations; keeping his head always well covered; refraining from icy drinks, but not from good wine; and "[taking] several morsels of theriac, the only medicine [*farmaco*] in which he accidentally had some faith, which, as he used to say, he judged a good antidote to the evil of the earth's evaporations."[29] Similarly, "from time to time" Marquis Romualdo de Sterlich (1712–1788) used a theriacal water, or theriacal spirit, which he expressly ordered from Venice. "I do not know how it is made, it is a sort of *aquavita,* which smells a lot like theriac, and in my experience of several years I see that it does good to the stomach."[30] When used preventively, the recommended dose was usually a scruple, to be taken once a week or once a month.[31]

In the early modern period, prevention was as important as treatment, if not more so. Like Magliabecchi and de Sterlich, early modern patients felt a sense of command over their health, seeking advice from and sharing knowledge with both physicians and their social circles. In seventeenth-century Bologna, buying theriac without prescription was considered a "usual" behavior. Apothecaries were allowed to dispense theriac without prescription in case of "necessity," although how one might define necessity was never established.[32] The growing interest in remedies such as theriac and the concomitant expansion of the market implied an increased focus on health in general, without necessarily indicating a shift from a preventive paradigm to a curative one, or the decline of preventive medicine and the rise of curative medicine.[33]

Patients often kept a few doses of theriac for safekeeping, especially when traveling or heading to dangerous places. Swiss naturalist Moritz Hoffmann advised colleagues undertaking botanical expeditions to take a root cutter and other useful instruments for preserving specimens, along with a little bit of theriac for protection from poisonous bites.[34] According to Bartolomeo Maranta, theriac was especially important for those traveling through misty regions: by virtue of its heating qualities, theriac was believed to warm the body better than "good clothes."[35] Conversely, traveling without theriac could be unpleasant. French poet Vincent Voiture (1597-1648) feared death when forced to face illness without theriac, and lamented having traveled without a stash. "I am suddenly breathless and I have unexpected weaknesses, without being able to find any theriac here, I am sicker than I ever was, in a place where there are no remedies for me. So that, Madame, I fear that [the city of] Nancy will be deadly to me as it was to the Duke of Bourgogne."[36] Keeping a little theriac handy was a form of reassurance. Faith in the remedy endured. Even in the nineteenth century the memory of theriac's heyday lived on—so much so that Venetian historian Girolamo Dian wrote that "faith in the effects of theriac was such that every family, even the poorest, would keep it thoroughly, as if it were a sure talisman to protect themselves from the hidden dangers of the thousand ailments that surround all humans."[37] At the very least, it seems that the mere availability of theriac had the power to soothe anxieties.

Making Theriac

Colloquially, preparing theriac was the epitome of complex tasks. In a letter to his dear friend Farinelli (Carlo Broschi, 1705-1782), the famous castrato singer, the poet Pietro Metastasio (1698-1782) ironically lamented how in Vienna it was easier to have the best cooks make a pot of theriac than a homey dish of macaroni with zucchini.[38] In the early modern period, making theriac was a significant undertaking, not limited to apothecaries. In 1687 the Bolognese Collegio Medico informed the Senate that "this year, since making theriac and other noble compositions requires it, the College will be occupied with great diligence throughout spring and summer."[39]

Making theriac demanded time and refined artisanal skills. Recent scholars have described the making of theriac as nothing less than "an artistic endeavor," recognizing the skills it demanded.[40] Early modern apothecaries approached production with reverence: it represented both the pinnacle of their various preparations and the culmination of their careers. As the editor of the Roman *Antidotario* declared, "After having discussed it, I was able to observe the composition of this antidote [theriac] many times. Yet, I only dared to attempt such composition at the age of forty-five, and not before."[41] Making theriac was a challenging process for many reasons: the sheer number of ingredients and their cost; the difficulties in sourcing several components; the uncertainty of identifying which plants to use; the uncommon skills and knowledge required to carry out the long and intricate compounding procedure; and the need for money, preparation, and a wide network of social connections. As we have seen, the successful production of "true theriac" was an apothecary's key to becoming regarded as a "learned apothecary." Recipes such as that of theriac needed interpretation by skilled artisans. Learned apothecaries became aware of and vocal about their artisanal competence, stressing the "universal rules of the apothecary art" over Galen's instructions, as Georg Melich described: "Practice [*l'esperimento*] has found a better way ... than what the Ancients wrote, and good apothecaries rely more on the general rules of the art and on experience than on the authority of Galen, although he is a great authority."[42] Melich's sense of pride and independence in his work, knowledge, and experience was shared by many learned apothecaries.[43]

Most Theriaca magna recipes used in Italy in the early modern period listed sixty-three ingredients, not sixty-four as is often stated.[44] More precisely, the recipe comprised sixty-one ingredients plus wine and honey, which served as the medium for blending. The ingredients were divided into six classes, and each had a usually fixed number of components: one, four, eight, seventeen, twenty-four, and seven. Class 1 comprised a single ingredient: 48 drachms (6 ounces) of squill *trocisci*—that is, small discs or thin circular tablets made with baked bulbs of maritime squill (*Drimia maritima*) mixed with the flower of bitter vetch (*Vicia ervilia*). Class 2 contained 24 drachms each (3 ounces) of four ingredients—opium, pepper, *trocisci hedicroi,* and *trocisci viperini*—for a total of 12 ounces. *Trocisci hedicroi* were a complex preparation in themselves, comprising eighteen ingredients, some of which were listed separately as ingredients for theriac. Class 3 contained 12 drachms each of its eight ingredients, for a total of 12 ounces. Classes 4 and 5 were the most crowded, with seventeen and twenty-four ingredients, respectively. Class 6 contained only seven ingredients. Three components of theriac—*trocisci hedicroi, scyllitici,* and *viperini*—were preparations that themselves involved several ingredients, so the actual number of ingredients totaled seventy-one (not counting repeats). However, the number of substances needed for the entire theriac manufacture was higher, because single components required other ingredients for production. For example, to make chalcitidis, apothecaries needed vitriol; to cook squill for *trocisci scyllitici*, they needed wheat flour; yet vitriol and wheat flour were not listed as ingredients of theriac.[45]

The ingredients of each class were added to the compound in fixed proportions: 48, 24, 12, 6, 4, and 2 drachms. Pharmacopoeias used the same scale for weights, but *systems* of weight differed greatly. Aldrovandi acknowledged the difficulties imposed by this variation: "As for the measures, we grope around and go blind in our understanding of Ancients' medicinal doses."[46] Apothecaries often compounded more than one batch at a time, multiplying each quantity to maintain the right proportions. Some pharmacopoeias, such as De Sgobbis's *Universale theatro farmaceutico,* provided specific instructions for producing theriac in bulk.[47]

The ingredients were as diverse as they were numerous. The recipe primarily involved ingredients of vegetable origin, including a mushroom (*Agaricum albissimum*) (which was then considered a plant), but also included earths (*Terra Lemnia*); minerals, such as chalcitis; one animal (viper); and one animal-derived component, castoreum, a secretion produced from beavers. Vegetable-derived ingredients required different parts of a plant, or indeed multiple parts: roots or rhizomes, such as gentian and iris; seeds, such as anise, fennel, and pennycress; flowers, such as red roses and *Teucrium scordium;* fruits, such as pepper; gums, such as gum arabic; extracts, such as licorice and *Cytinus hypocistis;* oleoresins, such as myrrh and *Commiphora opobalsamum;* woods and barks, such as cinnamon and *Cassia lignea;* and leaves, such as *folium* and *Origanum dictamnus.*[48]

This enormous variety required apothecaries to have good planning, timing, and organization—indeed, it sometimes took over a year to assemble the ingredients in their entirety. Because theriac had to ferment, it was good practice to make it early, before the summer, in May or June, so the fermentation could benefit from the season's natural heat.[49] This meant many herbs and roots had to be harvested a year before, during the previous summer, and then stored.[50] But then there was the risk of supplies becoming rotten, dusty, or moldy—especially *trocisci viperini,* which was notoriously susceptible to mold. For this reason, many apothecaries preferred to make theriac at a later date, in August. In 1577 the Collegio Medico in Florence decreed theriac-making season to run from June 1 and

August 31.[51] Apothecaries wishing to make theriac had to navigate recipes rife with contradictions, follow steps that were often ambiguous or downright obscure, then justify their decisions.

Many of the herbs and roots could be harvested locally, and entries about theriac in local pharmacopoeias provided detailed maps of where to find them. Apothecary Ippolito Ceccarelli, the editor of the 1612 edition of the official Roman pharmacopoeia, stated confidently, "Since we can locate numerous perfect simples for this purpose [making theriac] in our Roman countryside, I compiled a list to ensure we can gather them at the right time and place." He collected Roman turnip rape in the Horti Viminali and green horehound in the Horti Palatini, two gardens within the city; he picked Roman calaminta on the hills beyond Porta Angelica; and he sourced wall germander just outside Porta Appia. Then Ceccarelli bought licorice juice made in Ascoli and vipers from Tuscia. It took him a year to collect all the local simples for his theriac.[52]

Procuring ingredients that were available only farther afield proved far more challenging. In the sixteenth century, during the heyday of the quest for "true theriac," those embarking on production depended on an extensive network of friends and correspondents to acquire foreign ingredients. When Aldrovandi was preparing for production in 1574, he obtained *Acorus calamus* (sweet flag) from Istanbul through the patriarch of Aquileia; opobalsamum (oleoresin from *Commiphora opobalsamum*) from Marino Cavalli and Monsignor Daniele Barbani in Constantinople; cinnamon from Cardinal Paleotti in Spain; and castoreum from the Duke of Bavaria.[53]

Before the 1580s the rareness and scarcity of some ingredients meant that only a select few apothecaries would even attempt making "true theriac"—and modern scholars may experience similar difficulty. Danuta Raj, a pharmacist from Wrocław University looking to source all the ingredients necessary for reconstructing theriac, has reported having to write not only to international pharmaceutical and botanical suppliers, but also to zoological and botanical gardens, museums, missionaries, and ambassadors. Raj has affirmed that corresponding through well-connected friends and acquaintances was at times the only way to acquire some materia medica not in use today.[54] However, supplies for theriac became easier to source during the years 1590–1615, requiring a less privileged network. As making "true theriac" became even more common in the late seventeenth century, many apothecaries simply dispatched agents to Venice, the

Italian port where most exotic ingredients arrived from the East. Venetian apothecaries stabilized supplies as demand increased.

Until the mid-seventeenth century, knowledge of specific foreign ingredients was not widespread, even among apothecaries. According to Adriano Riccardi, a Bolognese apothecary and author, apothecaries should not rely solely on the integrity of the supply chain; individuals with first-hand knowledge should also exercise control: "Other things that are not in our country can be gathered by men of the highest intelligence, and [these ingredients] have to be examined with the writings of approved authors, who should have seen what they teach, and do not speak only following others' accounts, because it is easy to be trumped by these [accounts]."[55] To dispel any doubt about their authenticity, ingredients were accompanied on their travels by certifications (*fedi*) signed by university physicians or learned apothecaries. In 1594 Antonio Bertioli, apothecary to the Duke of Mantua, obtained his opobalsamum from the famous apothecary Giovanni Pona, along with a *fede* from Verona's Collegio Medico, which he duly published along with three more *fedi* to allay any possible skepticism.[56] By the mid-seventeenth century, knowledge about foreign simples became more widespread among apothecaries across Italy. Identifying simples and knowing their provenance became essential skills for any apothecary hoping to continue their production and protect their business from both inspectors and competing apothecaries.

Once all the ingredients were gathered, apothecaries hosted an exhibit, exposing the ingredients for three days or more for the approval of state officials, collegiate physicians, and other apothecaries. Inspectors had three concerns regarding the ingredients: quality, substitutes, and proper identification. Substitution was a common practice within Galenic pharmacy, codified since antiquity.[57] A substitute (in Latin, a *quid pro quo*) was a substance replacing a missing ingredient. Not all plants grew in every region, yet recipes dictated that most herbs be used while fresh, so substituting unavailable herbs with fresh ones with similar properties was considered beneficial to the patient. However, a compound with too many substitutes was deemed to be of lesser quality. In the case of theriac, Maranta considered substitution a "patch" (*rattoppamento*), and a theriac with too many substitutes "sick" (*ammalata*). It was acceptable to use as many as six substitutes, although Maranta was mindful to label as "lazy" (*poltrone*) the apothecary who was unwilling to look for simples that could be found with additional work.[58]

Once the apothecary had received the officials' approval, the concoction began. The equipment required for making theriac was considerable, illustrated by Bolognese state officials' appreciation for the workshop of Isabella Fontana's electuary, affirming that "the whole apparatus seemed more suitable for the preparation of theriac than that of a mere electuary."[59] The inventory list of theriac instruments in Bologna included numerous tools of iron and wood, as well as ladles, tongs, skimmers, a bellow, a shovel, large scissors, baking sheets, and two copper furnaces, each weighing 192 pounds.[60] This instrumentation was expensive and was kept highly secure. Depending on the kind of grinding needed, ingredients could be divided in mortars made of different materials, such as porphyry, marble, and bronze, and crushed with pestles made of metal or wood.[61] To avoid spoiling costly ingredients such as gums and oils, some apothecaries suggested melting them gently in a bain-marie, a type of heated bath.[62] Pharmacopoeias did not usually report what instruments apothecaries needed; so apothecaries were supposed to know what was required. Most procedures involved in theriac making were ordinary activities for apothecaries, but making "true theriac" posed new problems. During the heroic times of the quest for "true theriac," apothecaries and physicians exchanged useful information as they sought the best practices. Apothecary Francesco Accoramboni from Rimini detailed a number of subtle techniques, such as using oil when grinding *trocisci scyllitici*, which were especially hard, and cutting the opium with wood and soaking it in wine.[63] In the late seventeenth century these details became more commonly described in pharmacopoeias.

Grinding was particularly important, and demanded hard labor. Herbs, flowers, roots, seeds, and *trocisci* had to be finely ground through hours upon hours of ponderous crushing with large mortars and pestles. Yet this endeavor was imperative: as explained by Mantuan Filippo Costa (1550–1586), the author of a successful book on the most popular remedies, the quality of the grinding was fundamental to healing: "In order to heal well an internal ailment, it is necessary that the simples reach the disease effectively so that they can easily communicate their virtue where they should, which is troublesome with simples that are approximately ground."[64] In Venice the heavy work of crushing was traditionally carried out by laborers of poor origin hailing from inland Venetian dominions, such as Friuli or the provinces of Bergamo and Brescia (Figures 2.1, 2.2).[65]

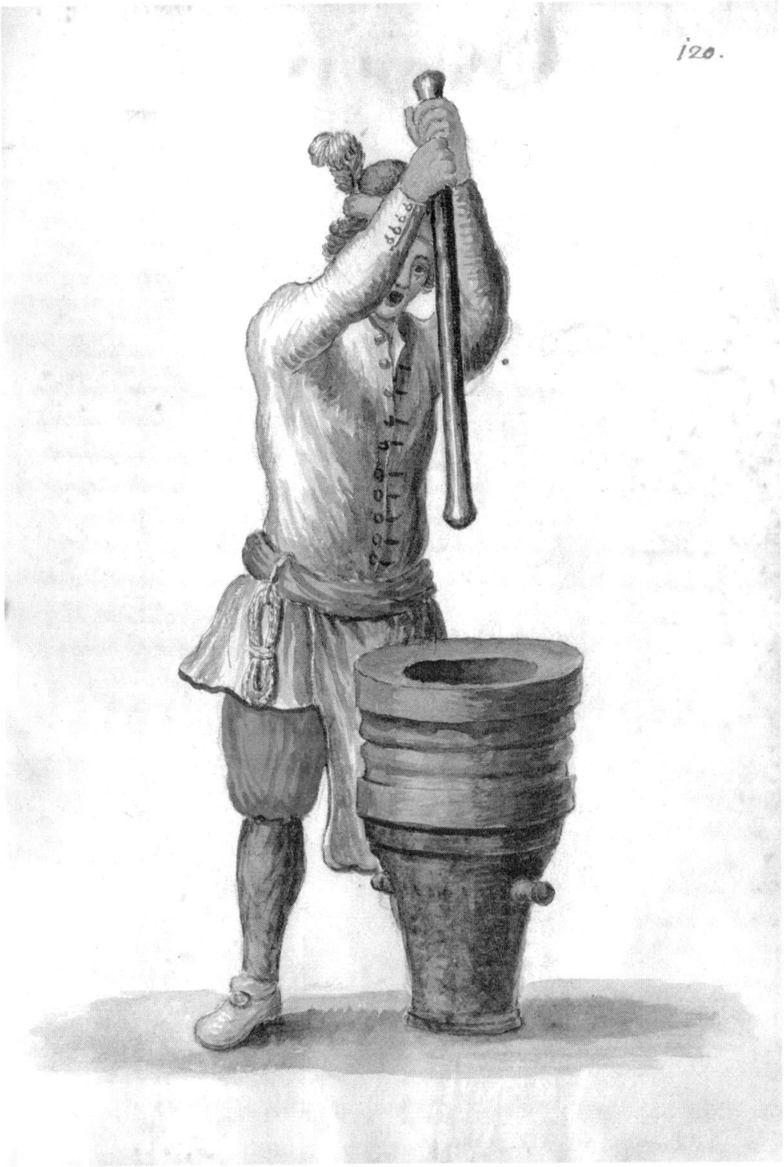

Fig. 2.1. Laborer grinding the ingredients for theriac in an eighteenth-century watercolor. Ms Gradenigo Dolfin 49.3 120, Gabinetto Stampe e Disegni, Museo Correr, Venice. 2024.
© Biblioteca Correr–Fondazione Musei Civici di Venezia.

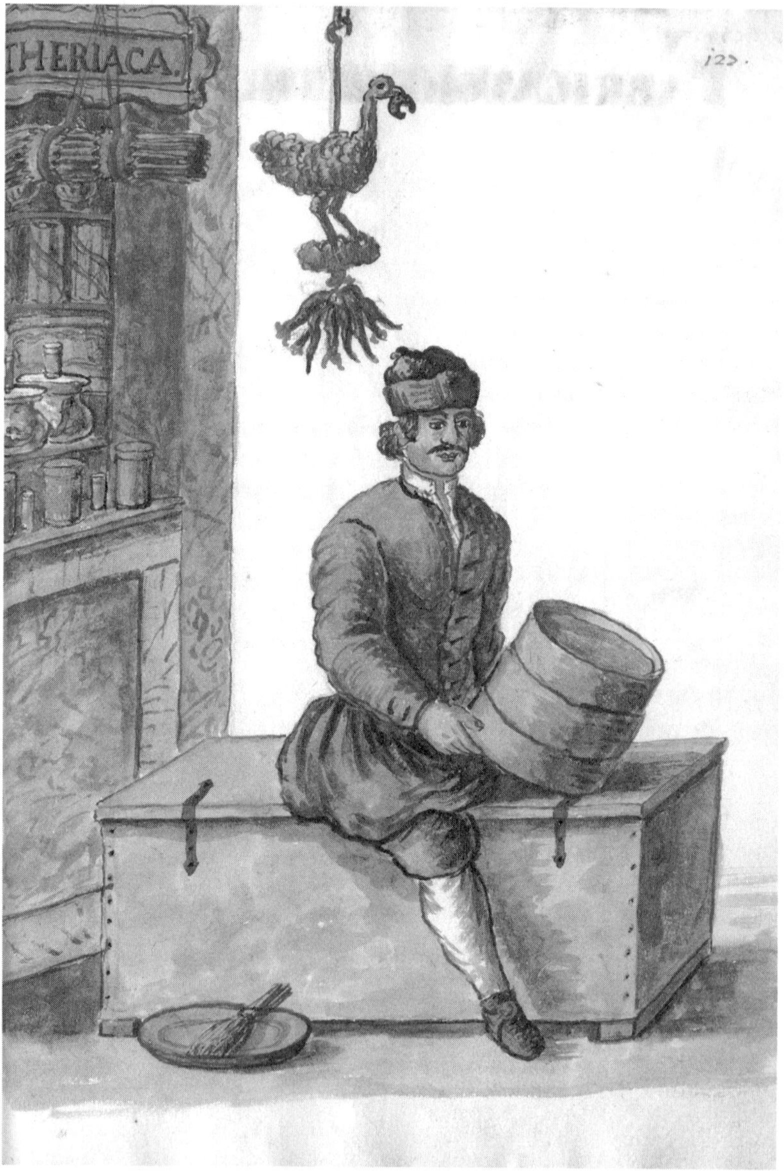

Fig. 2.2. Laborer sitting in an apothecary shop holding a sieve used to sift theriac ingredients. Ms Gradenigo Dolfin 49.3 120, Gabinetto Stampe e Disegni, Museo Correr, Venice. 2024.

© Biblioteca Correr—Fondazione Musei Civici di Venezia.

Once ground, minced, crushed, melted, and sifted, all the ingredients had to be carefully assembled in a precise order. Then the mixture had to be well stirred and put to rest. The final step was fermentation, which posed several problems. According to Ibn Sīnā, fermentation was fundamental to theriac production because it was during this time the compound developed its specific properties. Physicians also believed opium lost its narcotic effect when fermented. Maranta and most authors agreed that fermentation should last a year, during which the compound should be mixed regularly, which required much strength. Although the Milanese pharmacopoeia affirmed that fermentation "is infallibly practiced today," not all apothecaries respected the one-year fermentation: some put theriac on sale after six, three, or even just one month—and others skipped the process entirely.[66] Furthermore, during fermentation the compound was usually stored out of the public eye, and this was often when tampering and adulteration took place. We will never know how often theriac was placed into commerce without fermentation, or adulterated by the addition of honey for added volume, or tampered with in any number of other ways. These practices illuminate the hidden side of theriac production: illegalities and falsifications—collectively the diametric counterpart to theriac accountability.

An Open Recipe

Something that set theriac and mithridate apart from other medicaments was the transparency of their recipes and production. According to seventeenth-century apothecary Giuseppe Candrini, "[theriac] by tradition obtained the privilege to be made in public, almost as if the Sun of medicaments could not be born but in the patent light, giving clear proofs to the mundane tribunal just as daylight."[67] While guilds kept secret recipes in several artisanal trades, such as glassmaking, and families bequeathed pharmaceutical secrets in testaments, the recipes of Andromachus's theriac and Damocrates's mithridate were neither secret nor patented. This accessibility was considered a guarantee of quality compared to other medical preparations.[68]

From the sixteenth century onward, virtually every pharmacopoeia across Europe, official or otherwise, contained one or more versions of the recipe of Andromachus's Theriaca magna and Damocrates's mithridate, transmitted by the Galenic corpus. Tracing the transmission of these remedies' recipes is no less an undertaking than the making theriac of itself, and certainly beyond the purpose of this book.[69] During the Middle Ages, apothecaries could find these recipes in basic apothecary texts, such as the *Antidotarius Magnus*, pseudo-Mesue (the pharmacological corpus attributed to Mesue), and *Dispensarium Magistri Nicolai Prepositi ad aromatarios*, the most popular pharmacopoeia up to the sixteenth century, known as *Antidotarium Nicolai*.[70] Entries about theriac and mithridate varied in length: they were basic at first but increased in detail over time. Medieval pharmacopoeias such as *Antidotarium Nicolai* contained only a sweeping list of ingredients and quantities for theriac and mithridate. But as pharmacopoeias grew ever more discursive, entries about theriac included twenty-page descriptions of its ingredients, a discussion of procedures, an exploration of its history, and observations of or comments on other authors' versions. However, old-style pharmacopoeias published in the 1590s still reported only the list of ingredients and their quantities.[71]

In Italy the recipe for Theriaca magna was relatively stable. Comparing ten theriac recipes in Italian pharmacopoeias (including both Andromachus the Elder's and the Younger's) between 1556 and 1775 shows relatively few areas of disagreement.[72] Discrepancies involve the number of ingredients in classes 4 and 6, with a few ingredients switching classes over time. Official recipes either listed acceptable substitutes or directly listed substitutes in the place of the rare original ingredient—most commonly nutmeg oil for opobalsamum, *Spicae nardi* for *Nardo indicae*, and juniper berries for the fruits of balsam.

All apothecaries agreed that the quality of theriac depended primarily on the use of good and proper ingredients. Because individual apothecaries were obligated to use the local pharmacopoeia's recipe, they took pride in their own theriacs not for their recipes but for the quality of their procedures and ingredients. According to Galen, "a defect in one ingredient often spoils the whole thing."[73] Therefore, every production of theriac and mithridate was accompanied by a printed list of the ingredients and substitutes used and certified by the local medical college; I call these certified lists *formulas*. In Venice, formulas also had to include "the necessary declarations"—that is, validation by the authorities.[74] The bottom of an eighteenth-century handbill read: "This most famous antidote was produced according to the Venetian Senate decree and according to the art."[75]

When discussing the formulas of theriac and mithridate, I am referring specifically to documents longer than the standard handbills.[76] Theriac formulas included the list of ingredients, possible substitutes, the date of the production, the name of the apothecary, and sometimes the approval of the medical college.[77] Although often called *recipes,* formulas were a distinct *kind* of recipe. Recipes, of the most ancient medical genres, transmitted knowledge of how to make compounds, including ingredients, quantities, and instructions on how to compound them.[78] Meanwhile, theriac formulas listed only the ingredients, and never included instructions. They were also different from prescriptions—also called *recipes*—which were handwritten instructions for a single patient.

Theriac formulas primarily served a legal function, certifying that a specific production of theriac met the legal standards of the production process. In Venice the requirement to print theriac formulas dated to at least the 1565 statute of the apothecary guild, which referred to formulas as recipes. In an attempt to standardize production and "instruct" apothecaries on proper protocols, article 28 of the statute required apothecaries to print "recipes" at their own expense.[79] So when Giovan Battista Albricci, the apothecary at the sign of the Ostrich, printed recipes with his mark, he left the date blank so he could reuse the same form for subsequent productions. Theriac formulas were fundamentally different from the secrets of empirics and the recipes of charlatans. While these recipes were also a legal requirement, they were handwritten and included in the petitions charlatans sent to the authorities when asking for a license.[80] Meanwhile, although many secret recipes were published, empirics tried keeping their own undisclosed, as they were the core of their business, and even bequeathed them as family heirlooms. This was not the case for the recipe for theriac, which was published in pharmacopoeias and republished at every production in formulas.

Formulas constituted the paper trail of artisanal production, the tangible outcome of the collaboration between apothecaries and collegiate physicians. Printed formulas were used as checklists during productions of theriac (Figure 2.3). During the inspection, collegiate physicians and other officials checked the preprinted formulas against each ingredient. Furthermore, officials scribbled the total weight of each class to ensure

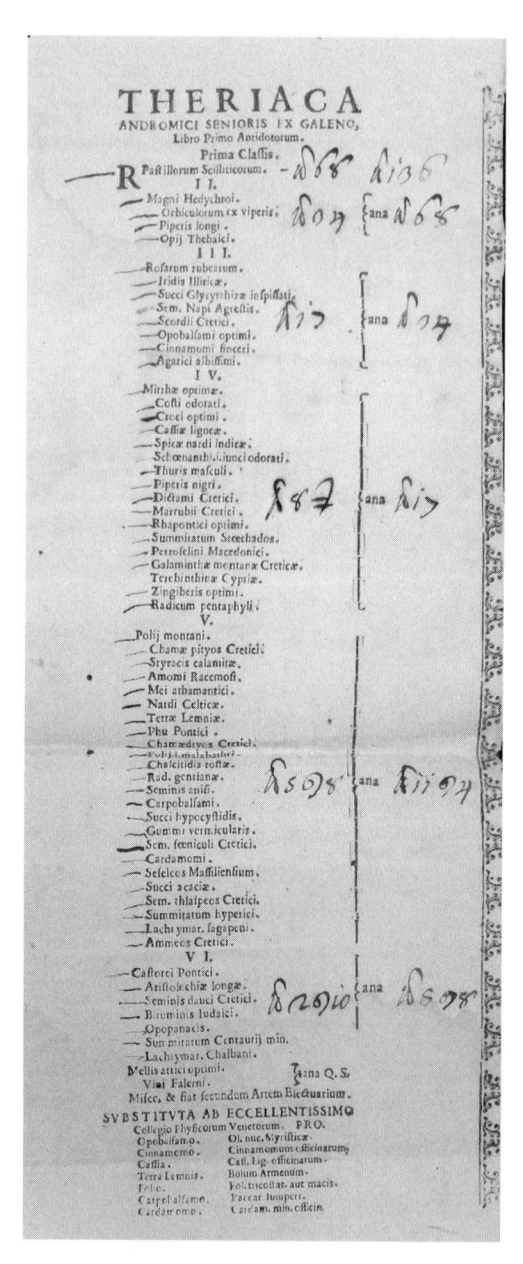

Fig. 2.3. Theriac formula with annotations. While composing theriac in 1661, an official controlling the ingredients checked each ingredient and scribbled the total weight of each class of ingredients. At the bottom is the list of substitutes approved by the College of Physicians; for example, *Bolum Armenum,* a red clay from Armenia, instead of *Terra Lemnia,* an earth from the island of Lemnos.

Giustizia vecchia, b. 211, Archivio di Stato, Venice.

apothecaries maintained the proper ratio between the classes. A few copies of each production formula circulated. While some remained in the archives of medical colleges for the benefit of historians, others were displayed in apothecary shops. It is unlikely that formulas were given to patients together with the actual medicine, as was the case with other publications describing the properties of theriac.

Apothecaries and physicians considered a good theriac one that was made following an official recipe and according to the rules of the art. This approach to evaluating products was common across Europe, where regulatory agencies such as guilds and state officers prioritized the process over the final product when assessing remedies. How a drug was made was of paramount importance.[81] However, goods entering the marketplace had to meet certain standards, which raised the question of how apothecaries and physicians could appraise an existing theriac.

The Sound of a "Good Theriac": Apothecaries' Sensory Knowledge

A trial involving a questionable jar of theriac provides rare insight into apothecaries' methods for evaluating theriac. On October 5, 1604, a routine inspection uncovered a suspicious jar of theriac in the Dominichini brothers' apothecary shop in Bologna at the sign of the Golden Vase. From the mid-sixteenth century, officials from the apothecary guild inspected apothecary shops every three months, along with the Protomedicato, a medical tribunal overseeing medical professions.[82] The brothers' theriac was deemed "too liquid," and its color "different from the color of good theriac." Several apothecaries were found to be at fault and were fined during the day's inspections, and remedies and substances deemed old, counterfeit, or unfit for sale were discarded or confiscated. The Dominichinis vehemently protested, asserting that their theriac had come from a legitimate batch. Nonetheless, the Protomedici confiscated their theriac and initiated a judicial case. Both the Protomedicato and the apothecary guild's officials summoned the brothers' appointed experts to evaluate the organoleptic qualities of three different jars of theriac (the Dominichinis' and two control jars).[83]

The trial provides an opening of the "black box," a glimpse into the sensory knowledge of physicians and apothecaries of this period, from which we gain an understanding of how this community expressed its expertise in compounds. Little of the apothecaries' sensory knowledge from this period survived the eighteenth century. As Lissa Roberts has highlighted, by the late eighteenth century chemists primarily used scientific instruments that relied on sight.[84] Although apothecary shop inspections were organoleptic examinations, few sensory experiences have reached us in a codified manner.[85] The Dominichinis' trial reveals how not just sight but all five senses were employed to assess a compound. The trial also highlights that apothecaries struggled to reach a consensus, possibly because of conflicting interests or loyalties, and showed they lacked a shared language on the subject.

Both the Collegio Medico and the apothecary guild stipulated that all theriac on the market should be reasonably similar and should produce on the senses the desired effect of "good theriac." This echoes what Jeremy Greene has called the enduring "challenge of making things the same"—that is, ensuring uniformity in pharmaceutical production, which predates the industrial era.[86] During the Dominichinis' trial, the Bolognese Protomedico seized the opportunity to not only assess a specific theriac but also generate a reliable description of what constituted a "good theriac." This knowledge centered around the organoleptic qualities of theriac—the Protomedici did not question theriac's medical properties, but instead assumed that these were already established. Intriguingly, the Protomedicato faced difficulties similar to those of modern sensory scientists when evaluating food products, such as wine and olive oil. Protomedici employed an organoleptic procedure and sought consensus among apothecaries to achieve intersubjective statements, shared judgments within the community.[87]

The Protomedicato conducted the trial by asking individual apothecaries to use their senses, judgment, and experience to compare the Dominichinis' theriac to two control samples.[88] The physicians formulated a questionnaire of thirty-two questions. Initially they sought to rate the three theriacs based on sensory descriptions. Then they attempted to ascertain what had occurred during the last collective production of theriac. Finally they endeavored to determine what had happened to the theriac in question during fermentation.

The first ten questions focused on comparing three theriac samples in terms of sensory qualities (color, taste, smell, density, even sound) and assess if they could be defined as "good." First the Protomedici queried whether it was even possible to distinguish between a good and bad theriac using the senses, to which all apothecaries responded positively. Then the Protomedici asked specific questions. For example, question two asked: "Should the color of a good four-year theriac be very dark tawny and akin to wet iron rust and similar to that in the small jar numbered 1?" Question four asked: "Should the taste of good theriac be sweet at first, then rather bitter, and finally aromatic and sharp [*acuto*], and does jar number 2 respond well to smell and taste?" Question five inquired whether theriac should stick and not fall out when its jar was turned upside-down.[89]

The Dominichinis' trial discloses the language of the senses and physicians' and apothecaries' understanding of compounds. However, it also places significant limits on our knowledge, for two main reasons. First, the Protomedici's questions were not open-ended, and they induced apothecaries to respond with the same words used in the questions. Physicians drew on the language of such classic texts as Galen's *De simplicium medicamentorum facultatibus* (The power of simple drugs) and pseudo-Mesue. Thus, the trial does not show whether apothecaries used language different from that of physicians to describe organoleptic qualities. Second, throughout the trial the Protomedici pressured apothecaries to agree on specific definitions. The apothecaries did not appreciate this, and ultimately this pressure made them refuse to dispense their knowledge and thereby come to an agreement. However, apothecaries appear to have been simply unaccustomed to describing their sensory perceptions, while their knowledge was embodied it was neither conceptualized nor shared. This limits artisans' awareness of their own embodied knowledge, as described by Pamela Smith.[90]

The Protomedici crafted their questions with language derived from a long-standing textual tradition in pharmaceuticals intrinsic to apothecaries' education. From the 1460s to the 1590s there were more than one hundred editions of pseudo-Mesue, one of apothecaries' most frequently used texts.[91] Pseudo-Mesue's writings provided terms for describing sensory experiences—naming odors, colors, and tastes—as well as ways to recognize materia medica. Additionally, Galen's *De simplicium medicamentorum facultatibus*—an influential text widely available in Latin translation—abounded in vocabulary for evaluating sensory data.[92] None of these texts, however, addressed the question of how to recognize medicines once the ingredients had been compounded.

Even though the wording of the Protomedici's questions heavily influenced the answers, apothecaries responded in their own way, modifying, adding to, and contradicting the statements physicians presented to them. Discussing density, for example, apothecary Ludovico Comeli said that "good theriac ... does not go back to its site like liquid things do," possibly referring to the common Aristotelian idea that things move toward their natural site.[93] Furthermore, some apothecaries simply refused to comply with parts of the interrogation. Paolo Groppio declared he had "the nose too full" of the previous odor to judge another theriac.[94] Hercole Dal Buono asserted he was present to judge only one theriac, not three, and refused to examine other jars.[95] In this manner, apothecaries found both practical and procedural ways to limit the examination.

The Protomedici also posed questions regarding the documentation associated with every batch of theriac, such as the recipe employed and the journal used by the master of apothecaries. In Bologna, theriac was made in bulk in public productions in the courtyard of the university, stored for one year in large jars handled by the prior of the medical college, and finally distributed to apothecaries who contributed to the initial investment or sold to retailers. One issue the Protomedici encountered was exemplified by the Dominichinis' theriac, which was part of a valid batch but had been either altered or stored improperly. The liquidity of their theriac may have been due to it having come from the bottom of a badly stirred jar. If so, the brothers' theriac would have acquired a curious classification: legally produced, but not fit for sale.

During the interrogations, apothecaries easily agreed on questions about the color and smell of theriac, and even the noise it made when struck with a spatula. They concurred that, when struck, a "good theriac" produced a deep resonance, followed by a sharp, piercing sound. They also agreed on which of the three theriacs was finest, and that the third was sweeter and more liquid. However, they diverged on what the discrepancies between the theriacs implied regarding the theriacs' quality. For physicians, an acceptable theriac should be comparable to what they all considered a "good theriac," which was the sample in the first jar. But despite the compounds exhibiting significant disparities, several apothecaries refused to label as "bad" the theriac dissimilar to the one they had all agreed was best.

Apothecaries held conflicting views on the three theriacs. Those called to testify in defense of the Dominichinis noted differences between the jars, yet deemed them all equally good because, in the words of Domenico Leanciani, they were "one and the same thing."[96] Groppio also concurred: "Being part of one body, liquid or not, it [theriac] has the same virtues." Yet other apothecaries maintained that the third theriac was substandard because of its dissimilarity to the first. Bernardino di Formigine affirmed: "In my judgment, the theriac of the first jar is good and those that are not similar to that can be of lesser or no value, and those that sound the same will be of equal quality." Moreover, he added, the overly liquid theriac from the bottom of a jar of proper theriac had too much honey and "necessarily has less strength."[97] Ultimately the apothecaries' final verdicts on the jars split according to their loyalties. Those called by the Dominichinis accepted all three jars as marketable; the others declared the brothers' theriac (the third jar) unfit for sale.

More surprising was apothecaries' disagreement on the effects of stirring theriac, a fairly common practice. Bernardino da Formigine asserted, "I do not believe that moving theriac makes it more or less liquid than its nature."[98] According to Ludovico Comeli and Fabrizio Bonacin, stirring theriac made it more solid because the spices and honey blended better. Giovan Antonio Pastarino disagreed: "In my opinion and judgment, when theriac is not moved, it becomes more solid and dry . . . but if stirred, it keeps more tender and softer."[99] According to Hercole Dal Buono, "when not stirred, theriac makes a crust on top while the honey goes down to the bottom; when stirred, theriac becomes uniform."[100] These contradictory descriptions demonstrate that Bolognese apothecaries had no shared understanding of how stirring affected density. The topic was not covered in their books, nor had they formulated a common language to articulate their observations.[101]

During the Dominichinis' trial, the Protomedicato grappled with the challenge of determining the quality of theriac post-production. Establishing a standard required an intersubjective statement from all apothecaries and physicians. But such agreement remained elusive, leaving the Protomedicato without a definitive answer. Had the Dominichinis' theriac been tampered with? Or was it part of a legitimate batch that lacked the right characteristics? Was their theriac fit for sale or not? The Protomedicato's decision erred on the side of caution, fining the brothers only for a spoiled rosemary compound, not for the jar of theriac—although the latter was nevertheless confiscated, resulting in an economic loss for the Dominichinis. While their theriac was considered not fit for sale, the possibility that it came from a legal batch prevented the Protomedicato from making a harsher decision. In theory everyone agreed on what constituted a good theriac, but in practice the variability of matter and procedure posed insurmountable obstacles. Mistakes in the production such as insufficient stirring could lead to flawed products. By not reaching an agreement about the Dominichinis' theriac, apothecaries protected not only their autonomy but also one another. Although pharmacopoeias provided recipes for most compounds, and inspections gave physicians oversight over simples and remedies in apothecary shops, apothecaries still retained some control over their final products.

Spiritual and Material Vipers

The trial brought to light the rarely discussed topic of apothecaries' and physicians' sensory procedures. Far more common were interminable debates about theriac's numerous ingredients. Some of these, such as red roses, iris, and licorice, were widely accepted and understood and warranted little discussion; others were highly debated, owing to difficulty in their sourcing, uncertain identification, or contested quantities in the recipe. Disagreements did not necessarily revolve around uncommon species; for example, the identification of rapeseed sparked a dispute between Marco Oddo (1526–1591) from the University of Padua and the ever-present Mattioli.[102] The quality and quantity of honey and wine, the excipients used to make theriac, were also matters of deliberation. Meanwhile, a few ingredients remained elusive—especially opobalsamum, the oleoresin of *Commiphora opobalsamum,* which for centuries drew considerable attention from scholars and laypeople alike.

The most controversial ingredient of theriac certainly was viper flesh, the remedy's signature ingredient that set it apart from mithridate, made with the stomach of the less iconic skink. Snakes' significance in the Western medical and scientific traditions cannot be overstated. Snakes are so emblematic of medicine that the symbol of the World Health Organization (WHO) features a snake coiled over the rod of Asclepius, the Greco-Roman god of healing, and at least forty medical institutions in the United States alone use this same symbol.[103] As demonstrated by historian Jutta Schickore, it has even been possible to write a book on the scientific method in Western science focusing almost exclusively on debates on snake venom.[104]

During the early modern period, scholarly discussions on vipers invariably centered around theriac, poison, and the snakes' supposed medical properties. One of the first anatomical observations of vipers, published in 1589 and featuring beautiful engravings by Carlo Angelo Abati, physician to the Duke of Urbino, was titled *De admirabili viperae natura, et de mirificis ejusdem facultatibus liber*.[105] The first chapter explored the importance of Leoniceno's treatise on vipers, which opened up the possibility of remaking "true theriac." Evangelista Quattrami, Ulisse Aldrovandi, Francesco Redi (1626–1698), Marco Aurelio Severino (1580–1656), and many other early modern scholars also wrote about vipers in relation to theriac and the snakes' relevant medical "virtues." A variety of popular works, such as *Trattato de gl'effetti marauigliosi delle carni di vipere* (Treatise on the marvelous effects of vipers' flesh), informed the public of the purported curative properties of vipers.[106] Laypeople shared the belief in the vipers' healing properties. Consequently, apothecaries sold various viper-derived products for different purposes. For example, apothecary Hercole Dal Buono used vipers to create an oil for hair growth; Girolamo Zanella from Padua exported viper *trocisci* to Germany.[107]

Leaving debates on viper's poison for Chapter 4, this section tackles two aspects of the history of vipers directly related to their use as a component of theriac. The first aspect pertains to the snake's religious significance, which added credibility to the curative powers of theriac. The second regards the extensive harvesting of vipers for the production of Venetian theriac. Both illustrate how theriac served as a repository for both material and spiritual elements.

Christ and the Snake

The most reliable origin story of theriac, as reported by Galen, credits Andromachus the Elder with improving the mithridate recipe by adding viper's flesh and more opium. However, a different origin story emerged in Western medieval encyclopedias sometime before the eleventh century. In this alternative narrative, Andromachus disappeared and theriac assumed religious significance: healing was linked with religion, and theriac and the viper were associated with Christ. While this religious origin story of theriac found no place in medical books about the antidote, the remedy's association with salvation contributed to its popularity among patients. The medieval origin story is exemplified by a legend recounted in *Speculum naturale,* a prominent encyclopedia authored shortly after 1240 by the Dominican friar Vincent de Beauvais (ca. 1190-1264):

> Around Jericho in the desert of Jordan there is a snake, tyrus, fatal to birds, animals, and especially birds' eggs, which it eats and swallows together with the birds themselves. The meats of tyrus are combined with other ingredients to form a sort of electuary called *tyriaca,* which expels and eradicates toxic poisons. Some people say that, before the passion of Christ, nobody had a remedy against it, and tyrus was very harmful to men. But on the day of Christ's crucifixion, one of these very poisonous snakes was caught and hung on the side of Christ on the cross. From that day forward, every one of those snakes acquired great power against all venoms.[108]

In this tale, the healing properties of theriac were no longer derived from Andromachus, the resourceful imperial physician, but directly from God through his son's sacrifice. The narrative linked the therapeutic power of the tyrus snake to the passion of Christ, uniting spiritual and physical salvation. De Beauvais likely drew inspiration from the *Liber de natura rerum,* a popular encyclopedia by the Dominican theologian Tomas de Cantimpré (1201-1272).[109] In this far-reaching medieval legend, Christ and a snake share the same fate, representing the intertwining of spiritual and physical cures. The supreme cure emerged from the supreme sacrifice.

The connection between snakes, medicine, and religion has ancient roots, predating Christianity, appearing in works from the Middle East, ancient Greece, and East Asia. Sumerian pharmacopoeias from the first millennium BCE list snake powder as a remedy. Medical texts from the Library of Assurbanipal (668-626 BCE) feature remedies made with snake and wine.[110] In Rome during the first century CE, when Andromachus created theriac, snakes' healing properties were associated with the cult of Asclepius the Savior, the god of healing. Asclepius was often represented by a snake coiling around a staff, symbolizing deliverance from disease as well as the renewal and indestructibility of life.[111] By incorporating viper into the recipe, Andromachus capitalized on the popular association of Asclepius's healing powers with the curative potential of snakes. This symbolism introduced a religious—albeit heathen—dimension to the new drug, a connotation that the medieval legend maintained while Christianizing it.

The juxtaposition of snake and Christ within the Christian context might surprise some today, but such symbolism was unremarkable during the Renaissance. The association between snakes and Christ was first articulated in the Gospel of John, written in the first century CE, at the same time as Andromachus's creation of theriac. The gospel of John employed a metaphor (3:14–15): "And as Moses lifted up the serpent in the wilderness, even so must the Son of man be lifted up that whosoever believeth in him should not perish, but have eternal life."[112] This verse referred to the Book of Numbers (21:4–9) in the Jewish Bible, in which Moses erects a serpent of bronze on a rod to cure those afflicted by poison.

Drawing from both the Jewish Bible and the New Testament, several medieval authors used snakes as allegories for Christ. Some even referenced theriac in these allegories. The English abbot Alexander Neckam (1157–1217) drew an analogy between Christ, theriac, and the serpent: "Christ is also [*etiam*] theriac and antidote, to expel the evil spread by the ancient enemy . . . Christ is also serpent through his wisdom, when in his weakness he parried the evil of this world's prince."[113] For Neckam, Christ was snake and antidote at the same time. This Christ-snake metaphor persisted through the fourteenth century, with such figures as the alchemist Petrus Bonus (fl. 1330) and the physician Galvano from Levanto (d. 1340) using it.[114] Serpents acquired an additional, negative meaning during Late Antiquity and the Middle Ages, but in the sixteenth century the reformer John Calvin (1509–1564) nevertheless argued that "the metaphor [the serpent for Christ] is not inappropriate or far-fetched."[115]

By incorporating vipers' flesh into theriac, apothecaries introduced a religious allusion to healing as salvation, a signal not lost on patients. The connection between theriac, snakes, healing, and Christ was common during the transformation of theriac into "true theriac." The credibility of traditional cures was grounded in religious elements. For example, the *pauliani* were healers who claimed to cure snakebites with the powers inherited from their ancestor Paul the Apostle. In Germany in the mid-sixteenth century, several medals illustrated the geographical extent of the association between Christ and snakes. One side depicted Christ on the cross, the other depicted the bronze serpent on the pole, perfectly aligning with the image on the obverse.[116] In Italy, Vincenzo Valgrisi (1490–post-1572), the French-born Venetian publisher of Mattioli's works, adopted an illustration of a Jewish Bible verse as his mark, with one instance explicitly referencing the gospel of John. Seventeenth-century theologian Filippo Piccinelli (1604–1678) associated medicines with snakes in his *Symbolic World* (1669).[117]

Medicine and religion overlapped in the early modern period; patients saw no clear distinction between rational, magical, and religious approaches to illness and healing. Seeking a cure, patients of any social status might consult priests, rational doctors, popular healers, or empiric healers.[118] According to biblical teachings, the ultimate power of healing derived from God, which enabled any healer to claim divine traits, including apothecaries. In northern Europe, the theme of *Christus Medicus* or *Christ as apothecary* (*Christus als Apotheker*) gained popularity.[119] Theriac's lineage may have been Galenic and imperial, and therefore fully rational within the Galenic medical tradition, which considered cures and illnesses as natural, nondivine processes—but the medieval origin story theriac still resonated with religious beliefs.

The Hunt for Vipers and Its Consequences

Vipers, integral to theriac, had both spiritual and material meanings. The making of theriac involved catching vipers, identifying females, and certifying, shipping, killing, cutting, and cooking them before they could be incorporated into the compound. According to the apothecary Imperato, one viper yielded about two drachms of flesh, so a single batch of theriac required at least twelve vipers.[120] However, not all vipers were suitable. In *Echidnologia*, Aldrovandi cited Galen when clarifying that vipers had to be nonpregnant females from dry areas—and definitely not from marshes or maritime regions, as these were believed to induce thirst—and captured at the end of spring. *Echidnologia* quickly gained acceptance in Italy.[121]

Certification of the vipers' origin was paramount for a theriac's approval. For this reason, in 1577 the Florentine secretary Baccio Nascimbeni stipulated that a public officer must authenticate vipers with a *fede* (certification) confirming their origin before apothecaries could use them. Apothecaries were also prohibited from keeping irregular vipers in their shops.[122] Only certain regions were considered good for harvesting vipers. In Italy the optimal vipers for theriac came from the hills near Padua, the Colli Euganei, the mountains of Calabria, and Tuscia, north of Rome. In France, vipers for the production of *trocisci* came "in thousands" from the Poitiers region, packaged in sets of twelve, each weighing three and a half ounces.¹²³

The rise in theriac production strained the supply of vipers, and both scarcity and smuggling became tangible issues. In Bologna the Cardinal Legate, the highest political authority in the city, issued edicts in 1606, and again in 1663, 1666, and 1683, prohibiting the export of vipers, dead or alive, without permission. Bolognese apothecaries allegedly engaged in buying and selling vipers both within and outside the city, leading to a shortage. The cardinal was "thoroughly informed of how necessary theriac was to the city of Bologna," and emphasized the vital need for a steady supply of vipers.¹²⁴ However, the repetition of the edicts indicated the inadequacy of the measures they entailed.

The high demand for vipers put much pressure on viper hunters (*viperai*), whose profession had been known since antiquity and was inherited within families from the Apennines populations, especially the Marsi of Abruzzo. This tradition continues today in the town of Corcullo, where a festival celebrating Saint Domenico Abate features snakes freely moving through the streets. During the early modern period, the professions of *viperaio* and charlatan (*ciurmadore*, "seller of medicaments") often overlapped, so mistrust toward the *viperai* was the norm.¹²⁵ Most physicians were reluctant to acknowledge the snake catchers' vast knowledge, and rarely admitted their debts to them, such as when Aldrovandi recognized the fact that "all physicians knew" about venomous animals came from popular healers.¹²⁶ Similarly, Francesco Redi publicly commended the expertise of *viperaio* Jacopo Sozzi, who demonstrated the safety of ingesting viper poison by drinking it in front of an audience.¹²⁷ But these two acknowledgments were exceptional: physicians tended to be suspicious of the professions on which they depended for the supply of medicines or materia medica, including *viperai* and apothecaries.

Being a *viperaio* was perilous, and ensuring the supply of a large number of vipers posed various challenges. When the Neapolitan Protomedici ordered 500 vipers in 1795, their correspondent in Calabria informed them that he "did not have a suitable place to keep them" and thus arranged a transfer. The *viperaio* Santolillo Candariello from Ottaviano had to carry on his shoulders a wooden case of seventy live vipers—and only at night, as exposure to sunlight would kill them. One can imagine Candariello traveling with his poisonous load in the moonlight along the Tyrrhenian Sea.¹²⁸

Venetian apothecaries received live vipers in wooden cases from Padua, accompanied by documents certifying their origin.[129] The enchanting hills of the Colli Euganei near Padua were internationally renowned for their vipers. En route to the Monselice Castle, a Flemish traveler gazed upon the delightful hills "where they gather infinite numbers of Vipers, for the composing of that so much famed Venice Treacle."[130] The *trocisci* exported to Germany by the apothecary Geronimo Zanella were accompanied by both an elaborate certification signed by Paduan physicians and a label with an image of Colli Euganei with *viperai* hunting for vipers (Figures 2.4, 2.5).

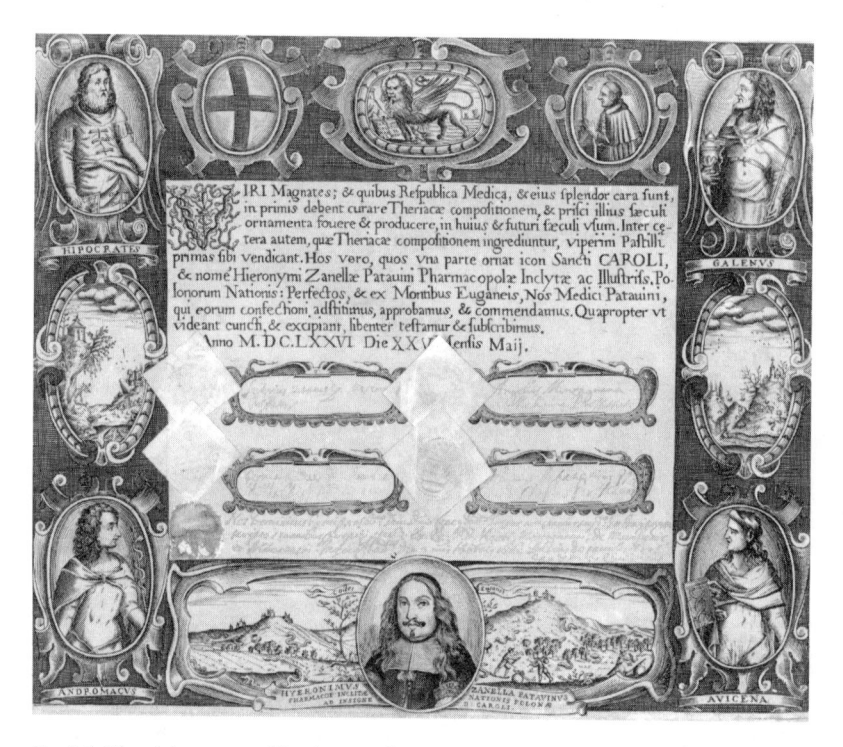

Fig. 2.4. The elaborate certification apothecary Girolamo Zanella from Padua included when he exported his viper *trocisci*, which reminded the recipient that this was a fundamental ingredient for theriac. Four physicians from Padua signed the document, dated May 25, 1676, declaring that they had assisted in the preparation of the *trocisci* and approved it. The Latin text is surrounded by the coat of arms of Padua (a red cross in a white field); the lion of Saint Mark; Saint Carl; and the portraits of Galen, Avicenna, Hippocrates, and Andromachus. Two oval medallions on the left and right of the image depict views of the Colli Euganei infested with oversized vipers.

Germanisches Nationalmuseum, Nürnberg.

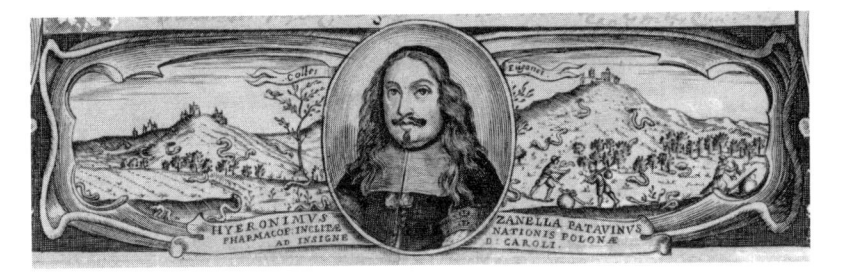

Fig. 2.5. This vignette from Figure 2.4 shows a portrait of Girolamo Zanella, apothecary at the sign of Saint Carl in Padua, flanked by images of the Colli Euganei with two *viperai* catching snakes in the countryside. The scenes are reminiscent of a more famous etching of *viperai* by Antonio Tempesta (1555-1630) in which the snake hunter is assisted by barking dogs. Zanella, author of *Della triaca et sue meravigliose virtù*, published in 1650, had close relations with Poland, a fact mentioned in the certification. Padua maintained long-standing relations with Polish universities and the Polish Crown.
Germanisches Nationalmuseum, Nürnberg.

The extensive harvesting of vipers in the Colli Euganei posed a threat to the species in the area. As early as 1606, Venetian apothecaries petitioned the Collegio Medico for permission to use vipers from outside the Colli Euganei; the apothecaries lamented that it was difficult to find vipers "due to a lack of availability, or greed of those who collect them."[131] The Collegio Medico initially rejected the request, but in 1628 allowed vipers from the hills of Verona and Vicenza. A similar issue arose in 1638, when too many vipers were arriving in Venice with fraudulent certificates. It took until 1716 for the Collegio Medico to permit vipers from the mountains of Treviso and Friuli.[132]

The preparation of *trocisci viperini* was gruesome, and kept away from public view. Apothecaries waited to kill the vipers in the presence of collegiate physicians. In the meantime, some fed the vipers only with wine, believing it purged them.[133] When theriac production increased considerably in the eighteenth century, the number of killings required became uncontrollable. Giuseppe Bolis, the prior of the Venetian Collegio Medico, observed in 1747 that the number of vipers killed in one day had become so high that physicians could not adequately check the process. Bolis reported that, between 1564 and 1630, apothecaries were killing 200 vipers at once. Quantities in other cities were lower. In 1606 a Bolognese apothecary noted killing somewhere between 25 and 50 vipers at once.[134] By 1670 the quantity killed in Venice reached 500—and continued to rise:

"After 1700, the number kept increasing, reaching 800, and then a thousand, and after 1735 they had reached approximately 1200, and in this last year, 1747, 2200 were cut, and in fact they [the apothecaries] were ready with 600 more, which would have brought the total to 3000, had it not been for a large number of them perishing."[135] Although it is not possible to ascertain these figures' accuracy, if nothing else they demonstrate contemporaries' impression that the process was out of control.

The viper species in the Colli Euganei (*Vipera aspis francisciredi*) was believed extinct until around 2015. Local experts concur that three centuries of intensive harvesting of females surely played a pivotal role in their disappearance. Female vipers become fertile at two years of age, reproduce annually with four to six offspring, and can occasionally live up to fifteen years. The continuous withdrawal of female vipers from the population was simply incompatible with the species' reproductive cycle, especially given the fact that the snakes also faced natural predators such as birds and hedgehogs. In recent years, animal associations in the area have reported one or two sightings of vipers annually, indicating a slow recovery of this wild population. Given that Venetian theriac with vipers was produced until the mid-1800s, it seems to have taken almost two centuries for the local viper population to recover from the damage caused by intensive theriac making, whose effects reverberated through countless animal, vegetal, and fungal species.[136]

Theriac afforded patients an intense sensory and emotional experience. Although theriac lacked standardization in the early modern period, the remedy had a distinctive taste, smell, and consistency, which apothecaries, physicians, and patients alike could identify. Throughout the early modern period, patients avidly consumed theriac for myriad reasons, and they knew what to expect. At the same time, when facing the challenge of deciding what was a good theriac and what was not, a pool of physicians and apothecaries in the seventeenth-century Dominichini trial could not reach a conclusion, hampered by professional and personal interests. The trial also showed that apothecaries' sensory experiences and language were not sufficiently codified and shared for it to be possible to collectively define what a good theriac should feel like—or even just agree on the meaning of basic apothecary practices, such as stirring.

While theriac incorporated ingredients from all over the world, it also conveyed a range of cultural meanings beyond the medical expectations of being an antidote with heating qualities. According to a medieval legend, a poisonous snake was hanged on the cross during the crucifixion of Christ, and as a result snakes gained powerful healing properties, which were transferred to theriac during preparation. Thus, when consuming theriac, early modern patients were ingesting not only the finest product of Galenic medicine, a rational tradition, but also a drug loaded with religious and institutional meanings. Such concentrated power, however, had a deflagrating ecological impact on at least one animal species. In eighteenth-century Venice, theriac production rose to such an extent that it produced a shortage of vipers in Veneto, and likely contributed to their near-extinction in the Colli Euganei, from which they took centuries to recover.

In this chapter we took a break from the chronology of the history of theriac to focus on the experience of theriac. Chapter 3 takes us to Italian courts, demonstrating that the "reinvention" of theriac was heavily influenced by the courtly culture of the Renaissance. Rulers, physicians, and court apothecaries focused on theriac's imperial legacy, referring to the origin story narrated by Galen.

II

Pharmacy and Statecraft

CHAPTER 3

Imperial Antidotes for Renaissance Rulers

*T*WO REMARKABLE gilded terra cotta jars, crafted around 1580 and credited to the Milanese artist Annibale Fontana, reflected the high status of their owners.[1] The reliefs adorning the jars picture the genesis of theriac and mithridate. One side of the theriac jar portrays Andromachus, sporting a characteristic physician's hat, cutting up vipers (Figure 3.1). The other side portrays Andromachus presenting a vessel of theriac to Emperor Nero (Figure 3.2). On the lid of the mithridate jar sits a statuette of Mithradates Eupator IV (120–63 BCE), king of Pontus.[2] According to a tradition tracing back to the third century BCE in the Middle East, Mithradates created mithridate, a legendary antidote.[3] Renowned for his knowledge of poisons and antidotes, Mithradates purportedly accustomed his body to poison by consuming it daily. This practice was so effective that his attempted suicide by self-poisoning proved unsuccessful—and, as illustrated on one side of the jar, he forced a servant to stab him. According to Pliny the Elder, Mithradates's medical commentaries and specimens were part of the spoils amassed by the Roman general Pompey (Gneus Pompeius Magnus, 106–48 BCE) following his conquest of Pontus. Commenting on his victory in Pompey and the

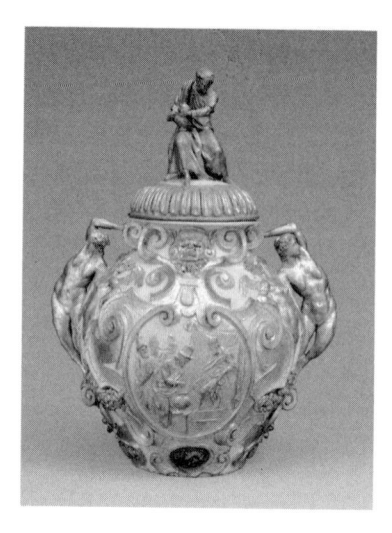

Fig. 3.1. Theriac jar in terracotta with white paint and glazed interior, attributed to Annibale Fontana, circa 1580. One side of the jar portrays the physician Andromachus at court, offering a pot to the Emperor Nero, sitting on the throne.

Getty Museum Collection, Los Angeles.

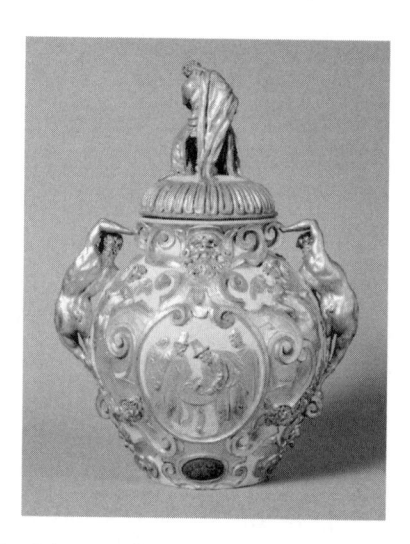

Fig. 3.2. The other side of the jar portrays the physician Andromachus, wearing a typical sixteenth-century physician's hat, cutting up vipers on a small table. The relief was inspired by a woodcut republished several times in the *Hortus Sanitatis,* depicting an apothecary or physician cutting vipers on a little table. Andromachus was credited with modifying mithridate's recipe and adding viper's flesh to it.

Getty Museum Center, Los Angeles.

booty, Pliny wrote: "This great victory therefore was as beneficent to life as it was to the state."[4]

The magnificence of these two jars is testament to the status of their owner, as well as to the importance of the Galenic origin story of theriac around 1580. Renaissance rulers were lured not only by theriac's promise of healing but also by its imperial legacy, which was deeply embedded in its history and materiality. In Chapter 1, I argued that theriac was especially relevant for the Venetian state because of its economic value and commercial reputation. Running chronologically parallel to Chapter 1, this chapter moves away from Venice to sketch the connections between theriac and state in other Italian cities. In several Italian Renaissance courts, "true theriac" became a *court object*—that is, an object that bolstered the prestige of rulers and courtiers. While physicians, collectors, and learned apothecaries were the main architects of the "reinvention of theriac," several rulers followed along or even prompted pharmacological research themselves. Theriac and mithridate were the perfect candidates to become state drugs. Furthermore, by analyzing sixteenth-century treatises on theriac, we can see how this subject led physicians to reflect on the organization of pharmacy in society. Theriac became a point of contention between physicians and apothecaries vying for their place in an emerging professional hierarchy. Most physicians considered pharmacy too valuable to be left in the hands of artisans such as apothecaries, especially when it came to the matter of theriac.

The first section of this chapter explores the imperial legacy that had been attached to theriac since antiquity, uncovering what this meant for Renaissance authors and rulers. The origin stories of theriac contained different notions of the birth of effective medicines. The medieval origin story discussed in Chapter 2 linked healing with salvation, whereas in the Galenic origin story healing (and theriac) stemmed from kings, generals, and emperors. This narrative resonated particularly well with Renaissance physicians and rulers, encouraging them to attribute political value to pharmacy. Moreover, the Galenic tale suggested that pharmacy was an occupation worthy of a prince, and theriac a remedy worthy of its position as a court drug.

The second section investigates the standing of theriac in mid-sixteenth-century Renaissance courts. Whether drawn by personal interest or the widespread and intense fear of poison, princes and rulers began framing pharmacy as a political enterprise, a tool for government, persuaded by the arguments of physicians or simply by their own political discernment. In cities where theriac trade was less developed than that of Venice, three factors drove the pursuit of and novel interest in pharmacy generally and theriac specifically: prestige, rivalries with neighboring cities, and the hope of making the most powerful antidote. Princes and their entourages conveyed their status by understanding "true theriac," as well as by making or sponsoring its production, and possessing, donating, or exchanging it. Sponsorship of theriac productions reinforced rulers' prestige and buttressed the official status of Galenic pharmacy.

In the concluding section I argue that theriac became a lightning rod for tensions between physicians and apothecaries seeking dominion over the professional hierarchy. Most notably, Giuseppe Olmi and Paula Findlen have demonstrated the centrality of theriac to disputes among collectors, physicians, and apothecaries, showing that questions of authority itself revolved around this one antidote.[5] I extend their argument to other cities by analyzing original treatises on theriac published in the 1570s.[6] These mainly discussed materia medica and the correct procedures for making theriac, but they also featured proposals about how the state could regulate pharmacy, how to reorganize relationships between physicians and apothecaries, and how rulers could lead and facilitate such reforms.

At a time when a profound restructuring of the medical professions was underway, writing about theriac meant writing about the hierarchy of the medical professional. I describe how several treatises on theriac fit into the context in which they were written. Rather than forming a uniform picture, such contextualization shows that authors influenced by their own ambitions responded to local relations of power between medical colleges and apothecary guilds. Nonetheless, whether the production of theriac was secured by medical colleges or by learned apothecaries, the creation of "true theriac" increased the hierarchization of the medical field.

The Birth of an Imperial Antidote

Sixteenth-century scholars could source historical information about theriac from several ancient texts. Chief among these was *De theriaca ad Pisonem*, attributed to Galen and probably written in the third century CE, which discussed the history, production, and functioning of theriac. This text also recounted Andromachus's poem-recipe, the offering of his creation to posterity, dedicated to the emperor: "Hear of the mighty strength of the antidote made of many herbs, O Caesar, giver of fearless freedom."[7] The poetic form aided memorization and helped those seeking to make theriac avoid mistakes. Over time, *Galene* ("tranquility," as Andromachus called the antidote) became known as *Theriaca magna of Andromachus*.

Repeated by hundreds of authors over the centuries, the origin story of theriac and mithridate told by *De theriaca ad Pisonem* explicitly outlined the relationship between the state and the two remedies. The state was both the creator and the recipient of such outstanding drugs: a king (Mithradates) created the antidote; a general (Pompey) secured powerful medicines; and an imperial physician (Andromachus) modified the king's antidote for his emperor (Nero). Furthermore, *De theriaca ad Pisonem* associated the remedy with other emperors, not just Nero: "We know that the divine Marcus Aurelius ... used the drug greedily and as if it were a food."[8] Emperors used, commissioned, and cherished theriac.

Theriac's imperial birth derived from its very materiality. Rare ingredients from across the known world entered its composition. Only a colossal empire at the peak of its power could plausibly expect to produce such a compound. A proper theriac demanded *Cyperus longus* from Africa, *Costus odoratus* from India, and licorice juice from Cappadocia, Turkey, to name just three ingredients. Such an antidote was the outcome of a productive, highly organized society with a vast and well-developed commercial network, the ability to set up complex supply chains, and wealthy patients willing to pay for expensive medicines.

The prestige of theriac and mithridate derived not only from their genealogy and materiality, but also from their consumption. Their complex formulation made these antidotes expensive, enhancing their prestige among the wealthy. During the reign of Marcus Aurelius (161–180 CE), "theriac was prepared by many rich people." The drug enjoyed great popularity among the upper classes, especially during the reigns of Septimius Severus (193–211 CE) and Caracalla (211–217 CE). In the first century, another physician, Damocrates, reformed mithridate, which also became favored among the wealthy.[9]

The imperial genealogy of theriac had another consequence: the ennoblement of this drug over all others. Throughout the Middle Ages and the early modern period, origin governed social position. Just as birth determined a person's standing, so origin established the quality and value of precious stones, plants, animals, and drugs. Wrote a sixteenth-century apothecary: "And what higher testimony of its [theriac's] excellency can anybody give than from looking at its provenance: originating with the most famous king Mithradates the knowledgeable, the foremost physician Andromachus created it with such art, with such success, with such happiness, that in the following times it has been embraced with admirable consent from the entire World, and with particular favor by great Princes and Emperors with good reason."[10] According to this apothecary, the simple fact of being compounded at court gave theriac an edge. Having the most noble pedigree destined theriac for its status as a drug suitable for emperors, sovereigns, and popes.

In their medical texts on theriac, early modern physicians and apothecaries cited its Galenic origin story, but they did not refer to Christian elements or the Christianized medieval legend discussed in Chapter 2. Renaissance physicians and learned apothecaries considered themselves rational doctors in a medical tradition based on Galen and Hippocrates. According to this learned tradition, medicine and pharmacy were rational enterprises, rooted in natural philosophy and theory, rather than empirical or religious undertakings.[11] Any reference to the supernatural by Renaissance authors was deemed not Christian but classic and mythical. Maranta noted in one of the most popular manuals on theriac, "I usually compare the two antidotes, one called *theriac*, the other *mithridate*, to two valiant captains, or we can say two strongest heroes, like Hercules and Theseus: both never had any other objective, nor engaged in anything other than to purge the world from all those things that with their enraged daring trouble miserable populations . . . And truly these two compositions resemble two great and most powerful kings."[12] For Maranta, theriac and mithridate were either semi-mythological figures or "powerful kings" whose task was to free the world from those evils grieving the population.

By choosing the origin story of Andromachus as told by *De theriaca ad Pisonem* and ruling out the medieval legend, physicians writing about theriac were historically accurate, considering that the former was more reliable than the latter. Furthermore, these physicians were introducing their interventions in healing matters into the rationalist tradition of learned medicine. In the wake of Galen and Hippocrates, they differentiated themselves both from religious healers and those without a degree or classical training.

In the Renaissance, the Galenic origin story of theriac offered a forceful precedent for the intervention of the prince in therapeutic affairs. Rather than representing a move toward secularization, the revival of the Galenic origin story afforded physicians and rulers a way to claim their own authority over the field of pharmacy. While the ultimate power of healing came from God, it was up to the state and physicians to ensure that people had access to powerful and reliable cures. If Roman emperors took on pharmacy, so too should the virtuous prince.

Theriac at Court

In the sixteenth century, the political map of the Italian peninsula simplified significantly. Power was concentrated in a few regional polities: Naples, Rome, Florence, Venice, and Milan. This was also a time of marginalization for Italy with respect to the rise of European monarchies and their overseas empires. Early in the sixteenth century, the Spanish crown conquered Naples and Milan and acquired indirect hegemony over Tuscany, Genoa, and the duchy of Savoy. With the exception of Venice and Lucca, republics disappeared. From the 1530s, old and new princes worked to stabilize their dominions and concentrate their power. They were not always successful. Administrative centralization met with resistance from country aristocracy and communal institutions.[13] But subjects leveraged the occasion to advance their own interests by siding with their rulers, which resulted in more stable institutions.[14] Italian regional states experienced different institutional solutions depending on the local forces at play. Regardless of regional differences, princes across the peninsula acted to legitimize and consolidate their power.

To centralize and maintain their authority in a changing environment, historical actors could either identify with existing popular symbols or create new symbols by sponsoring artistic and scientific works.[15] Influential members of society such as cardinals, aristocrats, princes, and wealthy merchants competed to sponsor cultural projects through the patronage system, in architecture, music, literature, poetry, visual arts, and natural philosophy. Patronage governed relations between patrons and clients, and favored the rise of new disciplines as well as the success of individuals.[16] For different yet ultimately concurring reasons, rulers, physicians, and learned apothecaries shared an interest in pursuing pharmaceutical studies, experimentation, and the making of theriac in particular.

In the sixteenth century, several princes took an interest in natural knowledge, together with court physicians and learned apothecaries. Princes and rulers collected *naturalia* and were conversant in alchemy and materia medica, and some had their own laboratories. Through pharmacy princes could pursue their fascination with poisons and counterpoisons.[17] Since Mithradates and throughout the Middle Ages, princes and their court physicians had sought antidotes, be they bezoar stones, scorpion oils, poison powders, or theriac. From the 1520s, rulers across Europe sponsored "experiences"—poison trials on people and animals, with the cooperation of high-status physicians. In the first part of the century, princes would offer prisoners sentenced to death the opportunity to undergo an experiment of ingesting a poison and an antidote. If the prisoner came out alive, they were free. In Germany, poison powders (*Giftpulver*) even circulated under princes' names.[18] A long-standing association between monarchical authority and the ability to heal was very much alive in the sixteenth century. If a prince had not inherited the royal touch, like French and English monarchs who still cured scrofula with the laying on of hands, he could turn to pharmacy.[19] When princes sponsored the quest for better remedies or practiced pharmacy themselves, they merged the sacralization of power and the ability to heal. In their hands was the power to give life—and, indeed, death.

The Grand Duke of Tuscany Cosimo I de' Medici (1519–1574) provides an early Italian example of princes' interest in antidotes, which did not fail to impress his contemporaries.[20] Cristina Bellorini has demonstrated Cosimo's early interest in pharmacy as a tool for consolidating the Tuscan state, which he attained in 1537 when the Medici's leadership was still contested.[21] Cosimo's interest in medicine and pharmacy sprang from a personal passion and the traditionally close association between the Medici family and the patron saints of medicine, Damian and Cosmas (after whom Cosimo was named).[22] Pharmacy was a component of Cosimo's cultural program, itself an integral part of the Medici's construction of their newly acquired status in 1532.[23] Cosimo and his wife Eleonora di

Toledo (1522–1562) used cosmetics and new medicinals to create patronage networks and distribute favors.[24]

Cosimo experimented with plants and metals using alchemy and other methods. He founded several laboratories, the *Fonderie* (foundries), and his passion for plants and medicine inspired other rulers. In his Fonderie, Cosimo distilled waters and produced Mattioli's counterpoison oil and mithridate "with so much perfection."[25] Florence was not at the forefront of the race for "true theriac," likely because Cosimo's experiments with his own scorpion oil (which contained theriac) had averted his interest from theriac, but the compound nevertheless remained a major concern. When the theriac craze blossomed in the 1570s, Cosimo and his heir Francesco discussed the possibility of permitting apothecaries to make theriac using the newly arrived New World balsam instead of the traditional opobalsamum.[26] Francesco and Ferdinando, Cosimo's successors, followed in his footsteps. He also set an example for other rulers.[27] In 1572 Pope Gregory XIII (r. 1572–1585) sought to set up a pharmaceutical and alchemical laboratory akin to Cosimo's.[28]

The state involvement in pharmaceutical matters came as a result of several solicitations from different sources. According to Machiavelli, a wise prince should prevent future dangers and guard against them.[29] Thus, the prince was responsible for his subjects' safety: "The greatest part of kingship is common safety." In this sense, Galen's *De theriaca ad Pisonem* offered both rulers and physicians a comprehensive medical-political program.[30] What better solution to generate results than theriac, the most powerful antidote? In his public production of theriac in 1586, the apothecary Vendramino Menegacci spelled out the connection between the "good prince," common health, and theriac: "If the duty of a good prince is to provide for the benefit [*giovare*] of his subjects as much as he can, what more good can be done to the people, and indeed to the entire world, than the gift of this happiest antidote, which can only serve to ensure the base of human life."[31] Menegacci delivered this address to the Collegio Medico of Vicenza, a city under Venetian rule, and the highest Venetian officials, who were there to profit from such claims as well as from the theriac pageant. Physicians and learned apothecaries offered theriac as a tool of authority to the prince, and claimed legitimacy for themselves as critical agents in preserving public health.

In the second half of the sixteenth century, rulers' interest in medicine was accompanied by a trespassing of medical language and methods into the political sphere and vice versa.[32] For example, after the St. Bartholomew's Day massacre, French physicians wrote about natural history as a tool "to help the king understand and 'heal'" the body of the injured kingdom.[33] As Samuel Cohn has shown, physicians included social causes and political remedies for the plague in tracts published in the 1570s.[34] In every field, scholars and artisans crafted their claims to direct their patrons toward worthy endeavors. Physicians and learned apothecaries prompted rulers to consider pharmacy a prerogative of political authority while expanding their own area of authority. Aldrovandi, for example, believed that the task of physicians was precisely to "excite" princes to undertake such endeavors as pharmacy (*farmaceptica*) rather than useless wars.[35]

To win the help of princes, physicians and apothecaries presented theriac as a civilizing object, a tool of government, and a product able to grant glory. According to political treatises, a prince's primary goal was to achieve "the greatest possible degree of honor, glory, and fame." The main way to achieve this objective, wrote Machiavelli—who aligned with other political writers on this subject—was to model one's efforts on a worthy figure of the past.[36] To be an "excellent" king, a prince had to emulate famous kings and emperors. In 1576 Parisian apothecary Nicolas Houel (1524?–1587) dedicated his *Treatise on Theriac and Mithridatium* to France's dauphin, Charles IX, using these words: "Following the example of these excellent kings and emperors [such as Adrian, Antoninus, Severus, and Marcus Aurelius], Your Highness would wish to dispense in the city of Paris the much-celebrated antidotes Theriac and Mithridate, which will help eternalize the memory of Your Majesty, and will bring to you and your subjects an inestimable profit."[37] Heirs to the throne, like all pupils receiving a humanistic education, would learn about theriac when reading about Pompeus, Mithradates, and Marcus Aurelius. To promote theriac, physicians suggested that by making it, a prince could emulate a Roman emperor. At the same time, such comparison raised the prince's physician to the rank of imperial archiater. Princes heeded this advice. In 1566 the apothecary Calzolari relayed that "many princes of our own times had theriac made in Bologna, (I say) in Padua, in Venice, in Ferrara, in Florence, in Rome, in Urbino."[38] Calzolari's use of the word "prince" leveled the difference between principalities and republics such as Rome and Venice, as well as between independent polities and their subjects, such as Venice and Padua, and Rome and Bologna. For Calzolari, the Duke of Urbino and the Bishop of Bologna were both "princes."

Emulation was far from the only benefit theriac offered to a prince—he could also use it to show his liberality, the quality of generous giving that distinguished aristocracy. The prince could show his largesse and foresight by sharing his theriac with his subjects, bestowing upon them health and protection. According to *De theriaca ad Pisonem*, "[The emperors] gladly give everyone a share [of theriac], getting as much joy themselves as those who are saved by them."[39] Knowing how to make theriac and donating it freely became part of a young prince's education. In Mantua the young Duke Francesco Gonzaga (1586-1612) was passionate about botany. With the assistance of his instructors, court apothecaries and collegiate physicians, the duke made "the most noble medicament of Theriac, of the highest and exquisite perfection for the use and the grace of the poor oppressed by poison to whom he distributes and donates it freely and with good disposition."[40]

Poet Torquato Tasso (1544-1595) was perhaps coveting the liberality of Ferdinando de' Medici when, sick and in dire straits, he wrote to the duke requesting theriac and other antidotes.[41] We do not know whether Tasso ever received the medicines he hoped for. Princes may have reserved such notable gifts for their peers, as a means of reinforcing their dynastic and political ties. In 1621 Duke Ferdinando I Gonzaga (1587-1626) sent his sick uncle, Grand Duke Cosimo II de' Medici (1590-1621), a container made of bezoar stone (another powerful antidote) with a six-year-old theriac, which he described as a drug "made in this house [the Duke's laboratory] and which responded fantastically to tests, there was no alteration in its description, great care was devoted to the preparation of some ingredients, as vipers and opium, and, since it received less honey, it will be worthwhile to take only a half-dose."[42] In this letter Duke Ferdinando exalted the quality of his gift to his uncle. Cosimo II had twice come to Ferdinando's rescue, sending money and armies against the Savoy military forces. Ferdinando's letter also showed that he was conversant with current medical literature: in the 1620s, the right quantity of honey in theriac was a subject of much debate.

Apothecaries and physicians depended on princes' liberality, too. Making theriac was expensive and complex; a "single poor apothecary" did not have the means to collect all the necessary ingredients from "faraway lands."[43] Apothecaries needed the princes' support because, as affirmed by Lauro de' Lavoranti, an apothecary from Pavia, making theriac was "such a difficult endeavor that it seems better suited for the highest puissance [*somma possanza*] of princes than for the little strengths of particulars."[44] In Mantua in the 1590s, the theriac made by court apothecaries was funded by the prince. Especially in the early days of "true theriac," princes' networks might have been integral to sourcing foreign ingredients. Their help was paramount because, as noted by Aldrovandi, they had "very long hands."[45] Without a large network, the kind only cardinals and princes could have, making "true theriac" was simply not possible.

Lastly, theriac was suitable as a court object because it held civilizing qualities. With its numerous ingredients, theriac represented the ability of humankind to reorganize and use natural resources to counter the dangers of nature. Bartolomeo Maranta exalted theriac's civilizing qualities alongside its medical ones: "And what else do these two most celebrated antidotes do if not free men from the wilderness [*fierezza*] of venomous animals, the betrayal of poisons, and the tyranny of diseases, and keep men in possession of their health?"[46] In the Renaissance, wilderness was not appreciated: it represented the opposite of civilization. In the sixteenth century, the vast popularity of poet Nicander of Colophon (fl. second cent. BCE) reflected a widespread gloomy view of nature.[47] In his *Theriaca* and *Alexipharmaca*, Nicander described the dangers nature posed to humankind.[48] Theriac was the antidote that could distance humans from untamed foes from the natural world, such as wild beasts, venoms, and diseases, and mitigate the wickedness of humans as manifested by betrayal by poison. As such, theriac came to the rescue of rulers, physicians, and learned apothecaries. Theriac was an ideal drug for a prince, as well as for physicians eager to demonstrate and strengthen their authority, not only because of its formidable healing qualities—encapsulating both a rational and a religious promise at once—but also for its illustrious genealogy, civilizing nature, and capacity to empower rulers to emulate Roman emperors.

Writing About Theriac, Reforming Pharmacy

New works about theriac began to be published in the 1570s, marking a move away from the form of comments on previous treatises to more lengthy discussions about ingredients, procedures, and terminology, while still referring back to previous authors.[49] In these works, scholars often added to the usual medical discussions their views on the reformation of the pharmaceutical field. Although the intertwining of medical and political discourses dates back to antiquity, most famously with the metaphor of the political body, the entrance of physicians into the political sphere became particularly evident beginning in the 1570s.[50] A telling example is Milanese physician Ludovico Settala (1550–1633), who authored a treatise about politics, on *ragion di stato* (which translates to "reasons of state), as well as medical treatises about theriac, the plague, skin diseases, and edited a Milanese edition of the *Antidotario Romano*.[51]

Theriac became a pivotal battleground for apothecaries and physicians. Treatises on theriac written in Italy in the 1570s to 1590s included political statements, often explicit, about how to organize the relationship between apothecary and physician, with their authors employing context-dependent strategies. Those writing from cities whose medical colleges had less influence, such as Venice and Naples, encouraged more collaborative relationships between learned apothecaries and physicians. In contrast, physicians operating in university towns such as Bologna and Padua proposed a hierarchical approach to pharmacy, and stressed the need for the state's involvement in pharmaceutical matters. Because of their superior knowledge and status, these physicians argued they should be in control of pharmacy for the public good, with "ignorant" apothecaries following their directions.

Affirming the superiority of physicians over apothecaries contrasted with the reality of business relations between the two professional groups. In the fifteenth century, apothecaries were richer and more numerous than physicians, not only in most Italian cities but also in other regions across the Alps. In the 1427 *catasto*, a detailed account of the financial state of Florentine citizens, apothecaries were second only to lawyers in wealth.[52] Furthermore, while medical colleges and apothecary guilds had been firmly established since the Middle Ages, these institutions did not necessarily mirror a well-defined division between medical professions.[53] Partnerships between apothecaries and physicians were common, and apothecaries often had the upper hand in such enterprises. Apothecaries commonly employed physicians and surgeons with a stipend, or created partnerships with physicians to manage apothecary shops. Additionally, apothecaries loaned physicians money, while physicians in turn sent customers to apothecary shops with costly prescriptions in exchange for medicines and prospective clients.[54] Historian Katherine Park has argued that ties between apothecaries and physicians in Florence constituted an "intricate social world," wherein strong bonds were forged through debts, partnerships, marriages, friendship, kinship, and contracts.[55] As Stefan Halikowski-Smith has suggested, while in theory apothecaries were the "physicians' hand," in practice the two professions went "hand in hand."[56]

In the fifteenth century, states sought to sever partnerships between apothecaries and physicians upon recognizing their potentially detrimental effects on patients. In 1410 a Venetian provision prohibited agreements between the two groups and set a penalty against them. This law was reinforced in 1480: the fine was increased fiftyfold, and physicians and apothecaries who violated the prohibition risked revocation of their practice licenses.[57] Despite these measures, partnerships between apothecaries and physicians persisted in Venice and throughout Italy.[58]

In the sixteenth century, physicians increasingly described the exuberance of the medical marketplace as hazardous to patients' health. Medical colleges issued a flurry of legislation, developed pharmacopoeias, and created a system of licenses and privileges to control empirics, charlatans, and makers of secrets operating for money or charity. Protomedicati (medical tribunals) were established as early as 1517 in the case of Bologna. Over the course of the century, the Protomedicati and medical colleges gained strength and intensified their control over apothecaries. In response, apothecaries reorganized their guilds to counter such pressure, in Venice as early as 1565.[59]

Although regulation of medical practice and pharmacy shared certain attributes across sixteenth-century Europe, Mary Lindemann has argued that "no single agency succeeded in monopolizing all ... functions."[60] Different forces were at play, and nowhere did they develop in exactly the same way. In England, medical corporatism—the "old medical regime"— had its greatest influence during the 1630s, but by the beginning of the eighteenth century physicians had lost their battle with apothecaries, who had gained the right to practice medicine.[61] In French cities, influence from the crown led to an intense corporatization of medical practice between 1500 and 1650. However, by the eighteenth century the rising number of practitioners, decreasing importance of universities as providers of medical education, and growing elitism of medical corporations had diminished the relevance of medical corporatism, which became an empty shell that cracked under revolutionary pressure.[62] The German region, divided into several states, presented various power dynamics. For example, physicians in Nuremberg presented medical reform as a top-down model. Within a few generations, they had won the favor of political authorities and established a "new order of medicine," leveraging writing as one of their main instruments.[63] The variety across the German lands at this time resembled that of the Italian states.

Apothecaries and Physicians in Naples and Padua

In Italy, institutional relationships between apothecaries and physicians followed patterns that did not necessarily coincide with political borders, but instead should be analyzed city by city. The case of Venice is more similar to that of Naples than to that of Padua, even though Padua was part of the Venetian state. Treatises on theriac provide valuable insights into such relationships, and the first such treatise takes us to Naples. Physician Bartolomeo Maranta's *Della theriaca et del mithridato* was published posthumously in Venice in 1572. Judging by the number of times it was cited, this treatise was the single most influential manual on theriac in all of Europe. Born in Venosa in southern Italy and mainly active in Naples, Rome, and the provincial town of Molfetta, Maranta was a favorite pupil of Luca Ghini (1490–1556), creator of the botanical garden of Pisa. Ghini was considered a teacher by an entire generation of physicians and collectors.[64] Maranta had previously published a book in Latin on how to recognize plants, disputed simples with Mattioli, and maintained a correspondence with eminent collectors and university professors such as Aldrovandi and Guilandino.

In his treatise Maranta challenged the conventional hierarchy of medical professions, at least at the elite end. He affectionately dedicated his bulky treatise to foremost collector and learned apothecary Ferrante Imperato. He also asserted that Imperato was the source of most of his knowledge of theriac and mithridate: "What else have I put in this book if not what I have observed and seen while you [Imperato] composed these two antidotes?"[65] Maranta even placed the learned apothecary above himself: "Finishing these two discourses, I well realize the difference between me and you, and I can see who was the Architect and who was the Mason, how the former is more noble than the latter, you more than me."[66] By comparing the "physician-architect" to the "apothecary-mason," Maranta clarified the hierarchy he perceived regarding his and Imperato's knowledge of making theriac—by inverting the actual hierarchy between their professions.

With this bold claim, Maranta did not mean to elevate an entire profession over another; instead he accepted and endorsed the difference between learned apothecaries and all other apothecaries. While recognizing Imperato's authority, he was also aware that most apothecaries "do not possess the same skills as physicians: apothecaries require a diluted language, a humble eloquence without frills." For this reason, Maranta made sure that his treatise was eminently clear and readable: "I wanted to extend my reasoning in every detail, maybe more than was necessary for comprehension. To be extremely clear so that apothecaries could understand me well."[67] However, Maranta believed his work could be beneficial not only to apothecaries but also to "erudite physicians" (*dotti medici*).[68] Hence, the expertise of learned apothecary Imperato could be useful to physicians, thus demonstrating how pharmacy could be improved by combining knowledge, skill, and experience. Maranta's treatise can be read as a manifesto on how to advance pharmacy.

Together with its practical approach, the book's success likely depended on the fact that no other manual of its kind had yet been published. Joachim Camerarius the Younger (1534–1598) translated it into Latin for a European public in 1576, and still today we can find copies of Maranta's treatise in several European libraries.[69] The book received a positive response, but approval was far from unanimous. Some physicians could not accept the recognition Maranta had intentionally granted to Imperato. In 1576 the Medical College of Padua appointed a committee of three professors—Marco Oddo, Paolo Crasso (?–1575), and Bernardino Trevisano (1506–1583)—to revise theriac-making procedures. The three physicians promptly published a Latin treatise on theriac titled *Meditationes doctissimae in theriacam & mithridaticam antidotum* (Very learned meditations about the antidotes theriac and mithridate).[70] They dedicated it to the Holy Roman Emperor Maximilian II, who was passionate about botanical studies.[71] From its very title and language, the Padua volume declared its audience loudly and unambiguously: learned physicians. *Meditationes doctissimae* reads as a resolute attack on physicians who had blurred the boundaries between the professions, like Maranta, and indeed on all apothecaries, regardless of whether they were learned like Imperato.

Remarkably, in *Meditationes doctissimae* the discussion of the relationship between physicians and apothecaries, past and present, spanned the first six chapters. Nearly all other books on theriac opened with a chapter on the meaning of the word and its origins, but *Meditationes doctissimae* did not touch this subject until chapter seven. Oddo and his colleagues' foremost aim was to reaffirm the hierarchal divide between physician and apothecary. Paduan authors disparaged apothecaries as ignorant, corrupt, and negligent, suggesting that they made medicines not with their skills (*ars*) but by accident (*fortuna*).[72] While the authors reiterated the various established reasons apothecaries should subordinate themselves to physicians, they also made it clear that physicians still relied on apothecaries and thus should be in control of them:

"These people [*pharmacopola*] stick to the Doctor like the helm to the ship; and as it happens when the helm is broken or in ill shape, the ship is tossed ... likewise if the Apothecary makes a medicine of an inappropriate sort, or gives the wrong medicine to a patient, not only does the doctor go further from his aim, but if the patient dies he loses his fame and authority."[73] Physicians needed to control apothecaries' productions to mitigate the risk to their own reputations and careers. Throughout the text, the Paduan physicians challenge Maranta directly—"Against Maranta, acacia juice is not a true ingredient of theriac"—and are consistently and unequivocally negative about Imperato.[74] Oddo, Crasso, and Trevisano harshly censured Maranta for having discussed some matters either only fleetingly or not at all, having deemed them unsuitable for his intended audience.

The Paduan attack on Maranta was too harsh for his Neapolitan circle to remain unresponsive. But since he had died in 1571, Maranta's cause was taken up by his pupil, Nicola Stigliola (1546-1623).[75] Stigliola's 1577 defense of Maranta, *Theriace, et mithridatia libellus*, written in collaboration with Imperato, included a system of references to Oddo's treatise in the margins to facilitate comparison.[76] Stigliola referred to Oddo's book as a series of calumnies and hallucinations (*calumniae et deliria*).[77] He dissected the Paduan treatise point by point, criticizing Oddo and his colleagues for their interpretations of both classical and modern authors, and ultimately accusing them of being ignorant of simples.[78] Stigliola intended his treatise to defend the memory of Maranta and his reputation as a scholar. He did not comment on the issue of who should regulate theriac or on the relationships between apothecaries and physicians. The fact that Stigliola did not mention apothecaries in his defense of Maranta, combined with the dearth of substantial archival documents on Neapolitan apothecaries, makes it difficult to reconstruct the connections between apothecaries and physicians in sixteenth-century Naples. However, what we know about the Neapolitan medical institutional structure suggests that physicians lacked the influence to rival apothecaries, who were both powerful and autonomous.

In most Italian states, control over apothecaries was mostly enforced through official pharmacopoeias, inspections of apothecary shops, and gatekeeping access to the profession. Maintaining this control was a prerogative of medical colleges and the Protomedicato, an institution that could be collegial, royal, or municipal, depending on the state.[79] In the Kingdom of Naples, the Protomedico, always a physician, was directly appointed by the king and independent of the local medical college. The Protomedico's decrees were sporadic and disorganized, preventing them from exercising centralized control over medical practice.[80] Additionally, the University of Naples had a lesser reputation than that of Salerno, causing many students to opt either for the latter or for private schools instead. Overall, physicians in the Kingdom of Naples were less esteemed than jurists.[81] Even the inspection of apothecary shops, which elsewhere was one of the collegiate physicians' main responsibilities, was carried out by representatives of the Counsel of the Eight, the powerful Neapolitan apothecary guild of which Imperato was a member.[82] As a result, apothecaries in sixteenth-century Naples were well rooted, and physicians were comparatively less established. Yet this imbalance produced an environment of collaboration between the two groups rather than hostility.

Meanwhile in Padua, under the rule of the Venetian Republic, the Collegio Medico was part of the University of Padua, one of Europe's most prestigious medical schools along with those of Bologna, Paris, and Montpellier. For a long time many of Europe's most renowned scholars, including Niccolò Copernicus and Andreas Vesalius, flocked to Padua to enrich their education or teach. The ancient Padua guild of apothecaries (called *fraglia*) was first established in 1260. In the sixteenth century it followed the example of the Venetian guild, separating *medicinalisti* from druggists in 1568 and establishing itself as a College in 1578.[83] Apothecaries in Padua were on good terms with the university; according to university statute they hung in their shops public notices of controversies at the university. Disputes among doctors were academically important, so the apothecaries' public notices provided yet another reason for scholars, artists, and students to congregate in Paduan apothecary shops to discuss medicine and science.[84]

However, the relationship between the University of Padua and its Collegio Medico was hostile, and interference from the nearby Venetian Collegio Medico made matters worse.[85] It is not surprising, then, that Oddo, Crasso, and Turrisani, writing for the local Collegio Medico, were so dismissive of apothecaries. Other Paduan professors emulated their approach, even in books with an explicitly educational intent, such as *La fabrica degli spetiali* (1566) by Prospero Borgarucci (1540–1578), a professor of anatomy at the University of Padua. Dedicated to the Dukes of Urbino, Guidobaldo II della Rovere (1514–1574) and Vittoria Farnese (1521–1602), this manual for apothecaries in the vernacular presented knowledge of pharmacy as a tool with which to govern, since "this thing [errors in the preparation of antidotes] is of such importance that Princes and Republics must vigorously provide for it."[86] Thus, Borgarucci offered his work as a normative instrument for the state. The manual proposed the idea of the "true apothecary," or "the good and wise apothecary," the ideal apothecary able to supply good medicines to the people. Borgarucci depicted actual apothecaries as being far from ideal, a rebellious bunch asserting themselves (*di nuovo rilevata la testa*), resisting control and education from above. The difference from Maranta's approach is striking. Nonetheless, in his manual Borgarucci could not avoid thanking several learned apothecaries, whom he called "rare intellects" compared to most apothecaries. These included Francesco Calzolari, Bonaventura Padovano, and Francesco Accoramboni from Gubbio but active in Rimini.[87]

Apothecaries and Physicians in Venice, Ferrara, and Bologna

Another learned apothecary Borgarucci praised was the German-born Georg Melich at the sign of the Ostrich in Venice. Melich authored the most popular book for apothecaries written by an apothecary, *Avertimenti nelle compositioni per uso della Spetiaria,* first published in Venice in 1575.

Avertimenti offers a peek into late-sixteenth-century relations between apothecaries and physicians in Venice, a topic we will revisit in later chapters. Along with Venice, in this section I also examine treatises on theriac by Evangelista Quattrami and Ulisse Aldrovandi, written, respectively, in Ferrara and Bologna, cities whose apothecary trades were quite different from that of Venice. As was the case when contrasting Padua with Naples, comparing theriac treatises shows that authors were extremely attentive to local relations while attempting to establish or enhance their authority.

Apothecaries in Venice were especially powerful because of the city's well-established trade in spices and materia medica. This centuries-old commerce continued unabated until at least the end of the sixteenth century.[88] In 1564 Venetian apothecaries successfully petitioned the Senate to form their own college. On this occasion, producers of remedies separated from druggists (*spezieri da grosso*) to institutionalize their different knowledge and responsibilities.[89] The reputation of Venice's learned apothecaries rested on their theriac, their knowledge of foreign materia medica, and their publications. Melich was an especially prominent apothecary because of his extensive travels, expertise in chemical and Galenic remedies, profitable commerce in his apothecary shop, and knowledge of simples acquired over the course of his long apprenticeship.[90] His reputation bolstered the popularity of both his theriac and *Avertimenti*, which had at least ten editions as well as a translation into Latin and an international circulation.[91] The editor of the 1596 posthumous edition remarked, "I remember having heard several times, not only from Italians, but also from ultramontanes, from many Turks, and from various people versed in pharmacy, that Melich . . . had the best theriac in the world."[92] Recognition by Turks underscored the fact that Melich's theriac had reached the quality of famous Egyptian theriac.

Dedicated to the prior and counselors of the Venetian apothecary guild, Melich's manual aimed to not only advance his reputation but also enhance apothecaries' knowledge. He did not subordinate apothecaries' knowledge to physicians' approval. In this way, *Avertimenti* can be read as a call for the dignity and autonomy of apothecaries. He acknowledged the rewarding collaborations he had enjoyed with physicians, especially Paolo Mongio, a learned commentator of Ibn Sīnā, and Andrea Marini, editor of Mesue. He even published a letter from Galeno Bellobuono from

Danzig.⁹³ "My physicians" encouraged Melich to publish his manual. Like Imperato, Melich admitted his limitations in writing—but while Imperato asked a physician (Maranta) to write in his place, Melich asked only for physicians' help in revising his work.

Besides some ritual affirmations regarding the submission of apothecaries to physicians, Melich addressed apothecaries as peers who might benefit from additional information. In comparison, Borgarucci's unofficial pharmacopoeia—also enjoying great popularity in Italy—approached the relationship between apothecary and physician with a top-down normative intent. Nonetheless, both works offered a novel approach to the textual transmission of knowledge and practice. Both exemplified a new kind of publication typical of this period, departing from the tradition of Mediterranean pharmacopoeias, such as the *Antidotarium Nicolai*, which offered only bare lists of medicaments and ingredients.⁹⁴ The two manuals also differed from early sixteenth-century pharmacopoeias, which took the form of commentaries on previous pharmacopoeias. Most importantly, this new breed of apothecary manual was in the vernacular, and altogether livelier. Authors presented accounts of their travels and apprenticeships in famous apothecary shops; related recipes with detailed discussions; and offered practical advice, anecdotes, and workshop practices. They both praised and criticized their colleagues, positioning their authors as learned within a burgeoning network of naturalists and scholars. Maranta's *Della theriaca* shared certain traits with pharmacopoeias while not actually being one, whereas most treatises on theriac, such as Quattrami's *Tractatus perutilis*, were more erudite.

Evangelista Quattrami was a well-known herbalist, at first apothecary to the Este family for thirty-seven years both in Rome and Ferrara, and then briefly at the service of the Gonzagas in Mantua and Farneses in Parma. Quattrami was in contact with foremost naturalists, including Ulisse Aldrovandi and Carolus Clusius. In 1597, at his own expense, Quattrami published *Tractatus perutilis atque necessarius ad Theriacam, Mitridaticumque Antidotum*, employing the usual structure of treatises on theriac by discussing every ingredient of theriac and mithridate one by one.⁹⁵ Quattrami's treatise was a veritable hybrid, directed both to apothecaries and physicians, a characteristic underlined by the fact it was written half in Latin and half in the vernacular. Quattrami wrote the dedication in Latin "for more urbanity," the discussion of local herbs and ingredients in the vernacular "for the satisfaction of apothecaries," and the exploration of foreign plants in Latin "for the satisfaction of physicians."

Quattrami admitted that few apothecaries and physicians could manage to accumulate the direct knowledge of simples he and a few others such as Aldrovandi had gathered. He knew that physicians would not have time to learn about simples and acquire a solid knowledge in the field by themselves if they also wanted "to visit their patients at bedside, attend Colleges for lessons about diseases, philosophy, medicine and qualities of simples, and care for their Prince." Pursuing new knowledge of pharmacy required time and dedication, as well as access to literature and direct observation of materia medica. Few could afford it.[96] Quattrami's position is especially interesting because it points to the practical difficulties experienced by both apothecaries and physicians in the face of the increasing complexity of their profession, which now demanded greater knowledge of simples and extensive familiarity with the classics. Physicians were too busy, and apothecaries lacked the means, to acquire new knowledge of simples. As a result, Quattrami believed, apothecaries should be actively policed—indeed, he himself did not disdain this task. In 1597, for example, while still in service in Ferrara, Quattrami wrote to Sigismundo Dondini, an apothecary in Cento, a small nearby city that was part of the Este dominions: "(Considering all the errors) your conscience will force you to agree to defer without the need to receive a formal order, so as to avoid compounding [theriac] with the same confusion as we used to years ago."[97] The herbalist called on the apothecary's conscience, while also threatening him with his authority. A few years later in Parma, Quattrami worked to ensure that his views would be incorporated into medical regulations by addressing his patron and ruler. Soon after the publication of his treatise, the herbalist sent a copy to Ranuccio I Farnese (1569–1622), Duke of Parma. In the accompanying letter, Quattrami proposed that Ranuccio use the treatise as a blueprint for regulating pharmacy in his dominions. In adopting the naturalist's own treatise, the prince would act in the interest of the "common good."[98]

Bolognese naturalist Ulisse Aldrovandi was even more outspoken than Quattrami when pushing for his views to be enshrined in law. An aristocrat with means, reputation, and a chair at the university, Aldrovandi was better positioned than Quattrami to effectively intervene in the public life of his city. He was an indefatigable advocate of medical regulatory effort, and historians have shown the especially close connection between his scientific research, theriac, and his involvement in pharmaceutical regulation.[99] Regulating pharmacy in Bologna was a contested process that put Aldrovandi at odds with both the city's apothecary guild and its Collegio Medico. Unlike other physicians, Aldrovandi criticized not only apothecaries' ignorance and greediness, but also their inappropriate ties with physicians, declaring that the economic interests of the two groups should be separated. "Physicians," Aldrovandi wrote, were moved by "particular passion and hate to follow their extraordinary and iniquitous appetite, governed only by their affection and interest."[100] In his view it was necessary to reinforce boundaries between medical professions in order to protect the interest of patients.

Written after 1597, toward the end of his life, Aldrovandi's unpublished treatise *Avertimenti sopra la Teriaca et Mithridato* not only contained his final word on the subject of theriac, but also outlined a comprehensive, visionary, and grandiose project for pharmacy (*farmaceptica*).[101] It is unsurprising that Aldrovandi consigned his mature reflections on pharmacy to a treatise on theriac. He had dedicated more than half a century to studying the drug, and his popularity beyond Bologna was partly due to his "true theriac" made in 1574. Yet it was also because of theriac that he suffered one of the darkest moments of his career: expulsion from the Collegio Medico.[102]

Pharmacy, wrote Aldrovandi, "is the most important business that anybody can do in the world" because its tools "are the instruments to preserve health and to heal."[103] In his unpublished treatise he offered a utilitarian justification for the study of natural knowledge. For Aldrovandi, the path to improving pharmacy was to understand the natural world and materia medica. Given that knowing the natural world was an immense task that no single individual could undertake by himself, scholars should collaborate. He envisioned natural knowledge as a collaborative endeavor for the common good, financed and coordinated by all the "princes of Christian Europe," whom he saw as bearing a responsibility to reform pharmacy. Princes should appoint the most learned individuals from Italy and Europe, following the lead of the councils against heretics.[104] A specific example Aldrovandi had in mind for the reform of materia medica was the 1582 reformation of the Gregorian calendar, which unified the calendar of Catholic Europe.[105] He also urged princes to pursue the betterment of pharmacy and the study of natural knowledge rather than destructive military campaigns: "The emperor [Habsburg], the King of France, of Spain, and many others spend millions of ducats in great wars which cause the death of thousands of men, and destroy castles, cities, and places with little gain not proportioned to the expense and not knowing exactly the end of the war. But in this endeavor to reform pharmacy, I know for sure that they will accomplish a very useful objective."[106] On the one hand, war was expensive, whereas pharmacy was both cheaper and certain to secure better results. On the other, ancient medical knowledge was lost "because of the negligence and the little care Princes had paid ... so that it is easy to see how the responsibility has to be given to the former magistrates who have reduced such sciences to a barbaric state."[107] To make up for their past mistakes and negligence, wrote Aldrovandi, princes should endorse and finance the study of plants, medicine, and the natural world to ensure the well-being of their subjects. Similar statements on the necessity of the states' involvement in pharmacy can be found elsewhere in Aldrovandi's writings.[108] It is telling that *Avertimenti sopra la Teriaca* was not addressed to a single patron. Aldrovandi longed for an ideal patron, "such as I desire him"—but he never found one.[109]

Every author considered in this chapter—Maranta, Oddo and his Paduan colleagues, Quattrami, Aldrovandi, Borgarucci, even Melich—formally agreed that apothecaries needed educating on materia medica through a top-down process directed by physicians. However, the degree to which this control was exerted was determined by local power dynamics. In cities with better-established medical colleges and universities, such as Padua and Bologna, physicians called for a steep hierarchy and advocated for a clear-cut separation of the two professions. According to Oddo, Crasso, and Trevisano, physicians' credibility depended on the quality of the remedies they prescribed, which in turn depended on the quality of the medicaments apothecaries made. Thus, controlling apothecaries was vital not just for preserving patients' health but also for maintaining their trust in physicians. By contrast, in cities whose apothecaries were wealthier and more independent, such as Venice and Naples, apothecaries and physicians presented pharmacy as a collaborative enterprise demanding the complementary knowledge and expertise of both professional groups.

In the sixteenth century, pharmaceutical concerns were increasingly on the agenda of Renaissance rulers. The origin story of theriac illuminated the usefulness of pharmacy, serving as a potent reminder to the state that healing had been a matter of state concern since the Roman Empire. Embedded in the concept and materiality of theriac were ideas of glory, genealogy, largesse, civilization, and empire. Physicians and learned apothecaries used persuasive arguments to present theriac to princes while bolstering their own relevance to the state.

In several Italian Renaissance courts, princes studied, sponsored, possessed, and donated theriac. A court object, theriac possessed civilizing qualities that resonated with life at court and offered a solution to poison, epidemics, and unsettling views of nature. Princes asserted their political prestige by financing the costly refashioning of theriac. Having "true theriac" became another means to compete with neighboring states.

The renewed eminence of theriac prompted authors to express their views on the social organization of pharmacy in their treatises on the drug. Even though all these authors—physicians and learned apothecaries alike—formally agreed to a hierarchical relationship between the two groups, they proposed markedly different ideas about what form this relationship should take. In Italy, projects of medical reorganization mirrored the social forces at play in single cities, and cannot be generalized even within polities, as exemplified by the differences between Padua and Venice. Local conditions, such as the presence of universities and the authority of medical colleges and apothecary guilds, shaped the initial plans physicians presented to regulate medicine, as well as the outcome of medical regulation.

CHAPTER 4

A Public Health Measure Against Poison and Plague

In discorso sopra la peste (1577), Bolognese physician Baldassarre Pisanelli (?-1587) opened his discussion of remedies for the plague by summarizing a commonly accepted belief: "The first remedy to be used among the most useful is Theriaca magna, which is the Queen of precious medicaments; it has the strength to obstruct and resist poison that might come, as well as to remove poison that already is [in the body]."[1] Medieval and early modern physicians and patients often conceptualized plague as poison—and they considered theriac, with its powerful antidotal properties, the best preservative and curative against it.

The plague epidemic that afflicted most of the Italian peninsula in the years 1575–1577 marked a turning point in the history of theriac. The outbreak of "exceptional gravity" devastated Sicily, Venice, Padua, Verona, Mantua, Brescia, Milan, and Genoa and took approximately 300,000 lives—more than 45,000 in Venice alone.[2] During such times it became increasingly urgent for authorities to uphold their promise to protect their subjects from threats both external and internal—or at the very least demonstrate their commitment to fulfilling those promises as best they could. Now that even Mattioli held that achieving "true theriac" was possible, theriac began featuring more prominently in physicians' discourses as a means to combat the plague. Consequently, theriac became integrated into the array of public health measures employed by the states, alongside other practices such as fumigation and quarantine—during the later plague of 1630, for example, theriac was commonly used in lazarettos (quarantine sites).

Moreover, apothecaries transformed theriac productions into grand ceremonies, sponsored and endorsed by magistrates and medical professionals to underscore their dedication to public health. These public performances served to visually represent the healing power of theriac, as well as the fact that this power had ultimately been granted by the state through medical colleges, physicians, and the medical knowledge they acquired in universities. When the plague or other scares were approaching, these ceremonies became nothing less than urban medical rituals for the protection of the community, generative pageants for the creation of an effective remedy, for an audience of patients and curious public alike, gathered around those who could produce and approve of theriac. Alongside restrictive measures such as lazarettos and *cordons sanitaires*, theriac productions functioned as cathartic rites that collectively exorcized the fear of disease, exhibited the unity of the social body, and promised to protect the city's population.

In the first section of this chapter I review the connection between poison, plague, and theriac. In the second section I argue that theriac entered the arsenal of dependable public health measures as a consequence of both the plague of 1575–1577 and the novel credibility it acquired when refashioned into "true theriac." Unlike other public health measures against plague, such as quarantine, theriac provided hope rather than confinement. For decades, often prompted by rulers, physicians discussed its effectiveness against epidemics. During the plague of 1630, treating patients with theriac became standard practice in lazarettos. In the third section I offer an account of the medical debates that followed 1630, when some physicians realized that theriac was simply not delivering the effects they had hoped for—although by then its position as state drug was well rooted.

In the fourth section I discuss public productions of theriac in Venice, Bologna, Vicenza, and Mantua, showcasing the different meanings these medical events took on, depending on the urban context.

Theriac ceremonies grew in complexity over time, progressively crystallizing apothecaries' prestige and social position. The final section analyzes the pamphlets that accompanied theriac productions. These prints—which I call *theriac celebrations*—recorded these performative events and offer a unique perspective on not only theriac-making ceremonies, but also the life of the early modern apothecary, and the interplay between the medical hierarchy and the medical marketplace.

An Antidote for All Poisons

Because theriac was primarily understood as an antidote, its connection with the fear of poison is well established in literature. Already in 1745 physician William Heberden had identified this fear as the main reason for theriac's popularity over the centuries: "In the ruder ages of the world, before experience had furnished mankind with any considerable knowledge of nature, they seem to have been under perpetual alarms from apprehension of poisons."[3] In 1966 historian Gilbert Watson also suggested that theriac's appeal in the sixteenth century was related to an increasing fear of poisons. Watson did not offer any evidence, but instead relied on the assumption that poisons were especially feared and used during the Renaissance in Italy.[4] However, more recently Frank Collard has dismantled the myth that poisons were more popular in the Renaissance than in the Middle Ages, and Alessandro Pastore has suggested that the stereotype of poison conspiracies overstated actual practices.[5]

Recent evidence demonstrates high demand for antidotes in the second half of the sixteenth century, when theriac became fashionable again. David Gentilcore's study of charlatanism has shown that, between 1550 and 1800, antidotes constituted 15 percent of all charlatans' remedies licensed for sale, and that 50 percent of all remedies sold by charlatans in 1560–1569 were counterpoisons, suggesting a peak in the demand for antidotes at that time.[6] Similarly, Sabrina Minuzzi's data on the petitions for licenses for medical secrets presented to the Venetian Magistrate for Public Health reveals that antidotes outnumbered other types of medical secrets in the sixteenth century. Antidotes' popularity declined slowly in the seventeenth century, then precipitously in the eighteenth century.[7] According to Gianna Pomata, the fear of poison was the precise meeting point of charlatanism and learned medical culture.[8]

Theriac was a synonym for *antidote*. Throughout the early modern period, metaphors of poison and theriac were commonly used in letters and conversation, tribunals and literature. In 1567 an Italian correspondent informed the Grand Duke of Tuscany that in Flanders the Duke of Alba had created a magistrate to serve "as theriac" against heresy.[9] All over Europe and beyond, titles of nonmedical books exemplified the flexibility of the metaphor: spiritual, as in *Theriaca del alma* (Theriac of the soul) (Grenada, 1542); moral, as in *Theriaca fina contra il pestifero veleno delle comedie mercenarie lascive e impudiche de' nostri tempi* (Fine theriac against the pestiferous poison of mercenary and lascivious comedies) (Cremona, 1614), and *A treacle fetch'd out of a viper: A brief essay upon falls into sins* (Boston, 1707); religious, as in *Theriaca Judaica* (Hanau, 1615) and *A preservative, or triacle, agaynst the poyson of Pelagius lately renued, by the furious secte of the Annabaptistes* (London, 1551); juridical, as in *Sueños ay, que verdad son, y punto en contra de los astrologos: triaca magna contra el veleno de la astrologia judiciaria* (Ah, dreams, how true they are, and a point against the astrologers: great theriac against the poison of judicial astrology) (1739); and political, musical, and literary.[10] Poison was a capacious metaphor: it could connote heresy, sin, obscenity, political enmity, even lust. As a consequence, any entity able to expel poison—object or person, whether pamphlet or magistrate—was understood to function as "theriac," for it restored balance in the physical, political, or social body.[11]

A Measure of Public Health Against the Plague

The plague was one of the most feared phenomena in early modern society.[12] Aldrovandi described it as "a blind, wandering, inexorable beast ... without law."[13] Beyond the fear of death, plague elicited the fear of living in a society without order, wherein social relations became confused, unsafe, and unsettling. Since antiquity, rulers and statesmen had feared the cataclysmic power of the plague, as an epidemic would invariably break down the rule of law, both human and divine. Thucydides (ca. 460–396? BCE) and many later political thinkers described the potential of plague epidemics to destabilize trade, morals, and personal and social ties within the city.[14] Cities were especially hit by the plague, as mortality in urban areas was higher than in the countryside. Plague created the conditions for the deviancy and disorder abhorred by authority. Colin Jones has argued that plague treatises, when taken as a body of literature, show that the disease "spectacularly severed the normal relationship between sacred and profane." Plague disrupted the social and religious collective body. Churches had to interrupt their services; mass was held periodically in the streets; and people were buried in mass graves, leaving survivors unable to preserve the dignity of individuals or even entire communities.[15]

States and princes responded to demands for protection and security against the plague by issuing regulations and enforcing public health measures. After the Black Death, in several Italian states the management of plague epidemics was placed under the jurisdiction of nonphysicians, such as the Venetian Health Board, which became a permanent institution in 1486. Popular understanding of the plague and how to combat it usually stemmed from the observations of health officials rather than the theories of physicians. Health offices were in constant contact to monitor the spread of contagion, opening or closing borders in response to new information. Lazarettos, quarantines, and the issuance of health certificates restricted mobility by regulating the points of entry to a city or region.[16] Jones has also noted that these measures preserved the integrity of the social body as "rituals of closure."[17]

It was common for civil order to deteriorate during epidemics, not only because of the plague, but also because of the public health measures themselves. Most state measures to contain epidemics restricted the movement of people and goods. Draconian measures taken to contain the spread of disease often exacerbated class divides.[18] Other actions fomented discontent and incited fresh fears, such as the slaughter of plague-carrying animals and the fumigations of goods and homes. Among others, physician Leonardo Fioravanti was critical of several actions that seemed to produce more problems than they solved: "When the plague reigns, princes and their ministers should . . . comfort their subjects . . . The first thing is not to instill fear in them, or apprehension, as now everyone does, frightfully forcing them out of their houses, and sending them out of their lands to the lazaretto."[19] Fear, according to Fioravanti, came not only from the epidemic itself, but also from the responses to it.

In such a confused and unsettling situation, many—physicians, health officers, bishops, priests, gentlemen, notaries, and artisans—felt the need to express their opinions and put forward solutions. As Samuel Cohn has shown, the veritable wave of plague tracts printed just in the three years

1575–1578 demonstrated society-wide engagement: people from all walks of life were attending to the social effects of plague.[20] Demanded by their profession to discuss medicaments and etiology (the study of the causes of disease), physicians recognized that, of all the aforementioned groups, they bore a particular responsibility for finding measures to combat epidemics.

Early medical theories were not confined to the medical books and could have significant consequences during epidemics. In search of effective anti-plague measures, political authorities sought reliable medical knowledge from physicians and health officials. Although learned physicians embraced the Galenic humoral paradigm, their prescriptions depended on the classification of the disease, not just the patient's humoral imbalance. Authorities' public responses to epidemics might depend on medical debates on etiology. For example, at the onset of the plague epidemic in 1575, the Venetian Senate held a hearing to define the nature of the disease: Was it or was it not "true plague"? According to a medical tradition dominant since Hippocrates, "true plague" derived from corrupt air. The air that everyone breathed had to be the cause of a disease that killed so many. Two respected professors from Padua, Girolamo Mercuriale (1530–1606) and Girolamo Capodivacca (1523–1589), disagreed with the Venetian Health Board on the nature of the epidemic, claiming it was not "true plague," and thus opposed the drastic measures used in these cases. Possibly also because traditional public health measures had been suspended, the death toll rose mercilessly soon after the two physicians left the city.[21] In dire need of more physicians, the Senate released the physician Girolamo Donzellini (1513–1587) from prison, where he was serving out a sentence for heterodoxy. Donzellini opined that, "in truth, since plague is a poison, pestiferous people are poisoned." He then prescribed several measures, including theriac.[22] By postulating that the plague was caused by poison, physicians such as Donzellini maintained and enhanced the usefulness of powerful counterpoisons such as theriac and mithridate.

Although historians may have studied medicines less than other anti-plague measures, in the early modern period medicines had their place in the toolkit of public health authorities. Fearing the arrival of the plague epidemic hitting nearby cities in 1564, the Bolognese Collegio Medico ruled that apothecaries could not export any theriac beyond the city walls;

every ounce had to be kept for the city.²³ A few years later in 1576, Aldrovandi anxiously wrote: "Cities nearby, such as Venice and Mantua, have been visited [by the plague], and the poison has penetrated the most noble cities of Lombardy . . . the first thing is to keep out people infected with the plague . . . every city should prepare many remedies to prescribe and medicate."²⁴ Because a direct link between plague and poison was commonplace in medical theory, theriac was considered and offered as a public health measure against the plague. Aldrovandi noted that, "in these dangerous times suspected of that terrible and frightening plague," the city that owned such a perfect antidote "can be said to be happy."²⁵ He argued that producing theriac served "the good [*utile*] of the city," as well as the "universal honor of the Medical College." A perfect theriac was invaluable because it was a "certain" medicament to counter the fear (*sospetto*) of plague, which "kills thousands of men in a moment."²⁶

In addition to theriac and mithridate, other medicines were considered suitable responses to the plague. In 1574 a physician in service at the Venetian lazaretto received compensation for a remedy he invented. The health office publicized this cure, and thirteen apothecaries obtained a license to sell it.²⁷ Similarly, in Modena in 1630 the Duke ordered health officials "to make a good provision of medicaments for the city at this suspicious time of plague." Purchases were to be made in a timely manner, before the "mountain pass might be closed." The Duke also issued bills of exchange, and sent an apothecary to gather supplies in Venice.²⁸ Having good medicaments and especially theriac might make all the difference between having a "happy city" or one devastated by epidemics.

Physicians believed their profession should involve researching remedies to equip the state with the knowledge necessary for effective public health measures. In a 1578 letter to Aldrovandi, Andrea Bacci (1524–1600), the physician to Cardinal Felice Peretti (then Pope Sixtus V), commended the effort made by "princes and republics" to find solutions to the plague. Bacci, himself the author of a treatise on venoms and antidotes, praised the hefty corpus of literature devoted to the "contagion," and lauded the Bolognese medical college headed by Aldrovandi for its indefatigable attempt to liberate theriac from obscurity. For Bacci, Aldrovandi's botanical research had yielded knowledge pivotal in defining the "true" ingredients of theriac, and he commended his colleague for having made one of the best theriacs in circulation, decisive in countering epidemics.²⁹

In parallel to the research into remaking "true theriac," in the 1570s physicians began debating the usefulness of theriac during epidemics. Most physicians believed that theriac worked against "true plague" but was not effective against all epidemics. Whether a fever was considered to be caused by poison or corrupt air, theriac was accepted as a medicament, and so medical controversies surrounding the use of therapeutics during epidemics centered around the question of poison. In 1570 an outbreak of pestilential fevers devastated the region of Brescia, and also impacted Milan and Bergamo. This epidemic allegedly caused 13,000 deaths.[30] That same year, physician Giuseppe Valdagni (?-post-1595) published *De theriacae usu in febribus pestilentibus*, in which he argued that the epidemic had been caused by "putrescent internal humors"—that is, by the production of poison within the patient's body rather than by "corrupt airs."[31] As poison loomed so large in his diagnoses, Valdagni advocated theriac as a treatment.[32] Physician Girolamo Donzellini sided with Valdagni, promoting the fact that "true theriac" was now available to patients.[33] Conversely, Vincenzo Calzaveglia (1500-1573), a physician representing the opinion of the medical college of Brescia, argued against Valdagni: because nearly everyone got sick, these fevers must have an external cause, so using theriac would be an "abuse."[34] Calzaveglia observed that patients who took theriac sometimes actually died faster. The dispute bubbled acrimoniously across several publications before turning violent: Valdagni and Donzellini had to leave Brescia, and Calzaveglia later hired a soldier who stabbed Donzellini in the face.[35]

In 1581 Giulio Alessandrini (1506-1590), physician to Emperor Rudolph II and a towering figure in the medical landscape, also contributed to the discussion, with his treatise anticlimactically titled *In Galeni praecipua scripta annotationes, quae commentariorum loco esse possunt* (Annotations on Galen's most important writings, which can replace commentaries).[36] Alessandrini was one of the finest and most erudite translators and interpreters of Galen. According to him, Galen's *De theriaca ad Pisonem*—arguably the single most important treatise on theriac—was spurious. Alessandrini believed that "it is appropriate to reject the use of theriac completely."[37] Despite its authoritativeness, this definitive statement did not settle the debate.

By asking for advice about the effectiveness of theriac, political authorities sometimes were the very cause of these medical arguments.

During a "malignant influenza of putrid fevers" in the region of Pesaro in 1591, the Duke of Urbino, Francesco Maria II della Rovere (1549-1631), asked the University of Padua for a consultation on how to best contain such fevers. His request instigated a dispute regarding theriac among several professors. Ercole Sassonia (1551-1607), a student of Mercuriale, proposed to cure the fevers with the ingestion of theriac and the use of cataplasms—*vescicatori,* poultices placed over the skin—which caused irritation.[38] Conversely, Alessandro Massaria (1510-1598) and other doctors— Girolamo Fabrici d'Acquapendente, Emilio Campolongo, and Albertino Bottoni—vehemently opposed the use of theriac except in the case of "true plague."[39] Political and medical authorities were called into action by their responsibilities during outbreaks, yet at the same time were just as personally affected as anyone else, which might help explain the level of ferocity these disputes often reached—although such vehemence was also not unusual in the Renaissance, when personal rivalries often escalated. These debates were testament to the widespread belief that poison was the cause of the plague, and that theriac could serve the physical as well as the social body.

Notwithstanding the medical disputes, the value of theriac in preventing plague went largely uncontested through the first half of the seventeenth century, when using it to ward off the disease became standard practice in hospitals. Most early seventeenth-century physicians agreed with Milanese Protomedico Ludovico Settala, who in his *Preservatione dalla peste* (1630) affirmed: "Theriac, thus, among those [all remedies] will keep the first place among the modifiers (*alteranti*), and those that tame virulence, or pestiferous poison. I have discussed at length ... citing many authors, and with many arguments I proved that nothing is more certain than theriac for preservation."[40] Although theriac would not "heal putrescence," it was effective against the plague because it acted against its "venenosity."[41]

From 1629 to 1633, French and German armies fighting in Mantua possibly caused an outbreak of bubonic plague in Northern Italy and Tuscany, which killed 10 to 57 percent of the population depending on the areas.[42] During the 1630 plague outbreak, theriac figured among standard therapeutic practices in the lazarettos of Venice.[43] In Florence the advice from the Sanità (Health Board) to peasants was to take theriac in the morning or, if it was unavailable, to eat dry figs, walnuts, and rue.[44] At the lazaretto of San Miniato, the morning routine started with an application of an ointment of theriac to the region around the heart, together with bloodletting and a bitter lemon cordial. A dose of theriac was administered in the evening with barley water and ointments of clay (*terra sigillata*). In 1630 Florentine apothecaries affirmed that they had plentiful remedies, including 200 pounds of "counterpoison oil," 2,000 pounds of theriac, and a "large enough quantity of mithridate." By December, theriac was being used less frequently, possibly because of a supply shortage. Then in 1631 the apothecaries of Pietro and Paolo supplied the lazaretto with theriac.[45]

Also during the 1630 plague outbreak in Bologna, theriac was one of the standard remedies in the local lazaretto. Once admitted, patients were visited by barber-surgeons for an initial assessment, then given a bed. After the physician's visit, the patient would receive a solutive medicament (a laxative), then a syrup. Patients also received an electuary, either Hyacinthus, Alkermes, *Theriaca magna,* or a generic cordial powder. Theriac was used both internally and externally as ointment for *carboni*, small pustules with black centers. Giovanni Polani, one of the physicians in service at the lazaretto, tried a secret remedy made primarily with theriac.[46] As in Florence, Bologna struggled with supply shortages during epidemics. The Jesuit Angelo Orimbelli, in charge of all the lazarettos of Bologna, took the news of the theriac shortage to Cardinal Bernardino Spada (1594–1661), Papal Legate *a latere:* "We would need four or five pounds of theriac, which we already asked for but never received, and there is no time to wait for it to be made."[47] The long, laborious production of theriac negated the possibility of quickly replenishing the supply chain and ensuring widespread availability of the drug during such times.

Theriac was widely used throughout the plague of 1630, by which time it was more accessible than during the previous epidemic of the 1570s. However, some physicians, having experienced its effects firsthand, noted that it did not always perform as expected. During the plague outbreak in Palermo, Father Virgilio Spada observed that theriac, mithridate, "and other hot medicaments" were in fact harmful.[48] When serving during the 1630 epidemic as director of the lazaretto of Lucca, Francesco Maria Fiorentini (1603–1673) started using theriac with enthusiasm. But he soon shelved this ineffective remedy in favor of *vescicatori,* poultices to which he attributed many recoveries.[49]

Old Objections and New Doubts

After the test of the 1630 plague and decades of use of "true theriac," the old objection to theriac's effectiveness resurfaced. Critiques had traditionally focused on its composition rather than its efficacy. Similarly, physician Giovanni Cinelli Calvoli (1626–1706) expressed his distrust of Venetian theriac, albeit mildly: "I have no doubt that the theriac of Venice, like that of Rome and Florence, is made with the same recipe. But I have seen the theriac manipulated in Florence, where I was Protomedico five times, ... and the one made in Venice in 1683 . . . and I say that the one from Florence is better manipulated, and this is why Fantasti . . . who is ours from Firenze . . . published a treatise."[50] Apparently Calvoli's critique stemmed more from a typical parochial attitude than from doubts about the concept of theriac itself. Others, such as Florentine physician Baldo Baldi (?–1644), more openly admitted that many were still disappointed by the "virtues" of theriac, whose effects they considered weak compared to those described by the ancients. As in the past, Baldi ascribed theriac's weakness to the lack of "true" ingredients, opobalsamum above all.[51]

As a matter of fact, the last major dispute over theriac in Italy took place in Rome in the 1640s, and centered around the appropriateness of the ingredients used in a specific production. In 1639 two Roman apothecaries under the protection of the pope's nephew Cardinal Barberini had made a ceremonial production of theriac with great pomp. However, the local college of apothecaries opposed the approval of opobalsamum made by the Roman Collegio Medico, and by extension opposed the newly made theriac in its entirety. Opobalsamum, the oleoresin of a bush called *balsam* whose supply was extremely scarce in Europe, had been known since antiquity and used for both religious and medical purposes.[52] Between 1638 and 1644, both the Roman Collegio Medico and the apothecary college requested counsel from medical authorities across Italy and beyond on the quality of the opobalsamum used in the production. Letters and prints circulated in Rome, Florence, Venice, Padua, Messina, Naples, and even Nuremberg. An entire network of physicians and learned apothecaries became embroiled in the dispute, triggering the publication of no fewer than twenty-five texts over six years.[53] On one side, Roman apothecaries tried disqualifying the opobalsamum used in Rome. On the other side, physicians and learned apothecaries unanimously defended it against the Roman apothecaries' challenge. Strikingly, a dispute over opobalsamum had morphed into an opportunity to attack the authority of the Barberinis, thus gaining readers beyond the medical milieu, as demonstrated by the circulation of several popular publications in the vernacular. The controversy ended abruptly in 1644 when the pope died and the Barberinis fell into disgrace.

In the years following this dispute, the scientific debate focused more on understanding and testing poison, although theriac remained prominent in the discourse. Most notably, starting in Florence in the early 1660s at the Accademia del Cimento, Francesco Redi carried out numerous experiments on vipers, and tested their venom on other animals. These experiments were of public interest for both practical and medical reasons, such as finding antidotes against snakebites and exploiting vipers' medical properties. They also regarded broader scientific discussions on the nature of disease and the body, chemical and mechanical philosophy, and the functioning of substances in the body. Furthermore, Redi's experiments in Florence were typical of courtly science, showcasing wealth and resources, and expectations surrounding courtly demonstrations in front of an aristocratic audience who had been called to ascertain the outcome.[54]

Redi engaged with classical literature and images as much as with contemporaries, such as Marco Aurelio Severino and Moyse Charas (1619–1698).[55] A student of Nicola Antonio Stigliola, Severino was a Neapolitan physician, surgeon, and philosopher. In 1660 he published *Vipera Pythia,* a book on vipers filled with literary citations, digressions about symbolism, anatomical observations and speculations, and therapeutic information, including some recipes. Two substantial chapters discussed which parts of the viper were suitable for theriac.[56] Severino argued that viper's black bile contained the principle that made theriac effective.[57] Redi recognized Severino's authority, but remained critical, claiming that Severino had not performed enough "experiences": "With all this, a single experience could not effect to alter the opinion of such consolidated and principal Doctors."[58] Experiments mattered to Redi.

Theriac and viper's venom were also at the core of an acrimonious dispute that lasted several years between Redi and French apothecary

Moyse Charas. Historian Jutta Schickore has primarily framed this dispute as a disagreement about how to define a reliable experimental method, arguing for the importance of these scholars' concerns about methodology, particularly when it came to distinguishing replication from repetition.[59] Both Redi's and Charas's writings demonstrated a substantial interest in establishing proper experimental procedures. They agreed on several points, including that knowledge should be based on matters of fact and that experiments should be careful, varied, and repeated.[60] However, they diverged on how to interpret and explain their experiments, and they held conflicting perspectives on viper's venom. For Redi, the venenosity of the viper stemmed from the yellow bile found in the head, which acted only when it came into contact with the blood of another creature. In contrast, Charas argued that the yellow bile was harmless unless the viper was angry, a state that endowed its poison with "infinite power."[61]

Redi and Charas also disagreed on the antidotal effects of viper. In his *Lettera sopra alcune opposizioni fatte alle sue osservazioni intorno alle vipere*, Redi reported that his experiments indicated that viper head did not serve as an antidote to viper bites (killing no less than "eight cockerels, two young cats, two little hares, and six tower pigeons," implicitly challenging theriac's efficacy.[62] Meanwhile Charas was a staunch advocate of theriac's therapeutic value. Despite overseeing the Grand Duke's production of theriac in his capacity as court physician, Redi seldom mentioned theriac in his writings, and prescribed it only once in his consultations.[63] Yet his skepticism was not widely embraced at the Medici court. For example, witnesses to Redi's demonstration of a snake handler drinking viper venom were dubious, either convinced it was harmless or suspecting the handler had protected himself by taking theriac.[64] Thus, these aristocrats still trusted theriac. Conversely, Redi probably shared Fiorentini's incredulity toward theriac: in 1671, now a renowned clinician and iatrochemist, Fiorentini called for more experiments: "Good Lord willing, if the famous *Theriaca Andromachi* underwent all due and diligent tests [*prove*], it would produce those effects on all sorts of poisons that many piously believe in."[65]

Unlike Redi, Moyse Charas's career jump was tied to theriac. In 1668 he published an ambitious treatise on theriac titled *Histoire naturelle des animaux, des plantes, et des minéraux qui entrent dans la composition de la Theri-*

aque d'Andromachus, in which he affirmed that, while theriac composition might seem "chaotic," if well prepared it was proven to be effective by an "infinity of experiences."[66] That same year Charas also staged a grandiose production of theriac in Paris, making 300 pounds of compound, followed by a second production in 1669. Both productions were endorsed by the highest medical authorities.[67]

By the mid-seventeenth century, some physicians' enthusiasm for "true theriac" had waned, and several had been casting doubts on the efficacy of theriac more broadly. But as we shall see in Chapter 7, up until the end of the century these doubts were expressed with only the utmost caution. In the meantime, reliance on theriac continued unabated for most of the seventeenth century. In fact, the drug's popularity even grew, sustained by medical and political institutions' sponsorship and made visible through public productions.

From Public Productions to Ceremonies

In the mid-sixteenth century the making of theriac increasingly involved elaborate public ceremonies brimming with music, poetry recitations, decorations, and choreographies. Apothecaries staged exhibits, either displaying the individual ingredients of theriac in similarly sized piles or stacks, or presenting them in order in same-size plates or vessels, placed on simple shelves or tables covered with drapes and ribbons or in elaborate architectures laden with paintings and statues (Figure 4.1).[68] With such staging, apothecaries transformed a medieval public administrative act—the checking and approving of the ingredients by physicians—into a festive, ritual event. In the Renaissance the certification process of theriac was hardly novel: procedures related to the making of theriac and other electuaries had been in place since at least the thirteenth century.[69] Across medieval Europe, apothecaries invited physicians and public officials to their shops to witness preparation. In this sense, then, the production of theriac was already public. In 1495, for example, apothecaries in Montpellier declared that apothecaries making theriac had to exhibit ingredients publicly to physicians and everybody else, "as they did previously," with a view to minimizing forgeries.[70] Similarly, all theriac produced in Venice in 1437 had to be made in one of only two central apothecary shops, where anyone could see it.[71] It is possible

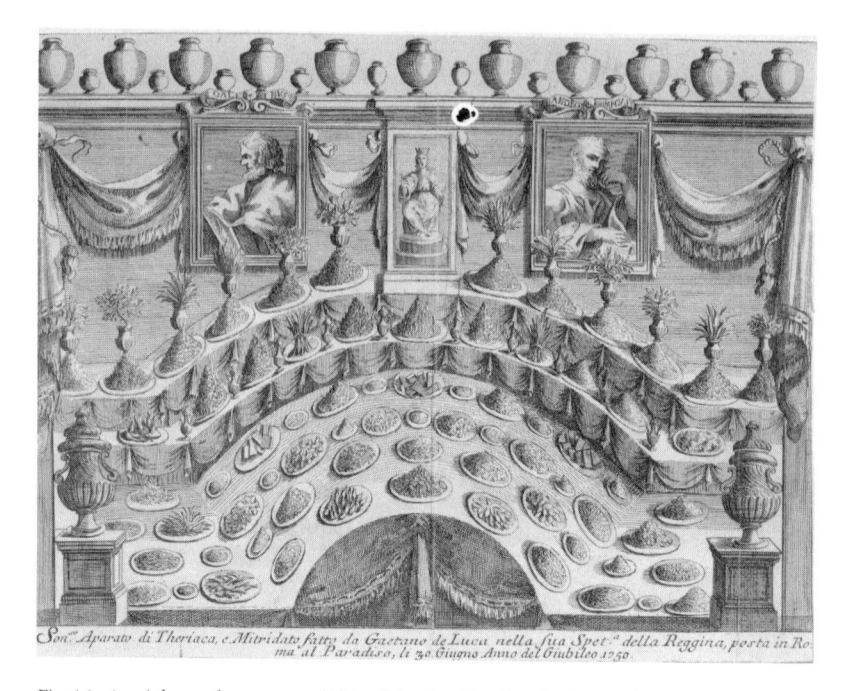

Fig. 4.1. An eighteenth-century exhibit of theriac. The description reads: *Sumptuous display of Theriac and Mithridatium prepared by Gaetano de Luca in his pharmacy at the sign of the Queen, located in Rome at the Paradise, on June 30, in the Year of the Jubilee, 1750.* The display took place under the auspices of the eponymous Queen (center), Galen (left), and Andromachus (right).
Getty Research Institute, Los Angeles (910002).

there were also early public productions of theriac in Germany: a 1512 woodcut is sometimes cited as a depiction of such a production in a German square (Figure 4.2). However, a careful examination shows that this woodcut portrays a sale of Venetian theriac in a German city, not a production.[72]

From the 1560s to the 1790s, ceremonies of theriac grew in complexity, length, and richness, evolving into a veritable triumph of the senses. Yet their fundamental structure appeared remarkably similar throughout the early modern period. Ceremonies centered around physicians' inspection and subsequent certification of the ingredients, and enhanced the prestige of the apothecary or apothecary guild. Nonetheless, the next sections analyze how the connotations of theriac-making ceremonies varied significantly in different cities.

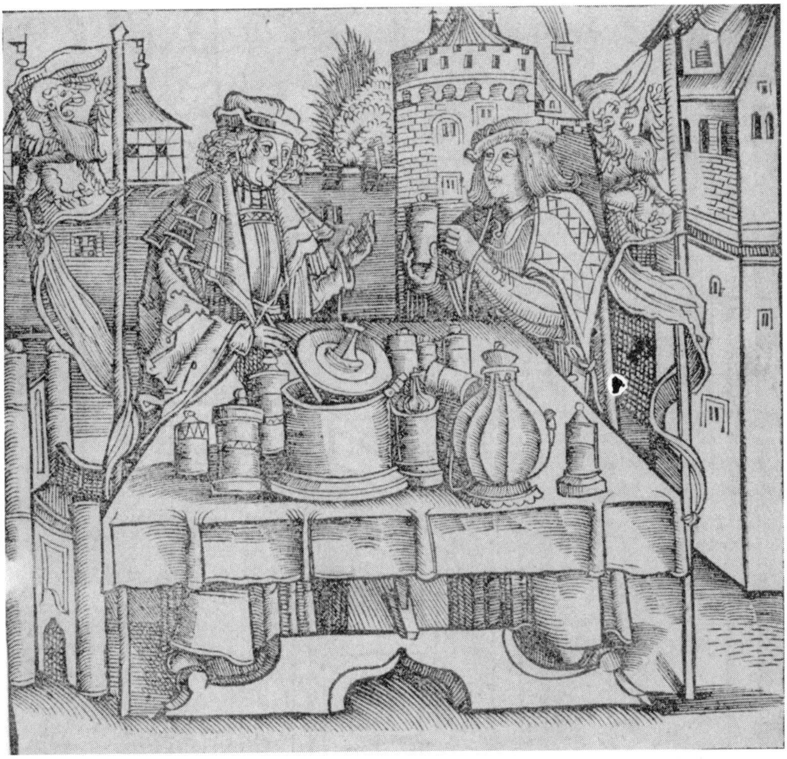

Fig. 4.2. Two men stand by an apothecary stall. Venetian flags of St. Mark's lion, the symbol of the Venetian Republic, indicate the provenance of the apothecaries. The descriptive architecture in the background sets the scene in a German city, perhaps Nuremberg, or maybe Strasbourg, where Brunschwig's text was published. One of the men removes something from a larger container with a dipper, while the other holds a smaller container. The text accompanying the image offers confusing information about the scene. The presence of many containers in different sizes and shapes on the table, rather than the pestles and cauldrons apothecaries used to make theriac, suggests that this image represented a sale rather than a production of theriac. Woodcut from Hieronymus Brunschwig, *Liber de Arte Distilandi* (1512) Ch. 36, 93r, reprinted in the 1519 edition, Ch. 36, 196v.
Wellcome Collection.

Venice: An Apothecary Event

Public productions of theriac likely started in Venice, with the city's apothecaries influenced by ceremonial productions of theriac in the Eastern Mediterranean.[73] In Italy the ceremonial and public character of these Egyptian productions was common knowledge. A map of Cairo indicated

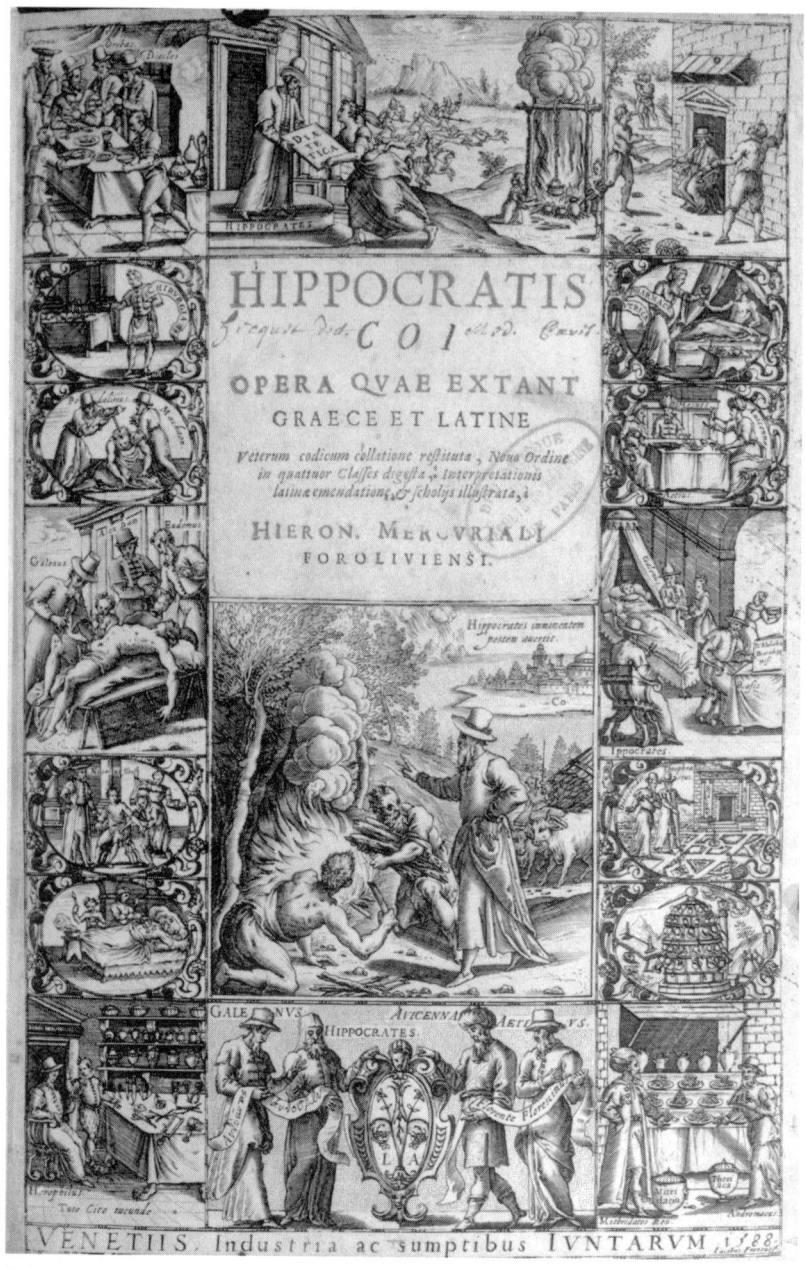

HIPPOCRATIS COI OPERA QVAE EXTANT GRAECE ET LATINE

Veterum codicum collatione restituta, Noua Ordine in quattuor Classes digesta, Interpretationis latinæ emendatione, & scholijs illustrata, à

HIERON. MERCVRIALI FOROLIVIENSI.

VENETIIS, Industria ac sumptibus IVNTARVM, 1588.

(a.)

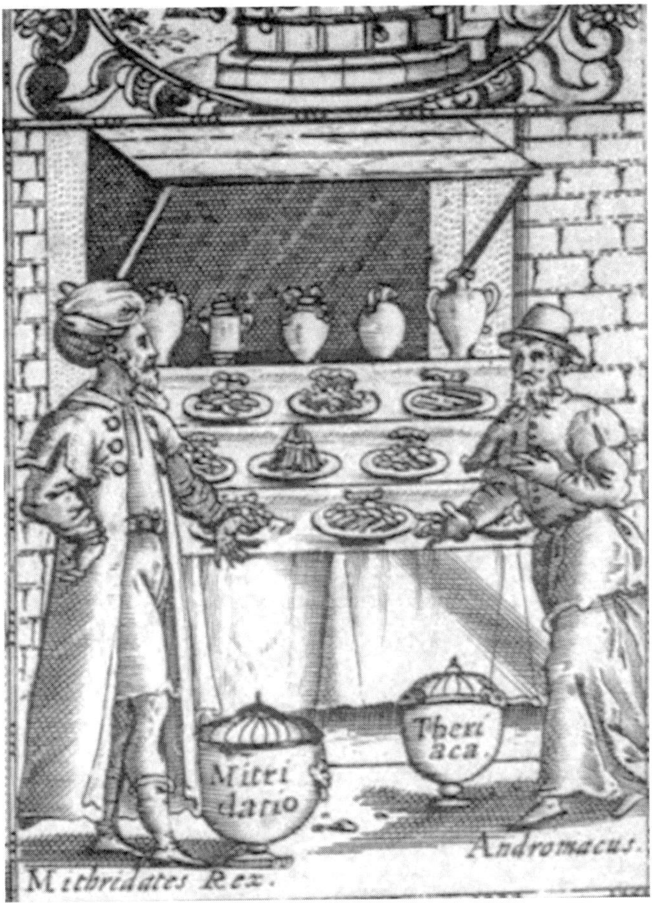

(b.)

Fig. 4.3. (*a.*) Frontispiece of *Hippocratis COI: Opera quae extant graece et latine*, edited by Geronimo Mercuriale and published in 1588, engraved by Giacomo Franco with a burin. The whole comprises several images detailing the foundations of medicine, including surgery, *dietetica*, and pharmacy. The publishers Giunti reused this frontispiece several times.
BIU Santé (Paris), Université Paris Cité.
(*b.*) Detail (bottom right) showing two men under a canopy of an apothecary shop looking at an exhibit of theriac's ingredients. On the left is Mithradates, king of Pontus, wearing a Turkish robe and a turban. On the right is Andromachus, dressed like an early modern doctor. On the floor are two large jars of theriac and mithridate.
BIU Santé (Paris), Université Paris Cité.

the place where theriac was made, and physician Prospero Alpini reported that theriac produced in Egypt was the only medicament expressly made in public for the sultan. At the Cairo Mosque "called Morestan," an appointed apothecary carried out the production in front of all the physicians who controlled it.[74]

Theriac was likely produced for the first time in Venice with "some publicity" at the apothecary shop of Galeazzo Corniani in 1565.[75] Although productions of theriac initially were held within apothecary shops, they might have later moved outside these establishments. The frontispiece of Hippocrates's works published in 1588 shows what an early exhibit of theriac might have looked like in Venice (Figure 4.3). The canopy of an apothecary shop protects the raw ingredients placed on shelves, on plates, or in little piles. King Mithradates and the physician Andromachus—political and medical authorities, respectively—inspect the simples to guarantee their quality.

Public exhibits of theriac became the defining feature of "true theriac"; they ensured that nothing was hidden, secret, illegal, or fraudulent. Reflecting on a famous production he had conducted in 1573 at the apothecary at the sign of the Ostrich, Georg Melich wrote:

> Now I am going to say about the theriac I made in Venice this year. I arranged in an orderly way all the simples necessary for the composition of both theriac and mithridate and, once the best were chosen among them, they were put in beautiful pots and placed in a public place greatly decorated for three days, so it could be a show for everybody, and they could examine the aforementioned things, and on the fourth day I summoned the excellent priors, and the officials of both physicians and apothecaries, who diligently inspected the ingredients.[76]

Melich stressed the quality ("the best were chosen"), the openness ("everyone could examine"), and the beauty of the display, and emphasized how his theriac was certified only after having been inspected by several authorities. The prior and the officials of the medical college, as well as officials of the Giustizia Vecchia and apothecary guild, ensured that each of the sixty-odd ingredients was properly identified. They checked the quality of the materia medica to verify that the herbs were neither old nor moldy, and approved any substitutes (*quid pro quo*) for unavailable ingredients.

Cunning merchants as they were, apothecaries developed theriac ceremonies as an elegant answer to both stringent medical regulations and increasing market competition. Especially in Venice, the ceremonial character of these public productions was apothecaries' commercial response to the growing presence of charlatans, who had become part of the urban landscape. Charlatans mounted impromptu stalls in public squares, sold their potentially harmful remedies, and performed with live snakes and bare chests. These scruffy yet flamboyant spectacles enlivened the markets, attracted many customers, and were popular with foreign travelers who looked forward to these performances when visiting Italian cities.[77] To compete with charlatans' and mountebanks' performances, which were both makeshift and self-sponsored, apothecaries offered grandiose, well-organized, certified, and official medical attractions.

The festive character of Venetian theriac productions soon became popular with foreign travelers, and would remain so for two centuries. In 1590 an English traveler reported: "The Venetians make the best Treakell, which is transported throughout Europe and about the first of November, at which tyme they make it, those Artizans have a Feast, wherein they weare feathers, and have Trumpitts continually sounding, and during the tyme of this worke all the shops about Rialto resounde with the blowing thereof."[78]

When in Italy for their Grand Tour, travelers such as French philosopher Charles de Brosses (1709–1777) and German poet August von Platen-Hallermünde (1796–1835) enjoyed these joyful performances.[79] Venice also set an example for other cities. While visiting the Collegio Romano in Rome in 1658, Christina of Sweden (1626–1689) "went ... into the Apothecary shop, where she saw the preparation of the ingredients of herbs, plants, metals, gems, and other rare things for the making of Treacle."[80] With time, Venetian theriac ceremonies became increasingly elaborate, with a dozen livery-clad shop boys grinding the herbs in large mortars, beating and singing in rhythm (Figure 4.4).[81]

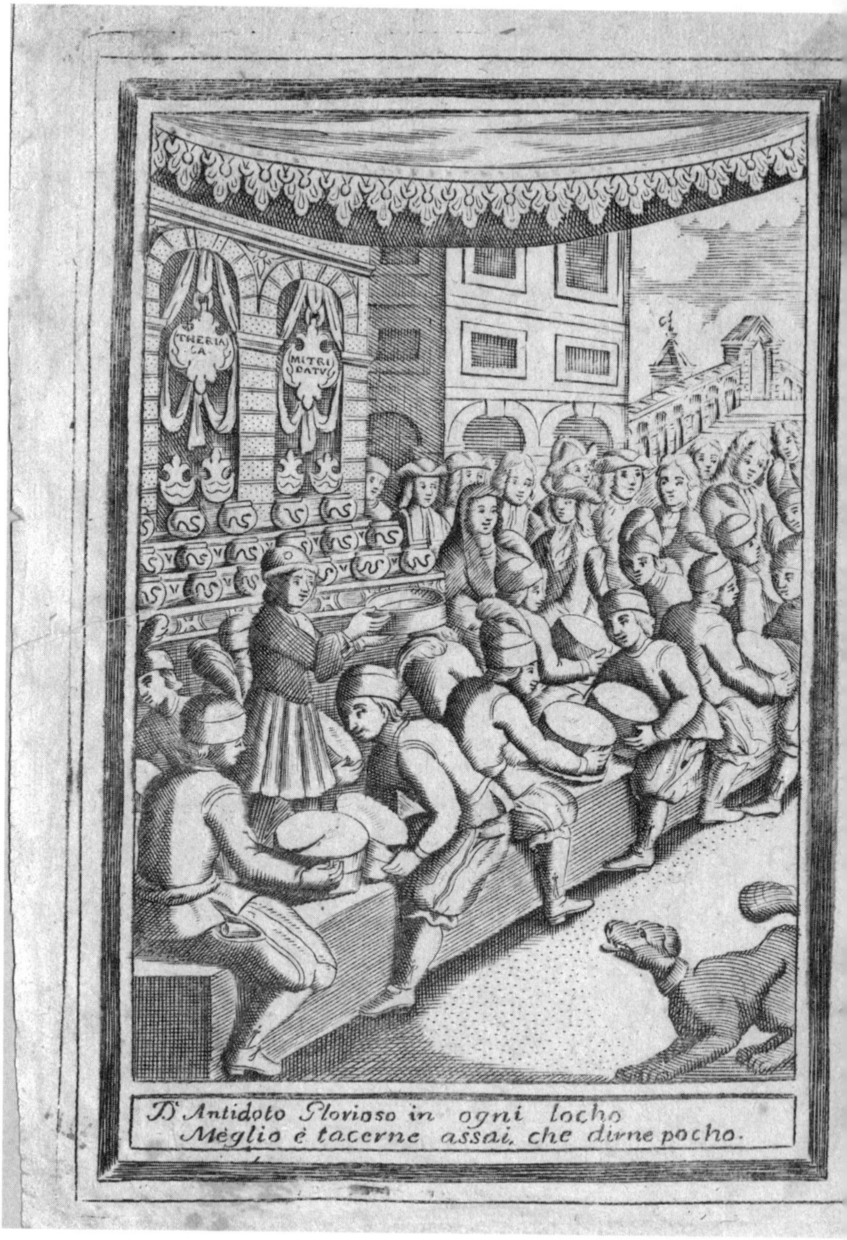

Fig. 4.4. A popular eighteenth-century print made with the two parts of a paper fan portrays a public making of theriac in front of the apothecary at the sign of the Golden Head (*Testa d'oro*) at the bottom of the Rialto Bridge (in the background), in Venice. The sign of the Golden Head is still on display today, above a clothing store. Numerous jars with the symbol of a snake are exposed on a wooden architecture built for the occasion. On the right, a dozen shop boys in livery grind the necessary herbs in large mortars, beating and singing in

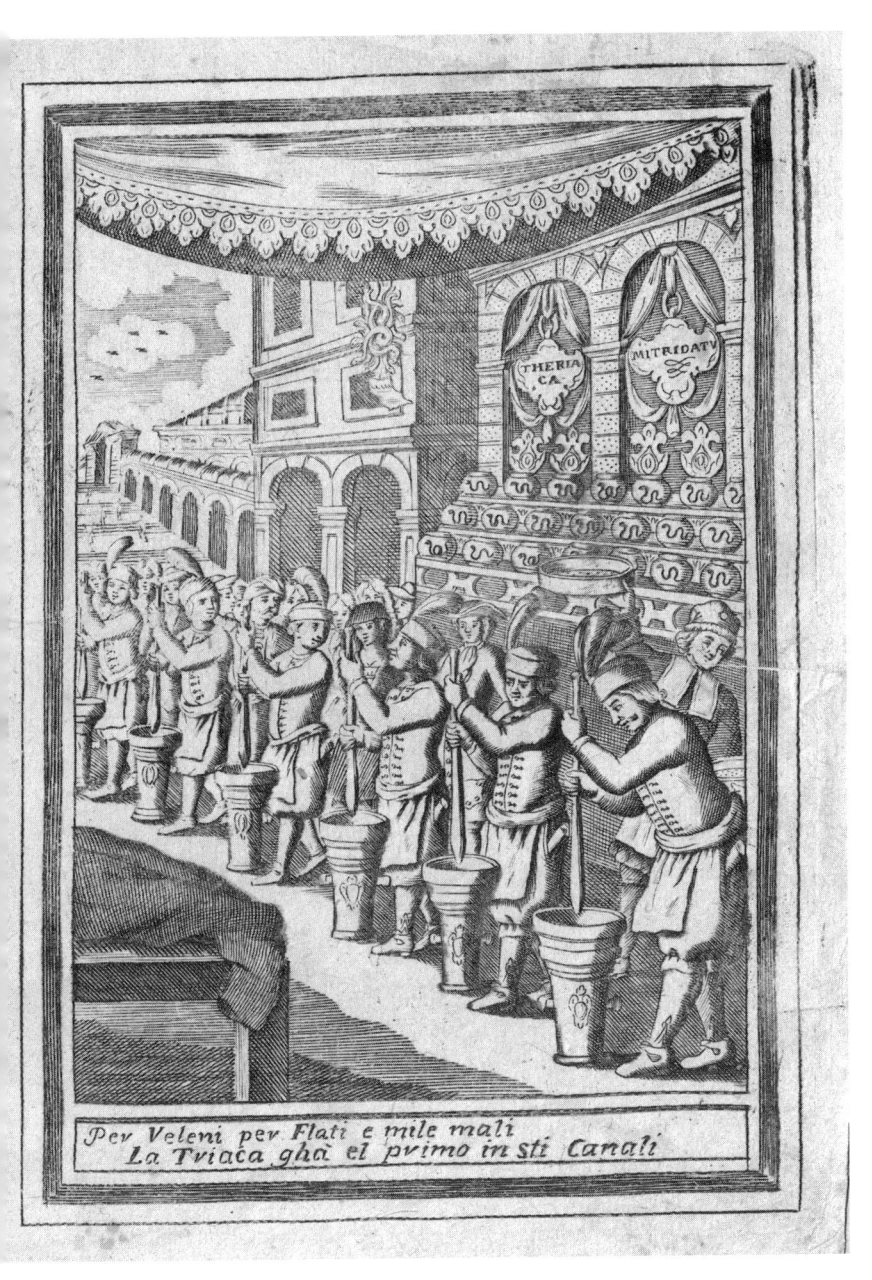

A PUBLIC HEALTH MEASURE AGAINST POISON AND PLAGUE 133

Per Veleni per Flati e mile mali
La Triaca gha el primo in sti Canali

rhythm, while others sift on the left. A festive public looks upon the scene, and a dog barks for the noise. At the bottom are a few rhymed verses that might have been sung by the shop boys: "A glorious antidote in every place, it is best to keep quiet than to say too little of it. For poisons, for gas, or for a thousand ailments, theriac is the best in these channels."

Civica Raccolta delle Stampe Achille Bertarelli, Castello Sforzesco, Milan. © Comune di Milano. All rights reserved.

Bologna: A Medical Performance

Bologna was not as renowned as Venice for its production of theriac, but the event was still integral to the medical life of the city. The first grandiose public performance was organized in 1574 by friar-apothecary Francesco Azzi and master Stefano di Silvestri, in the convent of San Salvatore in Bologna, supervised by Protomedici Aldrovandi and Alberghini.[82] The church of San Salvatore was one of the city's most sumptuous, chosen by Emperor Charles V for the celebrations of the Order of Santiago, a powerful religious and military order.[83] Aldrovandi boasted that this was a production of "true theriac" with only three substitutes. For the occasion, the *apparatus* (the public display of ingredients for the production) lasted eight days, and the apothecaries printed a broadsheet, *Le virtù et facoltà della theriaca di Andromaco Protomedico dell'imperatore Nerone*, explaining to patients how to use theriac (see Figure 5.5).[84]

The presence of political and religious authorities at the exhibit increased the solemnity of the ceremony and its importance to the city. Cardinal Gabriele Paleotti (1522–1597) inspected the ingredients with his secretary (*suffraganio*) and other religious officials. Bishop of Bologna until 1591 and a key figure at the Council of Trent, Paleotti was a humanist and intimately acquainted with the city's intellectual community.[85] Aldrovandi noted that Paleotti was knowledgeable about "these natural things" and knew "scientifically all the ingredients of theriac."[86] The next day Bolognese senator Camillo Paleotti (brother of the cardinal) visited the exhibit and conversed with Aldrovandi about each ingredient, "in the presence of... more than sixty people."[87]

Soon after the construction of the Archiginnasio, the new palace of the University of Bologna, theriac productions moved to its courtyard. In 1650 author Antonio Masini wrote:

> When the abovementioned apothecaries want to make theriac, they do it with great solemnity and magnificence in the Public Studio, and there everybody can see it, with apparatus, and in beautiful order they exhibit all the ingredients they use. Each is inspected and approved by the physicians of the Medical College, and there is no other place where there is so much diligence and mastery in doing such theriac. For this reason, this is the finest and most perfect [theriac] of any city. The

apothecaries started to make theriac in this way in 1550, while before they made it in their apothecary shops with the intervention of physicians. At present they make about 500 pounds, which after a period of rest is distributed among the apothecaries.[88]

Masini's proposed initial date of 1550 should be considered only approximate, as the construction of the Archiginnasio was not completed until 1563. In fact, public productions of theriac in Bologna probably began only after 1574.[89] During the eighteenth century, the city held ceremonies every three years.

Making theriac in the courtyard of the Archiginnasio underscored the fact that "true theriac" belonged to the University and the Collegio Medico. Flanking the famous anatomical dissections and the professors' disputes all in the same building, the public making of theriac with the exhibit of materia medica demonstrated the reliability of the Collegio Medico's control over the city's medical life.[90] Bolognese physicians hosted apothecaries in their courtyard, and the two professional groups made theriac for the city (Figure 4.5). This contrasted with Venice, where apothecaries made theriac in front of their shops and physicians traveled to inspect the ingredients. Insofar as locations delineated geographies of power, in Bologna physicians owned theriac, and in Venice apothecaries did.

Like public dissections and natural collections, theriac ceremonies evolved in response to the growing appetite for new natural knowledge. Holding a production of theriac was a source of scientific pride, and not only in Bologna. In 1637 apothecary Giovan Domenico Cardullo presented the first such production in Messina to elevate the status of the local university. The presence of physician Pietro Castelli (1570–1662) from Rome spurred an upswing in local medical studies, with both an anatomical dissection and the making of a "true theriac" occurring concomitantly.[91] Like dissections, theriac ceremonies were medical rituals, except reassuring, festive, and generative rather than gruesome and destructive. Vipers never actually appeared; their flesh was prepared in advance in little dry discs, *trocisci*. In their dissecting of the human body during anatomical ceremonies, physicians were disaggregating nature. Meanwhile, the display of over sixty ingredients reduced the natural world, an infinite

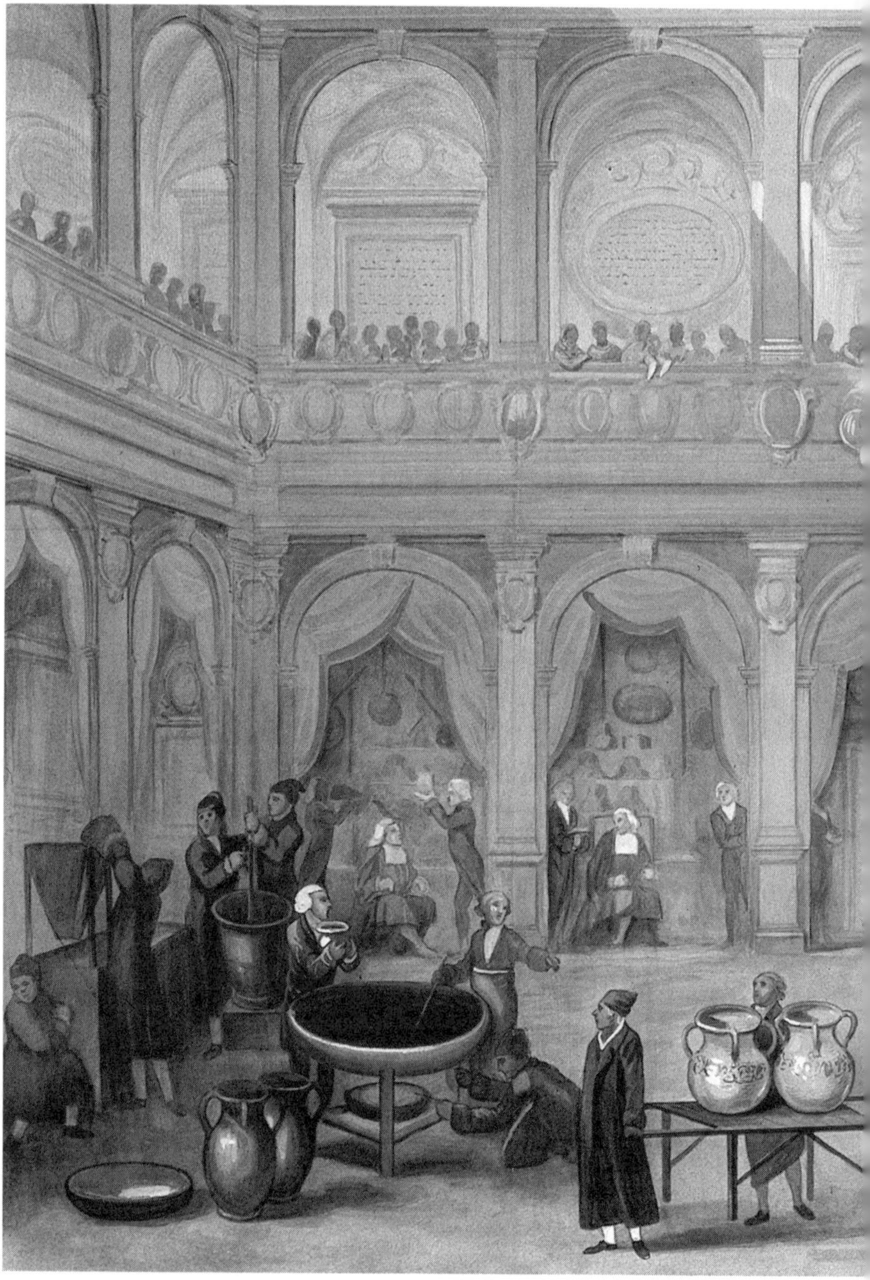

Fig. 4.5. Eighteenth-century manufacture of theriac in Bologna. Possibly the most detailed depiction of a theriac production, this gouache drawing by Aleardo Terzi, after an 1818 watercolor by Domenico Ramponi, shows the courtyard of the Archiginnasio transformed into an apothecary workshop. Some apothecaries and laborers sift, grind, and melt gums in cauldrons over braziers and bains-marie, while others mix and transport ingredients. On

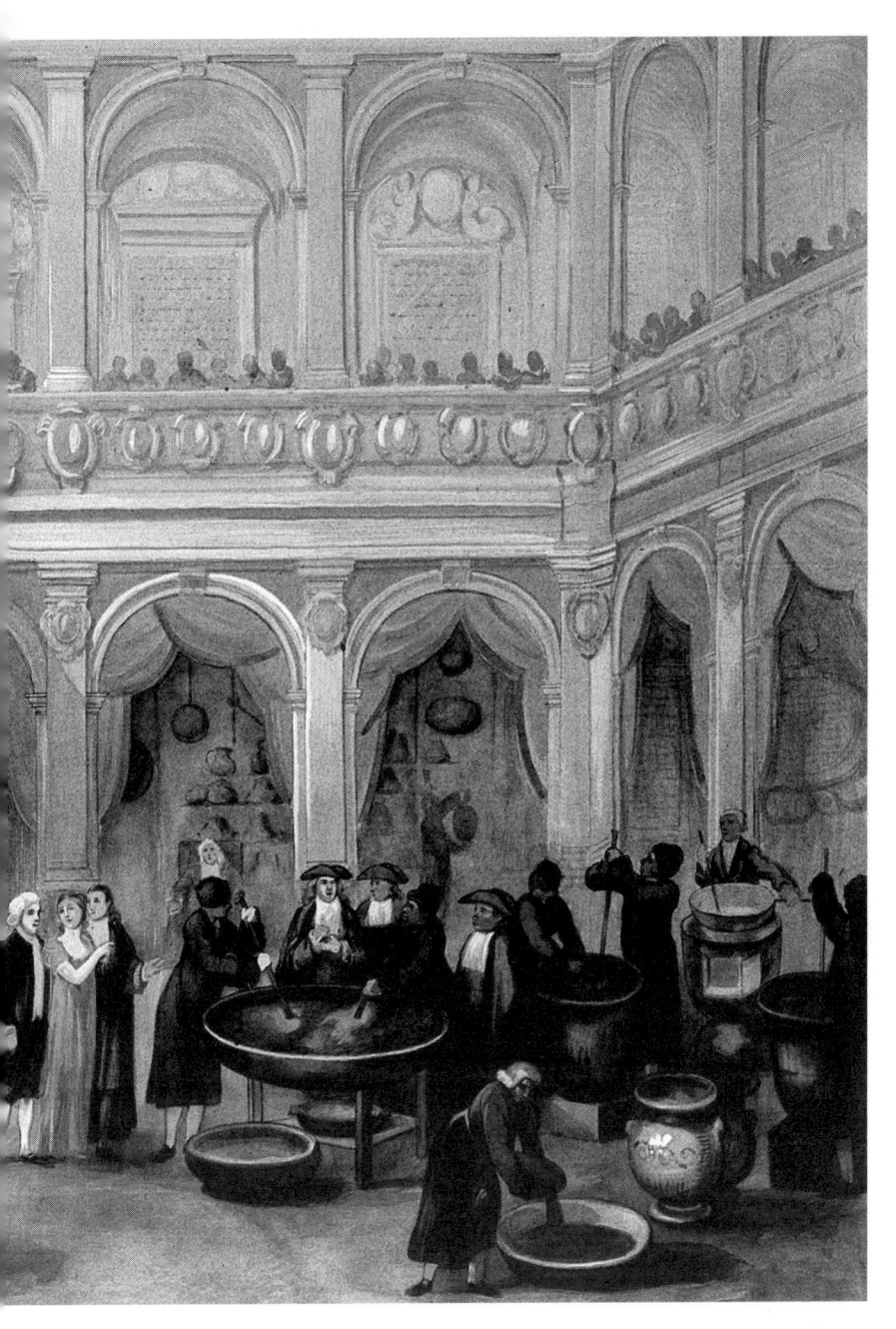

A PUBLIC HEALTH MEASURE AGAINST POISON AND PLAGUE 137

the left, in the background, physicians control the proceedings, and numerous utensils hang from the walls beneath the arcades. From the balcony the public could admire and observe the event. At the center of the scene, two men and a woman comment on the process.

Wellcome Collection (44599i).

source of venoms, diseases, and other mortal dangers, to agreeable and colorful specimens. Then, apothecaries making theriac would reaggregate the natural world in the form of a powerful antidote. When describing his 1612 exhibit at the hospital of Santa Maria della Morte in Bologna, apothecary Francesco Sartorio insisted on the "orderly manner" and reassuring display of nature: "The hospital was decorated with common ornaments, but in the men's infirmary in the middle of that stable were the ingredients, placed in an orderly manner over tables, on embroidered cloth as flowers in a delightful meadow, or stars in a delightful sky."[92] Similar to a natural history collection or museum of *naturalia*, theriac's exhibits conveyed a sense of harmony, beauty, and prosperity. Collectors of *naturalia* were proud of the "true theriac" ingredients displayed in their collections, which attracted a public of specialists and curious onlookers alike. Like a collection, these displays improved public perception of nature as something manageable, knowable, and beneficial to health.

Vicenza and Mantua: For the "Benefit and Ornament" of the City
The festive and public character of theriac productions might have been combined with explicit political meanings. In Mantua and Vicenza, the moving of apothecary shops to the central square transformed productions of theriac into civic festivities celebrating the prestige of the urban community and its rulers. In the sixteenth century, Mantua was a lively, intellectual city, bursting with natural collections, experimental gardens, and publishing houses. The Gonzagas, Dukes of Mantua, sponsored and favored naturalists, physicians such as Marcello Donati (1538–1602), alchemists, and learned apothecaries such as Filippo Costa and Antonio Bertioli. Mantuan apothecary shops were especially active places.[93] In 1594 the Bertioli brothers, apothecaries of the Gonzagas, produced "true theriac" in the square of the Duomo and the Ducal Palace, keeping the exhibit up for three days and nights.[94] Making "true theriac" in the main square of the city signaled both the scientific vitality of the Gonzagas and the availability of powerful antidotes in their dominions.

Through theriac, pharmacy became a way to make one's city and region more prestigious. A few years before the first production in Mantua, the first composition of theriac was made in Vicenza in 1586. The apparatus was put up "in public, at one end of the square [*à capo della piazza*]," and for ten days was accompanied by "music of voices, wind instruments, drums, trumpets, and fireworks."⁹⁵ The event was attended by the city's leaders and other important citizens, whose presence lent unanimous support to the apothecary Vendramino Menegacci. In 1586 the city was revamping its urban landscape by rebuilding the Palazzo della Ragione, a central edifice designed by architect Palladio and home to Vicenza's city magistrates. It would become Vicenza's pride and symbol.

Menegacci staged the production in an elaborate and costly temporary structure in front of the Palazzo della Ragione as it was being renovated. He declaimed for the onlookers, had a pamphlet published to celebrate the event, and presented the production as "benefit and ornament" to the city. Although Vicenza had the makings of a great city—illustrious citizens, good government, natural and cultural richness—Menegacci reminded his distinguished audience that the city lacked its own theriac. He was now providing Vicenza with an excellent theriac, which would bring the city both prestige and safety. This promise of security and esteem was echoed by an apothecary at the other end of the peninsula, Domenico Cardullo, who stated that producing theriac made "for the benefit of the people and the exaltation of Messina."⁹⁶ By remaking theriac after a long absence, both Menegacci and Cardullo were conspiring to enhance both their own prestige and that of their homeland. By taking over the main square, the heart of the religious, political, and economic life of these urban centers, theriac ceremonies elevated a city's reputation among its neighbors, and celebrated the farsightedness of its dukes or administrators and the skills of its physicians and apothecaries.

Theriac *Celebrations:* Pamphlets in Praise of the Apothecary

As we have seen, the making of Theriaca magna was a demanding enterprise that only a few apothecaries could afford, as it required a relatively high fixed capital cost for an artisan. In Bologna, members of the apothecary guild joined forces to take on the task. In 1762 the guild took a bill of exchange of 2,000 lire at 15 percent interest, to be paid back in ten years with the profits from sales.⁹⁷ In 1786, Venetian apothecary Giovan Battista Varè invested 13,037 lire, about the same as the total revenues from cheese exports of the entire province of Brescia.⁹⁸ In other cities, few apothecaries were able to make ceremonial productions of Theriaca magna and only a handful of times. For example, over the course of his thirty-year career, seventeenth-century apothecary Giuseppe Candrini from Modena organized only three public productions. Apparently he was familiar with how much other apothecaries were spending: "With Lombard splendidness, [a Milanese apothecary] spent 2,000 scudi for one theriac apparatus."[99]

One of the expenses of the theriac ceremony was the *celebrations*—pamphlets that outlined the remedy's composition and expounded on the significance of the event itself.[100] In Italy the "festival book" served as the blueprint for *celebrations*. Emerging as a recognizable genre in the 1520s, festival books described upcoming festivities, such as marriages, pageants, and processions, and constituted an expanding sector of publishing in the sixteenth and seventeenth centuries. Festival books exalted both the event and those who performed it to impress other courts. They were most elaborate when rulers most needed to affirm their rule.[101] And just as rulers leveraged festival books to improve their image, so apothecaries used *celebrations* to impress competitors and potential customers. In these pamphlets, apothecaries made explicit their ties with local aristocrats, state officials, and erudite physicians, and recorded their accomplishments for posterity. Like festival books, theriac *celebrations* became a tradition lasting until the late 1790s, not only in Italy but also Germany, Spain, France, Poland, and the Netherlands. To the best of my knowledge, the earliest example of a *celebration* still in existence was published in Reggio Emilia in 1578. The earliest surviving example from France was published in 1614 by Laurens Catelan, a prominent apothecary from Lyon. The earliest from the German-Polish region was published in 1630.[102]

While *celebrations* varied in content, Menegacci's *La theriaca e il mithridato,* published in Vicenza in 1587, is arguably the quintessence of this kind of apothecary print. The pamphlet had seven sections: dedications; a description of the event; poems composed for the occasion; Andromachus's poem-recipe both in Latin and translated into Italian; a woodcut of the apparatus; a list of the ingredients used in the production (*formula*); and certification pieces, such as *fedi* from other physicians approving individual ingredients or endorsements from the local college of physicians, sometimes called *privilegium* (although they were neither patents nor privileges).[103] Most theriac *celebrations* had only two or three sections, not the seven sections in Menegacci's.

With his theriac ceremony and accompanying pamphlet, the apothecary demonstrated his authority in the profession and his standing in the city. Some *celebrations'* frontispieces even featured the important citizens who participated in the ceremony, such as that of the pamphlet for a theriac made in Cesena in 1641, whose production was attended by the governor, the conservators, the entire college of physicians, "and foreign and local apothecaries."[104] Also displayed in the apparatus and described in the pamphlets were the coats of arms of the aristocrats and physicians of the medical college sponsoring the production. Especially hyperbolic was the apparatus organized by Giuseppe Candrini in Modena in 1677, which included no less than the coats of arms of the Este Dukes of Modena, the Protomedico, the prior of the medical college, and four local physicians.[105] These were visual stamps of approval from the medical and political hierarchies.

Theriac *celebrations* varied in use as well as content. Some were published as a memento of the magnificent production, and therefore included a description of the apparatus. In this case apothecaries printed invitations announcing the time and place of the ceremony, then published the *celebration* only after several months. Other *celebrations*, particularly in northern Europe, were published before the production as a means of advertising the event, mostly in the form of broadsheets. Hercolano Scalcina, a minor apothecary from Verona, left a rare description of his pamphlet, now lost, which he used as an invitation: "To promote the event, and to make it so the exhibition gained scrutiny from many, I printed several texts on this subject, enticing and inviting those who are fond of this matter to come and see the ingredients. And these texts were sent to different cities near and far, and many came to our satisfaction . . . gentlemen from Germany, Padua, Brescia, Vicenza, and Venice, and numerous other places."[106] Foreigners' appreciation of theriac productions, a common motif in *celebrations,* was further proof of the prestige these ceremonies brought to both the apothecary and the city. Demonstrating these international connections bolstered local status. As with festival books, when used in this way *celebrations* became part of the event itself, adding solemnity to productions.

As one would expect for a culture in which orality was still the primary means of communication, scholars and poets penned poems, couplets, and epigrams for theriac ceremonies as they did for other performative events such as marriages, deaths, births, and dignitaries' visits to the city. These verses were also printed as handbills or small pamphlets, such as *Corona d'applausi poetici in occasione di esporsi al pubblico la preparazione della triaca* (Crown of poetic applause on the occasion of publicly presenting the preparation of theriac), produced for a 1748 production held at the convent of the Santissima Nunziata in Florence, whose verses extolled both the theriac and the apothecary.[107] At least in one case the apothecary's first apprentice (*primo giovane*) seized the occasion to make himself known, having a poem composed at his own expense for a local notable: "hendecasyllables dedicated to the illustrious and most revered Lord Monsignor D. Alessio Falconieri, by Elia Mattia, the first youth in said Apothecary at the Queen's."[108]

Overloaded with classical knowledge and lacking humor (at least intended humor), these poems invariably pertained to a high linguistic register, their style directed to a select audience:

Spread thy immense evils from deep down below
Vase, full and overflown with woe
And as much poison thou have in you, field
Frozen Pontus, onto us miserable mortals.[109]

Convoluted phrases and stuffy puns often included the name of the apothecary—"the egregious art of a supreme Laurel" for an apothecary called Lauro—or compared the apothecary to Apollo: "I admire in you the virtues that others honor in the Physician of Delos."[110] In one instance two broadsheets containing verses were published to celebrate the same production, one in the vernacular and one in Latin, possibly signaling their markedly different audiences.[111] Theriac *celebrations* almost always included Latin, Greek, and vernacular versions of Andromachus's poem-recipe for Theriaca magna and Damocrates's recipe for mithridate. As the primary sources of the recipes, they perpetuated the myth of theriac as an imperial remedy. Consonant with the official solemnity of theriac, irony, satire, and jokes were banned from *celebrations*.

Narrative descriptions of the festivities became more frequent and detailed in the seventeenth century, sometimes accompanied by woodcuts. These images varied: some were symbolic, portraying an assortment of medical figures, ingredients, and decorations; others faithfully represented the exhibit of the ingredients. Menegacci's woodcut depicted a corner of

Vicenza's public square, although it curiously portrayed neither apothecary tools nor theriac ingredients.[112]

Unfortunately one of the most exhaustive accounts of a theriac apparatus was not accompanied by images. For his "theriacal theater" held in Parma in 1632, apothecary Simon Bocchi decorated the exhibit with, among other things, armors, columns, a carriage, a fake door, banners with writings, his coat of arms, a depiction of King Mithradates smashing a skull, a huge painting of a battle, a ship made of cotton with fake waves, a hydra mounted by a drake, "fake and monstrous animals" (possibly embalmed), and the skeletons of a woman and an ostrich. Each ingredient was accompanied by a sign noting its name and qualities (taken from Dioscorides), and decorated with snakes and "colorful flowers," with the top of the leafy branches colored silver.[113]

Every decorative element of a theriac apparatus was imbued with symbolism. The description of Giuseppe Candrini's exhibit held in Modena explained the meaning behind each decoration. The green of the background represented "the hope of the apothecary that his work would be appreciated."[114] The statue of Prudence holding a snake was a "sign of health, for it is a healthy animal, more than all those that crawl."[115] Even the grandiosity of the apparatus itself constituted a visual expression of theriac's magnificence, and the values underlying its production.

In their final pages, theriac *celebrations* featured "technical" pieces in the form of letters, *fedi*, and a list of substitutes. Menegacci included the latter for his 1586 production, along with the notarized approval issued by the Vicenza college of physicians.[116] These pieces certified the quality of the ingredients, as affirmed by local medical authorities or famous scholars from other cities. They also made explicit the apothecary's learned network. Apothecary Francesco Sartorio published a letter by Venetian apothecary Pompeo Sprechi, who testified (*Si fa fede*) to the quality of the "foreign" ingredients he provided for Sartorio.[117] In early modern Italy, *fede* was a term used to identify generic certifications. While typically issued by official authorities such as notaries or health boards, a *fede* could be issued simply by a neighbor, for example, to certify that a person was indeed whom they said they were.[118] Of course, the social value of the *fede* depended on the credibility of the issuing party.[119] Only an approved theriac might bring to the apothecary the prestige he sought. In the end, theriac *celebrations* reflected two hopes: the apothecary's hope to boost his prestige, and everyone else's hope that theriac might have some power to protect humanity from poisonous threats.

In this chapter I have argued that the plague of 1575–1577 was a watershed in the history of theriac in three ways. First, it increased theriac's use as a public health measure against the plague. Physicians and rulers promoted its production as a means to effectively oppose the plague, provided it was "true theriac." Second, the plague acted as a propellant for transforming theriac-making productions into urban medical rituals. Finally, the plague fueled decades-long etiological debates among physicians on the appropriateness of theriac as a treatment.

Theriac ceremonies came about primarily as a response to more stringent medical regulations and a competitive pharmaceutical market. Public officials had been monitoring theriac productions since the Middle Ages, but early modern productions spectacularized the approval of medical authorities. The first act of each ceremony was the exhibition of the ingredients for their certification by physicians. The making of theriac was a visual reaffirmation of the social and medical hierarchies, as well as a display of medical authority and the prestige of the apothecary. In times of plague, publicly creating a powerful antidote in a society obsessed with the fear of poison reinforced common beliefs and social cohesion.

The plague of 1630 presented physicians with another crisis in which to test theriac's effectiveness, and the drug was commonly used in lazarettos. Afterwards, doubts about theriac resurfaced in medical debates, but by then theriac had captured the general imagination.

CHAPTER 5

Theriaca Magna on the Marketplace

*I*N THE sixteenth century the commercialization of medicines grew along with the general proliferation of material goods and the rise of an international economy. Apothecaries invested more in their shops, which became distinctive for their spatial arrangements, elegantly furnished as they were with bespoke shelves of eye-catching jars, flasks, and boxes.[1] Bursting with new drugs arriving from other continents, chemical novelties, beauty products, and natural curiosities—including hanging alligators—apothecary shops became places of encounter to gossip, exchange international news, discuss natural knowledge, and whisper heterodox religious ideas.[2] In the public squares, empirics and charlatans who could not access guilds and medical colleges developed aggressive and innovative marketing techniques to sell their wares, including cheap prints and spectacular performances with snakes, fire, and poisons.[3] Nuns and friars increased their presence in the business of health by taking advantage of their religious sway and social networks, as well as by leveraging untapped market niches.[4] The ubiquitous demand from patients for medical knowledge, whether in the form of plague tracts, books of secrets, or guides to healthy living, was sustained for centuries.[5] In such a vibrant setting, *Theriaca magna Andromachi*—which we can consider the name of certified "true theriac"—was a relative newcomer.

In this chapter I show that in the seventeenth century "true theriac" and mithridate changed in terms of cost, availability, and diffusion on the pharmaceutical marketplace. A number of concurring factors discussed in previous chapters created the conditions for theriac's new popularity. What I called the "reinvention" of theriac inflated hopes for a decisive medicine as powerful as Galen's. In the wake of "true theriac," ruling and medical authorities promoted Theriaca magna as the official pharmaceutical response to anxieties arising from the threat of epidemics, uncontrolled medicaments, and poisons of all kinds. As entrepreneurs sensitive to changing trends, apothecaries took advantage of the situation. By staging regulated public ceremonial productions, they attracted patients' attention and confidence. Once it was fashionable again for the elites, theriac also became desirable to the lower classes. Exploiting the word and concept of *theriac*, apothecaries and other sellers of medicaments increasingly offered both forgeries and by-products, such as theriacal salt and theriacal water. Exuberant, polyphonic, and surprising, the concept of theriac was in tune with the dominant Baroque taste.

Alongside theriac ceremonies, apothecary publications played a fundamental part in building theriac's commercial growth. By the mid-seventeenth century, publications related to theriac ranged from legal handbills to promotional, celebratory, and informative pamphlets addressing diverse audiences and performing different functions. Apothecary prints achieved many ends at once: they enhanced apothecaries' prestige and authority, promoted their businesses, and informed patients. Through single-page leaflets called *virtues*, wherein they synthetized Galenic texts on theriac, apothecaries acted as brokers between patients and learned medical knowledge. Theriac was transformed once again, this time from an exquisitely elite drug into a drug accessible to patients at large.

In the first section of this chapter I show that "true theriac" was still a medicine for the wealthy at the end of the sixteenth century. Using quantitative as well as qualitative data, in the second section I demonstrate the growth of production of certified theriac in early seventeenth-century Venice. In the third section I challenge the long-held assumption that theriac was expensive at all times and in all places. Contrary to what is commonly believed, I argue that, in Italy, not just the wealthy but a wide range of patients—professionals, artisans, salaried workers—could afford a few doses of Theriaca magna, not to mention the plethora of theriac-related products, discussed in the fourth section. In the last section I examine the marketing strategies apothecaries developed, focusing on the prints and booklets that accompanied theriac. Apothecaries' communication strategies lay at the foundation of theriac's commercial success.

For the Aristocrats and the Wealthy: Theriac Consumption at the End of the Sixteenth Century

Until the end of the sixteenth century, despite the growing visibility of theriac and mithridate in urban contexts, patients' use of these remedies was limited. "True theriac" was exclusive to the elites. Its expense and limited production restricted both the product's availability and who could afford it. Physicians seldom prescribed theriac. In 1595 a Venetian physician lamented, "I cannot tolerate that [theriac] is so rarely used in Italy, and especially by some physicians of this city."[6] "Who would believe [that theriac] had also the power / to supersede the contagious pestilence / and that taken when the sky whitens / hinders corrupt airs," echoed an apothecary, acknowledging the skepticism of some.[7] A treatise on commonly prescribed medicaments published in 1576 and 1586, *Discorsi sopra le compositioni de gli antidoti & medicamenti, che più si costumano di dar per bocca*, did not mention theriac at all.[8] Yet the author, the Mantuan apothecary Filippo Costa, was a friend of Imperato and corresponded with Aldrovandi. He knew Maranta's book on theriac, and was himself a collector of *naturalia*.[9] Costa's *Discorsi* recorded that physicians most commonly prescribed preserves, syrups, and linctures (thick sugary syrups, dried to be licked and thus ingested slowly). The silence on theriac in Costa's work suggests that few patients used it regularly. Only occasionally would physicians prescribe theriac to their patients. In 1597 Epifanio Ferdinando (1569–1638), a physician active in Mesagne, a small town in Puglie, prescribed lemon juice with a little bit (*tantilla*) of theriac to a patient with a "deadly fever," but overall theriac featured only a handful of times in his lengthy collection of *observationes*.[10]

Similarly, shop inventories show that apothecaries did not necessarily keep theriac in stock, even in plague years. Between 1572 and 1587, for example, inventories of the apothecary of the Santo Spirito Hospital, one of Rome's most important medical institutions, showed no sign of theriac.[11] In Florence, apothecary al Giglio's inventory has no entries for theriac in 1567 and just one in 1568.[12] In the 1580s one could find only small quantities of "true theriac" in many Italian cities, including Bologna, Verona, Ferrara, Florence, Mantua, Venice, Padua, and Parma. In these cities, according to Aldrovandi, theriac "was made perfectly following my advice, so the aristocrats and the wealthy [*nobili et ricchi*] can find it and save it in their houses, and should the need of it arise they can have it ready."[13] Medical controversies over theriac, such as those described in Chapter 4, likely bolstered its popularity among both physicians and wealthy patients. Meanwhile, "true theriac" was not yet fashionable among or indeed accessible to patients with fewer means—but this was to change toward the beginning of the seventeenth century.

Increased Production of Theriac and Mithridate

Knowledge of how the early modern pharmaceutical market changed over time has been growing, but we still lack quantitative information on trends in prices, types of drug, and imports and exports, and we have little understanding of regional differences.[14] For example, with the exception of England we know little about how the sale of exotic drugs evolved or compared to those of local drugs. Patrick Wallis has shown that the English consumption of exotic drugs boomed in the 1610s and 1620s and gradually increased into the eighteenth century. The English and British markets for medicines are two of the most studied, but they appear quite different from continental markets.[15] Knowledge of the evolution of the pharmaceutical market would yield important insights into medical practice, as well as into the relationship between empires, commerce, and medicine.

Given its status and popularity, Theriaca magna can contribute to our understanding of how drugs—new and old, local and foreign—competed in the early modern marketplace. Using quantitative data from Venice, in this section I demonstrate that theriac production increased significantly beginning in the early seventeenth century. As we saw in the previous section, "true theriac" was not yet competitive in the late sixteenth century, but its prestige and overwhelming presence in medical literature might have led to an overestimate of its actual availability. Throughout this period, however, vendible theriac, often still certified by regulating bodies, remained available and habitually sold and exported. As "true theriac" acquired credibility, in several cities certified theriac and "true theriac" began to coincide.

In Venice the production of theriac expanded alongside the growth of the apothecary college. When the college was formed in 1565, the year of the first theriac-making ceremony, there were seventy-one apothecaries in Venice. By 1617 there were over one hundred.[16] According to the statute, "any" apothecary could compound theriac and mithridate if he obtained a license from the Giustizia Vecchia and the prior approval of the medical college.[17] Because the permission had to be renewed for each production, it should be interpreted more as an authorization than a license. Venetian records show that, from 1601, the quantity of legally manufactured theriac and mithridate increased considerably. Figure 5.1 shows apothecaries' output, as documented in both a copy of the *Book of Theriacs* and the apothecary college records (*Mariegola*).[18] These two sources confirm the number of producers of theriac and the quantities of compound manufactured by each. Production of theriac and mithridate more than doubled between 1596 and 1601, and production over these five years matched that of the last fifteen. Production doubled again over the ensuing three years, for a total of about 3,580 Venetian pounds. After 1605 the output averaged 1,500 Venetian pounds a year (453 kilograms). Every two years between 1606 and 1618, Venetian apothecaries produced as much certified theriac as they had in the fifteen years between 1580 and 1595.

In 1611 the total Venetian production of theriac was worth 11,868 ducats, about the cost of building a light galley.[19] This was not a sizable production when compared to the output of other Venetian artisanal trades, such as glassmaking. However, at this time only sixteen apothecaries were producing theriac officially, so this production was a considerable source of revenue for them.[20] Furthermore, the Venetian state considered theriac an important business. Exports of theriac brought substantial revenues to state coffers and generated satellite commercial activities.[21]

A look at foreign markets sheds light on the international trade of Venetian theriac. Better studied than other regions, England shows that

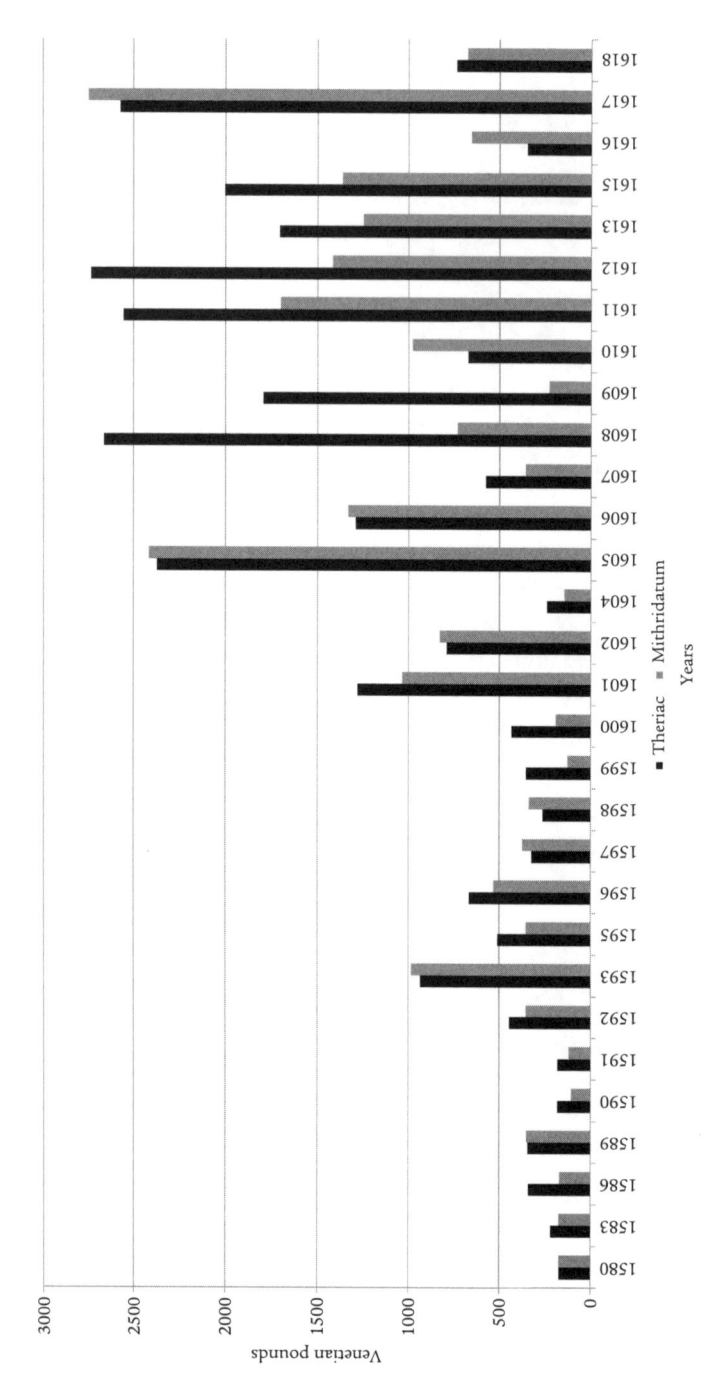

Fig. 5.1. Production of theriac and mithridate in Venice (1580–1617) in Venetian pounds. (1 Venetian pound = 302,229 grams.) (*Data sources:* ASV, Giustizia Vecchia, 211; MCV, Mariegola 209, 145r–168v.)

demand and production of theriac resisted the arrival of exotica. Between 1567 and 1610, theriac was the most imported foreign drug in England, and the only compounded medicinal—all others were simples.²² Until 1600 most theriac exported to England traveled through Antwerp, arriving under the name *treacle* or *treacle of Genoa*. The label *treacle of Venice* first appeared in English port books in 1600; after that time England imported almost no other form of theriac. *Treacle of Venice* came directly from Venice or Leghorn, or through nonspecified "streights"—Gibraltar—which usually meant it traveled via French ports.²³ Once in England, small quantities of theriac (6–15 pounds) were reexported to North America (New York, Virginia, and Maryland, as well as Barbados and Antigua), while more significant quantities were reexported to the Netherlands.²⁴

In England after 1610, imports of exotica (drugs imported from other continents) overtook theriac imports. The weight of theriac imported annually between 1600 and 1774 ranges from zero to 2,000 pounds, substantially less than the weight of exotic drugs reaching England.²⁵ This unevenness could be explained at least in part by smuggling, which was responsible for a great proportion of English commerce, most notably for "luxuries for consumption at home." It is therefore safe to assume that a portion of theriac imports entered this way, especially in the years when quantities recorded in the books were extremely low or null.²⁶

A low level of imports, even when accounting for undocumented smuggled imports, does not necessarily imply that English demand for theriac waned completely. Indeed, its prestige in England remained consistent and stimulated local production. In 1585, as part of the European movement of reforming materia medica, and possibly influenced by Italian theriac-making ceremonies, English apothecaries renovated their own production of mithridate. They admitted that "in this our time all things are called to a better examination" and produced their own reinvention of mithridate, claiming that "Mithridatium made in England is rather to [be] chosen, than that which is brought from Venice and other countryes beyond the Sea."²⁷ With support from their local college of physicians, London apothecaries produced a version of theriac called *Theriacae Londini* (London treacle).²⁸ In the following years Londoners made "great use of Methridatt Theriacha in this time of infection during the plague of 1625."[29] English patients attended public productions, which resembled those held in Italy. In London in 1659, John Evelyn (1620–1706) recorded: "I went to see the several drougs for the confection of Treacle, Dioscordium and other electuaries, which an ingenious Apothicarie had not onely prepared and rang'd on a large and very long table, but cover'd every ingredient with a sheet of paper, on which was very lively painted the thing in miniature, well to the life, were it plant, flower, animal, or other exotic drug."[30] Like elsewhere across Europe, apothecaries in England performed the medical ritual of public productions to reassure their customers of the quality of their production, and patients enjoyed the show.

Production of English theriac gained further traction when John Woodall (1570–1643), the first surgeon general of the East India Company, ordered a ready-made powder of London treacle for the surgeons-at-sea chest, which surgeons at sea could mix with honey.[31] London treacle was sold alongside Venetian theriac, whose higher quality continued to lure English patients. Several times in the seventeenth century, Richard Lassels (1603?–1668) visited Italy, where he saw "where them [sic] make their famous Treacle."[32] Similarly in 1646, Evelyn would leave Venice only after having packed some theriac among other riches: "Having pack'd up my purchases of books, pictures, castes, treacle &c. (the making and extraordinary ceremonie whereof I had been curious to observe, for 'tis extremely pompous and worth seeing) I departed from Venice."[33] Alongside Venetian and London treacle, the English marketplace carried counterfeit theriacs arriving from the continent, such as from the Netherlands. In *The Surgions Mate: The First Compendium of Naval Medicine, Surgery, and Drug Therapy* (1617), Woodall's advice was to favor London treacle over "the mithridate we buy from beyond the sea, for it is by the Hollander so uncharitably sophisticated that a man may feare to take it in his neede." In the Netherlands, Woodall spoke to a peasant ("a Bore") who produced "Mithridate and Treakell" with only nine simples. The forger "had pewter boxes so artificially [made] as no man could discover them to be other [than] right Venice ones."[34] By the 1610s theriac—whether from Venice, London, or the Netherlands—was a sought-after drug in England, and readily taken to sea for export to other continents, as we shall see in Chapter 7.

A Drug for All Pockets

Most historians report that theriac was an expensive drug, but this contention is problematic. Theriac has a long history, and its price changed innumerable times. In the fifteenth century, for example, its price was relatively low, whereas in Italy in the last quarter of the sixteenth century "true theriac" was expensive or even priceless, because often it could be obtained only through social connections. Theriaca magna was also expensive in seventeenth-century Thorn and Danzig (Polish Prussia), when a drachm of local "true theriac" cost 4 silver groschen, a considerable sum for the average worker.[35] Theriac's affordability should be appraised on a local basis, as well as by considering whether it was certified Theriaca magna, "true theriac" made at court, or simply vendible (*vendereccia*). I argue that, from the beginning of the seventeenth century in Venice and Bologna, official *Theriaca magna Andromachi* and *Mithridatium Democratis* were affordable except to the poor. Even artisans and salaried workers (middle-income ranks) could afford a few doses of theriac in times of need, considering that a single dose for acute conditions or poisoning varied from a scruple (1–1.2 grams depending on the system) to a drachm (3–4 grams), to be taken once or a few times as required. I base this argument on three considerations: the official prices of theriac, the discounts apothecaries consistently offered to patients, and the comparison of theriac prices with those of other drugs.

Italian state authorities had been controlling the prices of most goods since the Middle Ages, but only started fixing prices for medicines—including theriac and mithridate—in the mid-sixteenth century. Prices for drugs were first published in 1558 in Rome, 1566 in Venice, and 1557 in Bologna.[36] Venetian authorities even set prices for charlatans' remedies.[37] Dedicated commissions featuring apothecaries and physicians conducted annual reviews of medicament prices, and apothecaries had to display official prices in their shops.[38] Thus, the official price of theriac reflected neither its costly production, nor consumer demand, nor specific events that might inflate its price, such as plague outbreaks.

Prices for medicine were set at the "most convenient adjustment between sellers and buyers."[39] When setting prices and wages, "government actions aimed at implementing the common good" following two ethical principles: *aequitas* (distributive justice), through which authorities sought to maintain a disproportion between social groups, as this was considered to align with the natural order of things; and *aequalitas* (commutative justice), which "implied an equivalence between what was given and what was received in return." Governments had different interpretations not only of these ethical norms but also of notions of common good.[40] Prices of medicines therefore varied both across the Italian peninsula and within each state. Every price list, called a *tassa* or *tariffa*, was calibrated to mitigate short-term price changes and according to what the local population could afford.[41] In 1689 the Papal States simultaneously set at least three official lists of prices. Tariffs of cities such as Rome and Bologna listed expensive and fashionable medications, the likes of which were not even available in poorer regions such as Marche and Romagna.[42] Local tariffs reflected local customs, general wealth, new trends, and consumers' sophistication.

In Bologna, authorities curbed theriac prices so they would not "weigh on the population."[43] When apothecaries asked to sell their theriac at 10 soldi per drachm in 1607, the Collegio Medico and Cardinal Legate decided that instead it should be sold at a mere 4 soldi and 16 denari per drachm, less than half the proposed price. Furthermore, to make sure theriac was available to as many patients as possible, they agreed it "should be dispensed so that the public will not suffer, and each will be given only a small quantity."[44] Authorities' preoccupation with the prices and distribution of theriac and mithridate reflected the official status these drugs enjoyed. Medical institutions and political authorities vouched for the drugs' efficacy, and ensured they were trustworthy, available, and reasonably affordable.

A comparison of wages and the price of theriac in Bologna and Venice suggests that Theriaca magna was accessible to middle-income ranks, such as craftsmen, merchants, small landowners, and even laborers. Unlike other medicines, the official price of theriac remained relatively stable throughout the early modern period. The official price in Venice of 6 soldi per drachm barely changed for the entire seventeenth century (Figure 5.2). Even when general prices increased dramatically during the plague years of 1628–1629, apparently this was not the case for theriac and mithridate.[45] A box of theriac containing 4–5 drachms of theriac might cost 24–30 soldi. In seventeenth-century Venice, apprentices in the glass in-

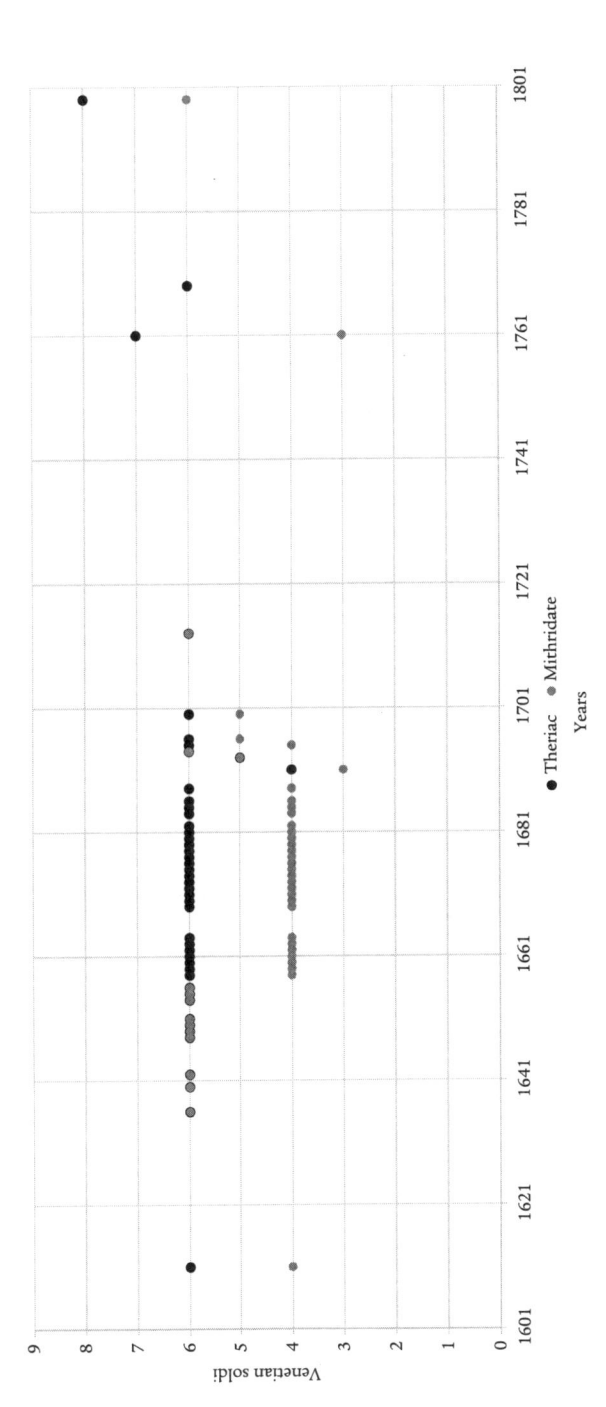

Fig. 5.2. Official prices of theriac and mithridate in Venice (1611–1799) in Venetian soldi per Venetian drachm.
(*Data source*: Archivi Storici Diocesani di Udine, Archivio dell'Ospedale S. Maria Della Misericordia, AOSMM, b. 1064 *Index pretia continens omnium rerum Medicinalium simplicium*, published in 1611, 1636, 1640, 1642, 1648-1651, 1654-1656, 1658-1664, 1669-1682, 1684-1686, 1688, 1691, 1693-1696, 1700, 1713, 1761, 1769, 1799.)

dustry earned 20–90 soldi per day, and masters 40–180 soldi per day.[46] Glassworkers were well paid compared to other waged workers: builders earned about 24 soldi per day before 1630.[47] Even laborers could just about afford a few doses of theriac in times of necessity, although they could not afford to use it regularly as a preventive.

In Bologna the price of theriac was less stable than in Venice (Figure 5.3). For example, within the space of a few months in 1584 it tripled from 2 to 6 soldi per drachm. This sudden and short-lived increase possibly reflected the stricter requirements for theriac ingredients as set by the new pharmacopoeia, first published in 1574. From 1587 until the mid-eighteenth century, the price of theriac in Bologna oscillated between 2 soldi and 6 denari and 4 soldi per drachm.[48] The rising prices of theriac and mithridate between 1613 and 1630 aligned with a general inflation in the region of Bologna and Modena following the famines of 1612–1622 and 1627–1630. During these years the price of wheat oscillated between

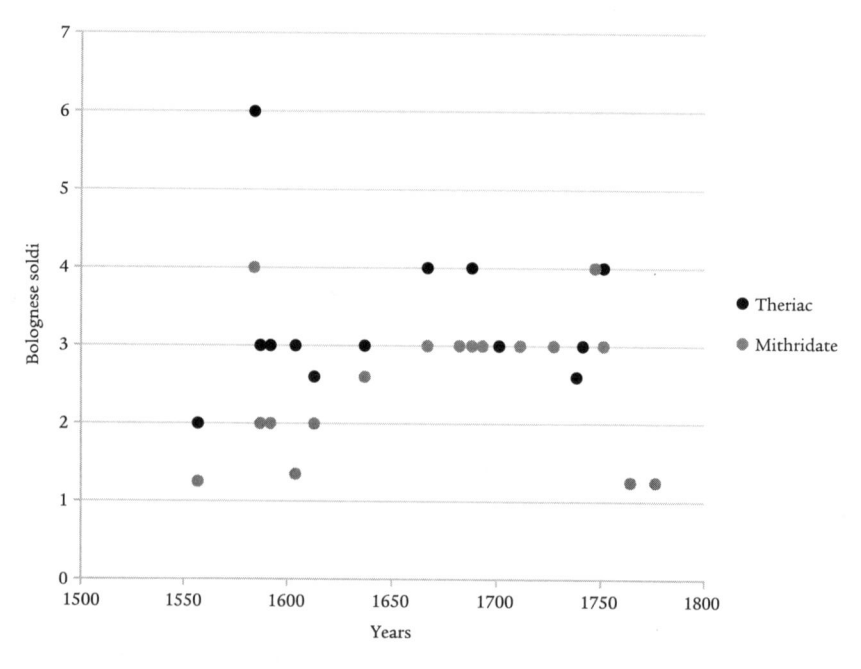

Fig. 5.3. Official prices of theriac and mithridate in Bologna (1557–1776) in Bolognese soldi per Bolognese drachm.

(*Data source: Tassa de Medicinali ultimamente stabilita dall'ecc. Collegio dei Medici e Honor. Compagnia degli Speziali,* published in 1557, 1584, 1587, 1592, 1604, 1613, 1637, 1667, 1682, 1688, 1693, 1711, 1727, 1738, 1741, 1747, 1751, 1764, 1776.)

5 and 15 soldi. In the next century, in Bologna in 1725 a generous 1-drachm dose of theriac (for an emergency) cost 3 soldi, equal to 36 denari, about the same price as 1 kilogram of bread (33.2 denari). According to Giovanni Vigo, between the late-sixteenth and late-eighteenth centuries, real wages of masons in Italy oscillated between the equivalent of 4 and 10 kg of bread per day.[49]

These calculations warrant cautious consideration, given the controversy surrounding the use of early modern wages to gauge levels of consumption. Some historians in the field denounce an irrational overdependence on highly imprecise datasets. The assessment of expenditure and consumption levels is constrained by three factors: a lack of consistent sources for constructing price series and household budgets, the exaggeration of the significance of wage labor, and neglect of the contribution of women and children to household income.[50] Relying solely on wages for such assessment most likely leads to significantly underestimating consumption levels. Consequently, theriac may have been even more affordable than previous calculations suggest. Low incomes did not necessarily equate to a stagnation in consumption, as households may have adapted their purchasing patterns and enhanced their living standards.[51] Furthermore, sufferers or their relatives might have been willing to go to great lengths to regain lost health, even resorting to taking loans at usurious rates, as noted by one early modern physician.[52]

Moreover, official prices across Italy were usually higher than actual prices. Patients rarely paid the official price, because apothecaries consistently offered them discounts. Officials in both Rome and Bologna inflated prices, and apothecaries offered discounts of one-quarter or even one-third off the official tariff.[53] This practice was so widespread that in 1690 the Venetian Senate ordered the Giustizia Vecchia to prohibit apothecaries from discounting their products by more than one-third, and to post the decree in a visible place in the shop.[54] Generally, households that bought medicines in large quantities paid less for drugs than individuals who bought single doses. Typically buyers paid apothecaries for their purchases every few years.[55] At the time of payment, prices were further discounted or might even change entirely. Fraud and mistakes were common, and from 1690 in Bologna every household's apothecary bill was inspected by an apothecary, the *tassatore*, appointed to manage tariffs.[56]

Another useful measure for assessing the relative expensiveness of theriac is comparing its price to that of other drugs. Theriac in the seventeenth century may not have been cheap, but it was more affordable than other fashionable drugs of the time. In 1637, when theriac in Bologna cost 3 soldi per drachm, it was more expensive to buy exotic drugs, such as those used against syphilis, including *China electa* (12 soldi per drachm), *Extractum guaiacum* (25 soldi per drachm), and *Extractum china* (40 soldi per drachm).[57] Levantine musk cost 160 times the price of theriac: 8 soldi for 1 grain. Theriac compared favorably not only to exotica but also to electuaries and pills made with precious stones. "Fragments of Hyacinthus prepared" cost twenty times more than theriac.[58] Apothecaries' drugs were usually more expensive than charlatans' remedies, but not necessarily. The prices reported for charlatans' wares in Venice (a range of 6–30 soldi) do not support the claim that apothecaries' drugs were always more expensive than charlatans'—although clearly apothecaries sold the most expensive drugs—nor does the fact that apothecaries rarely complained about charlatans' prices being competitive.[59] Theriac was priced more reasonably than some of the wares sold by charlatans. In 1769, for example, Fortunato Rossetti sold his antivenereal syrup at 10 soldi per teaspoon.[60]

Regardless of its price, throughout the seventeenth century theriac maintained both prestige and currency in Italian courts. In 1607, to alleviate a fever and swelling of her spleen, Eleonora de' Medici-Gonzaga took "various antidotes and external remedies, but especially mithridatium and fresh theriac, from which she gained considerable benefit."[61] Princes exchanged theriac with other courts and sent it as a "thank you" gift in the Republic of Letters. In 1677 Ferdinando Carlo Gonzaga Nevers (1652–1708), the last Duke of Mantua, sent to Florence a box of assorted remedies, including a theriacal water considered to be of "rare goodness."[62] In 1663 Leopoldo II de' Medici (1617–1675), an avid collector and counselor to his father the Grand Duke, sent theriac to astronomer Ismael Boulliau (1605–1694) in Paris to thank him for his help in finding a rare book.[63] Dukes and their peers continued experimenting with theriac. The Gonzagas of Mantua actively financed pharmaceutical research.[64] In 1621 Duke Ferdinando I Gonzaga sent a theriac he considered special to Florence. He specified that it was made with the utmost care with regard to vipers and opium and contained less honey than usual, and therefore it was necessary to take only half a dose. He also explained that it needed stirring only twice a year, because it "does not inflate or boil for the heat." This proved his technical knowledge of theriac, which often broke its glass container while fermenting.[65]

Since the Middle Ages it had been commonly known that not all theriacs were of the same quality. Together with its prestige, an important part of the appeal of Theriaca magna compared to other medicines was its accompanying legal certifications, which made it trustworthy. According to Aldrovandi, the poor especially suffered from illicit sales, as they "do not know" how to distinguish good from bad medicaments.[66] This concern reflected Aldrovandi's paternalistic attitude toward the lower classes. In fact, the poor were not the only ones who struggled to distinguish "true" from "fake" theriac. As we saw in Chapter 2, a 1605 Protomedicato trial to judge a suspicious theriac in Bologna ended without a verdict because the apothecaries and physicians were unable to reach a consensus on how to evaluate theriac once it was aged.[67]

Only purchasing from members of the apothecary guild supposedly guaranteed theriac's quality and reliability, which is why exports were recorded. In 1630, before sending to Nuremberg 20 lire of theriac "made in his shop and put in a vase with a tin band and his usual stamp of the ostrich," both apothecary Alberto Stecchini and the intermediary declared the sale in front of the officers at the Giustizia Vecchia.[68] However, it was no secret that even apothecaries might sell counterfeit theriacs made with much more honey than necessary or by substituting the most expensive ingredients with cheaper ones.[69] Despite the emphasis on trustworthiness, convenience also played a role in determining where customers obtained theriac. Bolognese tooth puller Scarnecchia petitioned the Protomedicato to be able to sell theriac: people in his profession commonly did so, he reasoned, and moreover patients in his shop would frequently ask for it.[70] Bolognese druggists were granted permission to sell theriac, but only in the eighteenth century.[71]

Apothecaries experienced frequent infringements upon their monopoly. In 1679 a peddler declared he did not know that by selling theriac in the countryside he was breaking the law. He promised he would stop, and pleaded with the Protomedicato to not revoke his license.[72] Similarly, in 1744 the Protomedicato interrogated a former soldier, Domenico Grandi of Modena, who admitted he had donated some "fake" theriac to friends upon their request. Admonished, he promised to neither sell nor donate any theriac again.[73] Itinerant healers either sold theriac to buyers who had too far to travel to buy theriac in an apothecary shop, or used their commercial abilities to compete with apothecaries. Take Giuseppe Pannei, who stamped jars with his own brand: "Jesus theriac" (*Triaca del Giesù*).[74] Most likely not a "true theriac," Jesus theriac would have been either made by the charlatan himself or bought from an apothecary or some other private producer.

Theriacs for All

Seventeenth-century patients had access not only to counterfeit theriac but also to many products derived from theriac or simply *labeled* "theriac": several variations of theriac, chemical theriac, and numerous by-products. Mithridate was always available. Some authors, including Maranta, favored it over theriac for a number of diseases.[75] Mithridate was less expensive than theriac because it contained mostly local plants and no vipers, although apothecaries still sold less of it than theriac. By the mid-seventeenth century, patients' choice of theriacal products increased. Antonio De Sgobbis's *Nuovo et universale theatro farmaceutico* (1667) proposed no fewer than seven different theriacs (besides two for Theriaca magna and one for mithridate): a "Common theriac from Aubsburg," London theriac, Poterio theriac, Augmented theriac (*Theriaca accresciuta*), and three alchemical theriacs by André Duchesne (1584–1640): Reformed and Blessed (*Benedetta*) theriac, and Celestial theriac (*Theriaca coelestis*).[76] De Sgobbis also added four recipes for theriacal waters (distillates of several ingredients, including theriac) and theriacal salt (also a chemical product including theriac), both of which were a popular alternative to theriac.[77] A theriacal essence to be taken in drops was considered "worth in all respect as Theriaca magna, but ... more efficient and handier."[78] Pharmaceutical operators took commercial advantage of the appeal carried by the label *theriac*, which increased throughout the seventeenth century.

To better position themselves in a crowded market, German and French apothecaries manufactured Celestial theriac, a chemical version of theriac, by introducing chemical procedures into the formulation of "true theriac." Celestial theriac was invented in 1608, when French physician and alchemist Joseph Du Chesne (ca. 1544–1609) added to Theriaca magna new ingredients—a few apothecary preparations and a good dose of opium essence—as outlined in his *La reformation des thériaques et antidotes opiatiques*.⁷⁹ This chemical theriac incorporated "the more substantive virtues" of Theriaca magna through *"ars spagyrica* or true chemistry." Such a procedure was supposed to separate good qualities (virtues) from "what is there of filthier and excess material." Rather than present his novel theriac as a new medicine, however, Du Chesne advertised it as a product of "the ancients," capitalizing on theriac's prestige.⁸⁰ Continuation of tradition granted efficacy and reliability, while his pharmaceutical innovation increased the product's appeal. Du Chesne assured readers that although in the eyes of novices Celestial theriac might appear to be a complex preparation, it "was nothing but a work for women, which means a work that a woman can do." But at the same time he contradicted himself by writing that only "true philosophers and sons of the art" would be able to follow the recipe for Celestial theriac—unless he meant that women were true philosophers.⁸¹

Apothecaries may have found the task a little daunting and the potential gains uncertain, as it was twenty-five years before anyone attempted a production of Celestial theriac. Frederic Greiff (fl. 1630), a daring apothecary from Tübingen, first made Du Chesne's Celestial theriac in 1634. Production was difficult, but it paid off: physicians and wealthy patients welcomed the novelty. Greiff produced Theriaca coelestis again in 1641 and 1652, changing the recipe and keeping it secret, with the complicity of the apothecaries of the house of Württemberg.⁸² The time span between each production testifies to its complexity and expense. By the 1660s apothecaries in other cities were producing their own chemical theriac: in Nuremberg (1664, 1675), Hanover (1668), Hanau (1670), Geneva (1674), Marburg (1674), Kassel (1676), Frankfurt (1680), and Giessen (1680). Theriaca coelestis was also made in Sweden and Denmark. Between 1641 and 1711 at least thirty-one productions of Theriaca coelestis, synchronous with Theriaca magna and mithridate, were celebrated in apothecaries' publications. To make these remedies, German apothecaries imported viper *troscisci* from Padua, which arrived with the decorated approval of Paduan physicians, as we saw in Chapter 2. These imports made theriac quite expensive in northern Europe. Celestial theriac entered the Strasbourg pharmacopoeia, and by 1760 cost sixty-two times more than the traditional Theriaca magna.⁸³

Not all could afford such expensive remedies. As poverty spread across Italy and Europe in the seventeenth century, practices of charity followed.[84] Besides more substantial interventions, physicians also conceived of medicaments explicitly for the needy, including new "theriacs for the poor." In 1654 Bolognese physician Ovidio Montalbani (1601–1671) published a booklet under the pseudonym Antonio Bumaldi on how to run the Opera de' Poveri Mendicanti, a charitable institution. Montalbani proposed the adoption of several cost-saving measures when treating the poor, including a "major theriac for the poor" made with ninety-five ingredients. The recipe followed the structure of Theriaca magna, but was made entirely with readily procured local herbs.[85] In 1726 Bolognese Protomedicato approved a "theriacal water" for the poor made with herbs and theriac.[86] Similarly, across Europe recipes for cheaper theriacs were appearing in compilations for those involved in charitable activities, such as country priests and urban aristocrats.[87]

Simpler antidotes called "theriacs for the poor" were not a seventeenth-century innovation. Since antiquity the word *theriac* had also been used as a generic noun meaning *antidote*. Galen allegedly used the locution "poor's theriac" for garlic, while other authors occasionally employed this same term for medicinal herbs such as rue.[88] Books of secrets exacerbated the confusion. Mario di Marino Galasso wrote both that "the theriac for the poor was the antidote of King Mithradates," and that "the theriac of the peasants" (*la tyriaca de' rustici*) was a glass of "untouched" child's urine with *eau de vie*.[89] The most popular theriac for the poor was *Theriaca diatessaron*, an old and respected compound made with four ingredients and attributed to Mesue.[90] The difference in price between Theriaca diatesseron and Theriaca magna was notable but not discouraging, especially when compared to other expensive medicines. In Bologna in 1711, *Theriaca diatessaron* cost 8 soldi per ounce, while Theriaca magna cost three times more, at 24 soldi per ounce.[91]

An episode reported by Johannes Faber (1574–1629) allows for a few reflections on the use of and customs surrounding theriac. Faber was a member of the Accademia dei Lincei, a physician at the hospital of Santo Spirito, and a professor at the University of Rome. He reported on a reaper who, while working in the field in 1603, was bitten on the hand by a viper. The reaper immediately sucked it out, only to become even more empoisoned. He took some orviétan with vinegar, as well as some "veal's bile"

(*bile vitellina*), which "the plebs generally carry with them and it is totally inefficient compared to theriac, but the populace uses it largely because it is sold at a cheaper price."[92] Orviétan, which contained theriac, was a popular alternative to Theriaca magna.[93] The reaper was brought to the hospital of Santo Spirito in bad condition, whereupon Faber forced him to "vomit his sins," then cured him by administering theriac both internally and externally, along with other medicaments. The next morning the man was healed.[94] This incident highlights just why peasants would carry antidotes, albeit cheap ones. Faber reported the episode "for the benefit of young physicians" to reaffirm the qualitative difference between theriac and cheaper antidotes. However, the incident also shows that even the poor who could not afford Theriaca magna might still sometimes benefit from it in hospital or through charity.

The outstanding success of theriac in the seventeenth century derived from the pull of "true theriac," as evidenced by the mushrooming of pseudo-theriacs, theriacal imitations, and by-products, and the availability of Theriaca magna in hospitals and apothecary shops, as well as at court. David Gentilcore has argued that charlatans contributed to the commodification of medicines by making cheaper versions of certain goods, which, depending on the context, oscillated between "populuxe goods" (imitations of costlier goods) and "semi-luxuries" (objects associated with values of civility, worth saving for).[95] For its peculiarity, sorting Theriaca magna into such categories is problematic. Theriac was at once a necessity, administered to the poor in public hospitals, a priceless luxury used at court, and a product whose price was strictly controlled so it would not "weigh on the population." Such vast diffusion was primarily contingent on its status as a state drug and the public productions of theriac, but the printed materials promoting theriac and forming part of its production ceremonies also played a key role, as explored in the next section.

Marketing the Virtues of Theriac

Theriaca magna boasted several advantages over other pharmaceutical products. With its millenary medical prestige and endorsement from the medical hierarchy, theriac was especially visible in urban contexts because of public ceremonies, and it came accompanied by a variety of printed materials. Theriaca magna was the only early modern medicament followed by such an extraordinary richness and diversity of prints, including recipes, visuals, certifications, accounts of productions, historical references, and information on dosage and ingredients. Compared to books of secrets, plague tracts, literature on healthy living, and the ubiquitous charlatans' handbills, apothecaries' materials on theriac were only a small percentage of nonscholarly medical publications. Yet of all printed materials dedicated specifically to medicines and their use, apothecaries' publications related to theriac constitute an especially consistent corpus.[96]

Apothecary publications on theriac were intended for local circulation. The quality of the publishing was mostly poor, and print runs were generally limited. These materials varied greatly in size, content, and purpose, and diverged in form as well, being pamphlets, broadsheets, leaflets, and paper objects such as cards. Although few survive today, at the time apothecary publications on theriac were much more numerous than scientific studies on theriac published in the same period, especially in the eighteenth century—but of course medical books on theriac were valued more highly and have therefore been better preserved. Furthermore, apothecary handbills or short pamphlets are often filed among archives' and libraries' miscellanea rather than individually catalogued. I found 140 publications on theriac by apothecaries—excluding paper objects and medical and botanical treatises—published between 1566 and 1799. By way of comparison, I identified three times more medical treatises on theriac published during this period, written primarily by physicians. The limited scope, use, and characteristics of apothecary publications related to theriac affected their conservation, and produced a selection that has impacted the material available to historians today. A similar pattern of conservation applies to exemplars within apothecary publications related to theriac, with high-quality pamphlets printed for special occasions remaining in a higher number than handbills. Thus, we can safely assume that the number of extant apothecary publications related to theriac does not mirror how many were actually circulated.

Chapter 2 discussed *formulas*, which certified the ingredients used in a specific production and were required by law. *Formulas* were bureaucratic vestiges of theriac productions. By contrast, Chapter 4 illustrated *celebrations*, pamphlets issued on the occasion of a specific production. With *celebrations*, learned apothecaries claimed authority and a position in the local medical and social hierarchies. Here I discuss a third kind of apothecary print related to theriac, *theriac virtues*. Directed to patients, *virtues* provided practical advice on how to use the antidote. Their content shows that, together with promoting theriac, apothecaries conveyed mostly standard Galenic knowledge; few apothecaries were genuine innovators. But exemplars from the eighteenth century suggest a gradual simplification of Galenic medicine and commercialization. In time, the content of *theriac virtues* came to resemble the *virtues* that accompanied charlatans' wares.

Virtues derive their name from the Latin *virtus,* meaning an "excellent quality" (for people), or "force" or "power" (for objects). The term had been widely used since the Middle Ages for the properties of simples and compounds, after Mesue, who refined Galen's concept of *dunamis*. Of Greek origin, the term *dunamis* named the power that made a drug act in a certain way.[97] In the early modern period, *virtue* was a word everybody understood. It was widely employed in the titles of learned medical treatises, such as Andreas Butner's *De theriaca et mitridato Graecorum: De usu et virtutibus veræ Theriacæ et Mithridati* (Venice, 1546), as well as in those of charlatans' handbills, such as *The Vertue and Operation of this Balsame* and *Virtues of the castor-bean preparation*.[98]

Theriac virtues came in two forms, long and short. The short were handbills, which were used to wrap containers of theriac, a practice also employed by charlatans for their wares.[99] Longer *virtues* came in the form of pamphlets. Apothecaries donated both long and short *virtues* to their customers. Apothecary De Sgobbis informed his readers: "In my shop it is custom to donate for free to buyers of theriac the description of its virtues printed with the most noteworthy peculiarities, so that anyone can comfortably use such fine antidote without setback."[100] *Virtues* therefore might have been especially useful to patients living where there were no doctors.[101] Moreover, Sabrina Minuzzi has shown that Venetian apothecaries in 1768 ascribed great importance to *virtues* because the practice of printing "recipes" to accompany remedies was a "very old and never-interrupted custom." Apothecaries even attributed the success of theriac over mithridate—which oddly was never accompanied by its own *virtues*—to the popularity of these printed materials.[102]

The content of the *virtues* derived mostly from Galen's *De theriaca ad Pisonem* and *De theriaca ad Pamphilianum*. One of the most widely circulated pamphlets on theriac's virtues was *Trattato delle mirabili virtù della theriaca,* first published in 1596. Poet and physician Orazio Guarguanti dedicated a short tripartite Latin treatise to Ludovico Taverna, Bishop of Lodi and Apostolic Nuncio in Venice, his patron and patient.[103] The treatise contained a discussion of the medical virtues of three remedies: eggs; the Michoacán root, imported from the Mexican region of the same name; and theriac. The part about theriac was translated into the vernacular and republished immediately. "This is the paraphrase of the virtues of theriac," declared the subtitle. Together with Galen's, Guarguanti's text served innumerable apothecaries as a source of inspiration (if not of plagiarism, as we would consider such a close emulation of a source today).

Guarguanti's connections in Venice were key to the popularization of the newly refashioned theriac. A student of Mercuriale in Padua, Guarguanti moved to Venice and joined the Collegio Medico. He was part of an intellectual circle that included health magistrate and historian Niccolò Doglioni (1548–1629), writer Moderata Fonte (1555–1592), musical publisher Giacomo Vincenti (d. 1619), and composer Giovanni Croce (1557–1609). In Venice this circle had a critical role in bringing theriac to the public attention. In 1595 Croce published *Triaca musicale*, a collection of musical pieces, in whose title *Triaca* referred to the variety of ingredients in theriac.[104] In 1596 Vincenti edited the second edition of Melich's *Avertimenti*, which included Guarguanti's treatise. The latter was republished with its own frontispiece at least eight times as the final part of Melich's pharmacopoeia.[105]

Guarguanti's pamphlet listed ailments following Galen and the traditional order, head to toe. According to Galen the antidote was to be taken against venoms (such as those of viper and rabid dog), but also as a preservative from any internal poison after three days of fasting. Theriac protected travelers during journeys across insalubrious areas and against the plague, and cured coughs old and new, as well as fevers, be they malignant, quartan, or pestilential. It cleared the head of fear and hypochondriac melancholy, dissolved migraines and vertigo, eradicated edema and vermin, and treated abdominal cramps. Theriac also helped the menses and to expel a dead fetus. Indeed, the listing of ailments cured or soothed by theriac appears endless.

With *virtues*, apothecaries communicated directly with patients. Handbills were always written in the vernacular. In the eighteenth century, apothecaries (or forgers) printed exemplars in English, German, Arab, and

Greek, to accompany theriac destined for export. *Virtues* were written in simple, accessible language, although they assumed an audience at least somewhat familiar with both medical terminology and concepts. Indeed, early modern patients possessed extensive medical knowledge and were acquainted with medical practices. Marginalia indicate that early modern readers corrected and added information to the texts they read. Similarly, the titles and content of early modern vernacular medical texts reflect the diverse intellectual curiosity of readers. Even street poetry sung by peddlers assumed a common baseline of medical knowledge.[106] However, when apothecaries printed the virtues of theriac, they tended to be quite practical. They did not mention, for example, that a single compound curing all these ailments contradicted both the general theory of humors and the basic tenets of Galenic pharmacy. Nor did they dwell on technicalities by explaining how physicians, from Ibn Sīnā to Peter Abanus, attempted to resolve theriac's contradictions by developing a rational explanation of its mechanisms.

Instead, longer *virtues* had the space that allowed apothecaries to be more precise regarding theory, dosage, and conditions. Pamphlets also enabled apothecaries to cajole and amuse patients by using emotional stories and historical examples. Most likely, apothecaries offered pamphlets to a select clientele, as they did with *celebrations*. A few *virtues* even contained engravings or woodcuts (Figure 5.4). In his thirty-two-page *Trionfi contro la morte overo le rare prerogative e virtù singolari della teriaca*, elegantly printed in 1655 in Piacenza along with the long list of ailments cured by theriac, apothecary Clemente Rutta offered his readers a few "wondrous triumphs against death."[107] One such "triumph" was the tearful story of a physician "shoveling violently a drachm of theriac" down the throat of a twelve-year old, saving her life. Another "triumph," drawn directly from Galen, featured the moving description of a plague epidemic that ended with the success of "Aelianus Meccius, master of Galen," who defeated the plague thanks to the use of theriac, thereby "freeing the whole Italy."[108] Although not all *virtues* were as dramatic as Rutta's, longer *virtues* informed and delighted their readers in equal measure.

The case was different with shorter *virtues*. These handbills were designed as clear and concise reference texts, intended for consultation in specific situations. To my knowledge, the earliest extant example of a *theriac virtue* was published in Bologna in 1574, for the production of San

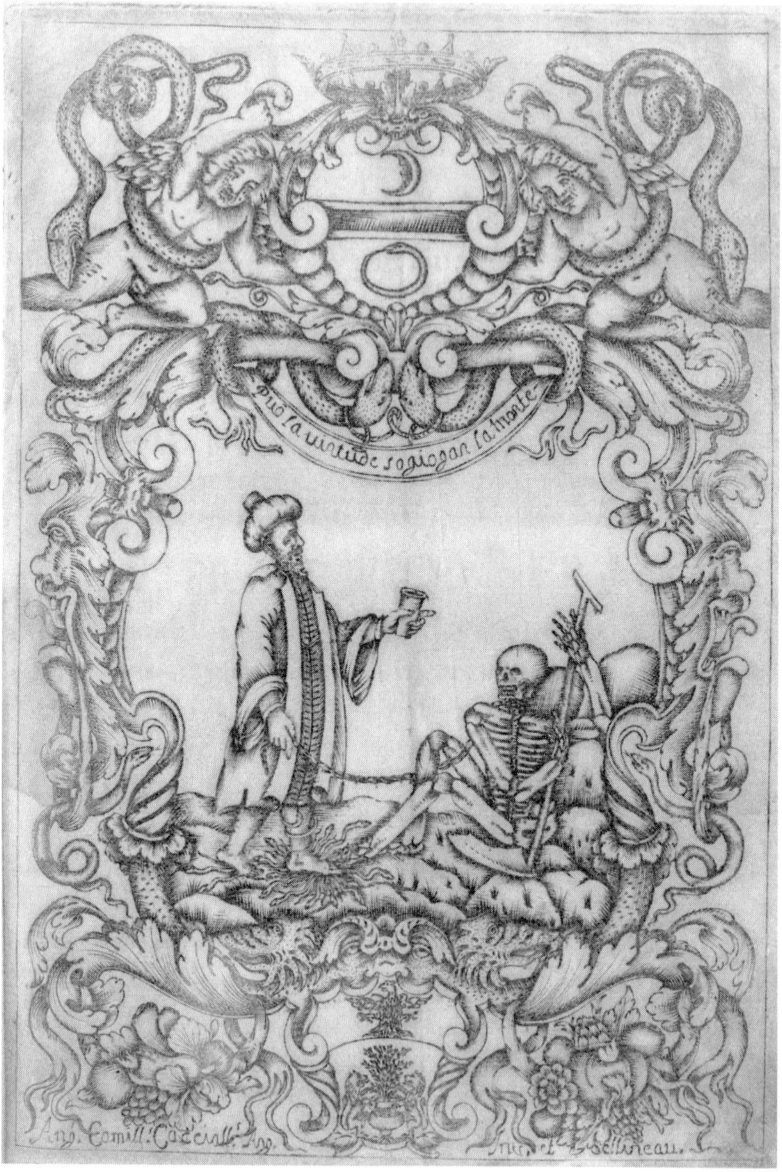

Fig. 5.4. The elaborate engraving of this *virtue* invokes theriac's capacity to dominate death. An ancient physician in a vaguely oriental robe, possibly Andromachus, keeps death in the form of a skeleton on a chained leash, while crushing snakes under his foot and holding a theriac jar. Two big snakes bite the mythological figures holding the baroque frame with the motto: "Virtue can subjugate Death."

Reproduced from Rutta, *I trionfi contro la morte* (Piacenza, 1655). Libri Pallastrelli 11, Biblioteca Comunale Passerini-Landi, Piacenza.

Salvatore.¹⁰⁹ Apothecaries likely began printing *virtues* in the form of handbills when they began staging public ceremonies in the second half of the sixteenth century. I believe the origin of apothecaries' *virtues* followed the custom initiated by charlatans and producers of secrets. At first the circulation of cheap prints was strongly associated with oral public performances. For example, news of war or treaties was broadcast through performances and leaflets in verse. *Cantastorie,* performers of chivalric tales, played a central role in the dissemination and production of books of battles (*libri di battaglie*). Likewise, peddlers, producers of secrets, and charlatans hawked their goods together with cheap prints from the late fifteenth century onward, and surviving handbills date to the 1550s.¹¹⁰ As Gentilcore has put it, "printed handbills and charlatans selling medicines have contemporary origins."¹¹¹ In Venice, any remedy sold by a charlatan was required by law to be accompanied by a *virtue*—in this case often called a "recipe"—from as early as 1547, when a charlatan was fined for selling one remedy with the *virtue* of another.¹¹² While to the best of my knowledge no similar requirement was ever enforced for theriac, it is likely that apothecaries also started printing *virtues* to accompany theriac in response to charlatans' performances.¹¹³ As others have noted, charlatans used theriac as a reference point when fashioning their bombastic claims about their remedies' efficacy. One charlatan affirmed that his remedy was "manufactured in the public square before the whole population of Varese," just like theriac.¹¹⁴ Although charlatans' *virtues* probably predated theriac *virtues,* it was theriac that became the gold standard to which remedy sellers compared their wares.

The evolution of the content of *virtues* in their shorter handbill form suggests that apothecaries experimented with different formats, then became less discursive, more concise, and progressively disconnected from humoral theory and individual conditions. Many *virtues* are undated, so it is not always possible to evaluate this transformation, but some comparisons are telling. Two *virtues* published in Bologna in 1574 and 1663 show apothecaries' innovation over time to better facilitate consultation and independent consumption. The 1574 *virtue* reported a list of ailments treatable by theriac, from head to toe (Figure 5.5). This handbill implicitly directed the patient to a doctor or apothecary, as it remained vague on dosage, stating that the benefits of theriac would be forthcoming only if it were "taken in the right way and proportionate quantity"—with no

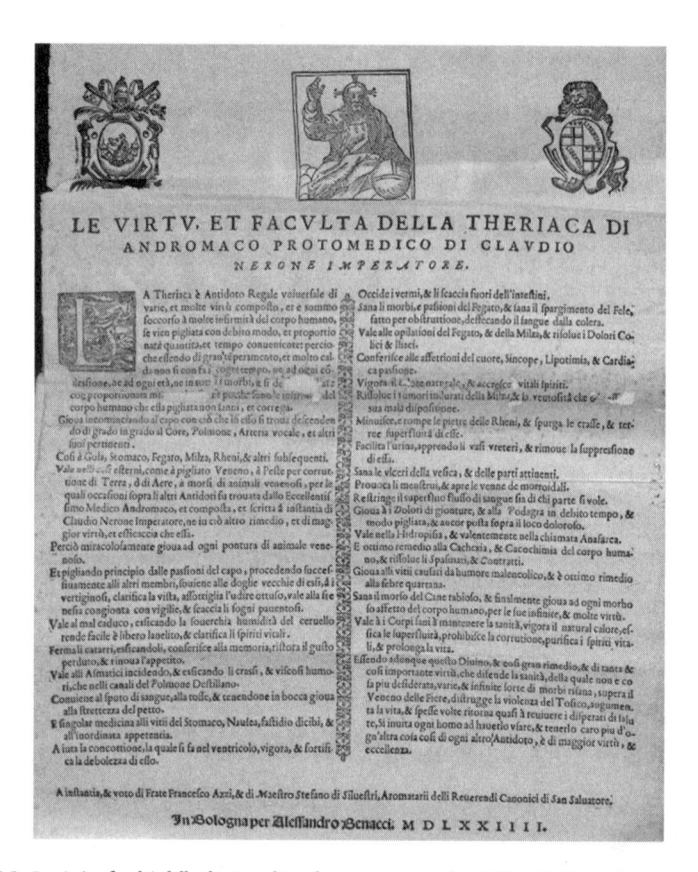

Fig. 5.5. Le virtù e facoltà della theriaca di Andromaco protomedico di Claudio Nerone imperatore. To the best of my knowledge, the oldest extant *virtue* of theriac was published in Bologna in 1574. Ms. Aldrovandi 91, 352.

© Alma Mater Studiorum Università di Bologna–Biblioteca Universitaria di Bologna. All rights reserved.

further specifications. The text of the 1663 *virtue*, however, was divided into two columns and carried precise instructions, presupposing the patient would use the remedy autonomously (Figure 5.6). The left side enumerated forty-three ailments and medical problems for which theriac was useful, such as "9. To furious deliriums" and "13. To Asthmatics." The right column explained how to take theriac for each illness. For "furious deliriums," the patient was to take theriac "with lettuce or endive water, and theriac not older than six years." "Asthmatics" should take 2 ounces of theriac with a quarter ounce of vinegar of squill. Instructions for other illnesses included consuming theriac with wine or broth, or combined with other ingredients.[115]

Le Virtù, e Facoltà Principali
DELLA TRIACA
DI ANDROMACO SENIORE,
ARCHIATRO DI CLAVDIO NERONE IMPERATORE,

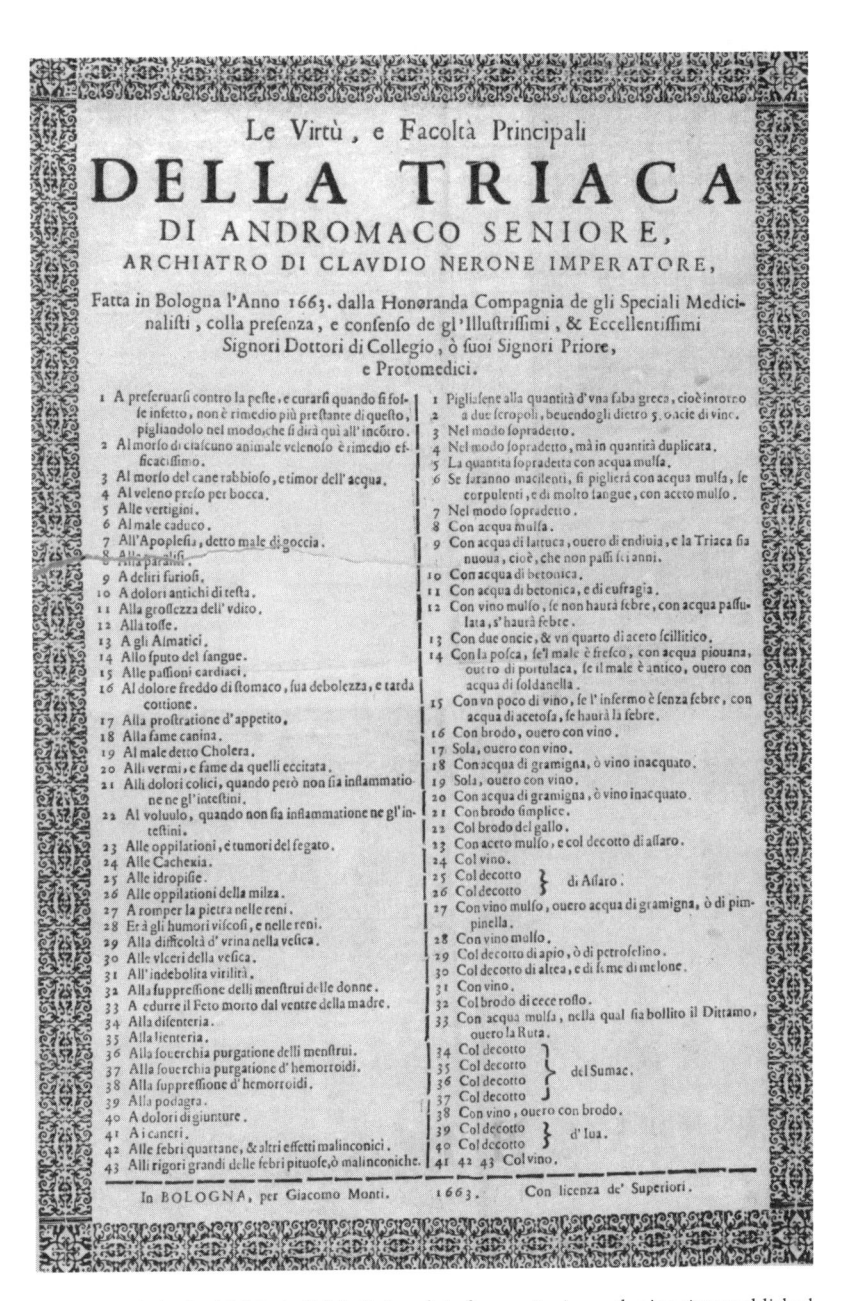

Fatta in Bologna l'Anno 1663. dalla Honoranda Compagnia de gli Speciali Medicinalisti, colla presenza, e consenso de gl'Illustrissimi, & Eccellentissimi Signori Dottori di Collegio, ò suoi Signori Priore, e Protomedici.

1. A preseruarsi contro la peste, e curarsi quando si fosse infetto, non è rimedio più prestante di questo, pigliandolo nel modo che si dirà qui all' incôtro.
2. Al morso di ciascuno animale velenoso è rimedio efficacissimo.
3. Al morso del cane rabbioso, e timor dell' acqua.
4. Al veleno preso per bocca.
5. Alle vertigini.
6. Al male caduco.
7. All'Apoplesia, detto male di goccia.
8. Alla paralisi.
9. A deliri furiosi.
10. A dolori antichi di testa.
11. Alla grossezza dell'vdito.
12. Alla tosse.
13. A gli Almatici.
14. Allo sputo del sangue.
15. Alle passioni cardiaci.
16. Al dolore freddo di stomaco, sua debolezza, e tarda cottione.
17. Alla prostratione d'appetito.
18. Alla fame canina.
19. Al male detto Cholera.
20. Alli vermi, e fame da quelli eccitata.
21. Alli dolori colici, quando però non sia inflammatione ne gl'intestini.
22. Al voluulo, quando non sia inflammatione ne gl'intestini.
23. Alle oppilationi, e tumori del fegato.
24. Alle Cachexia.
25. Alle idropisie.
26. Alle oppilationi della milza.
27. A romper la pietra nelle reni.
28. Et à gli humori viscosi, e nelle reni.
29. Alla difficoltà d' vrina nella vesica.
30. Alle vlceri della vesica.
31. All' indebolita virilità.
32. Alla suppressione delli menstrui delle donne.
33. A edurre il Feto morto dal ventre della madre.
34. Alla disenteria.
35. Alla lienteria.
36. Alla souerchia purgatione delli menstrui.
37. Alla souerchia purgatione d' hemorroidi.
38. Alla suppressione d' hemorroidi.
39. Alla podagra.
40. A dolori di giunture.
41. A i cancri.
42. Alle febri quartane, & altri effetti malinconici.
43. Alli rigori grandi delle febri pituose, ò malinconiche.

1. Pigliasene alla quantità d' vna faba greca, cioè intorno a due scropoli, beuendogli dietro 5. oncie di vino.
2. Nel modo sopradetto.
3. Nel modo sopradetto, mà in quantità duplicata.
4. La quantità sopradetta con acqua mulsa.
5. Se saranno macilenti, si piglierà con acqua mulsa, se corpulenti, e di molto sangue, con aceto mulso.
6. Nel modo sopradetto.
7. Con acqua mulsa.
8. Con acqua di lattuca, ouero di endiuia, e la Triaca sia nuoua, cioè, che non passi sei anni.
9. Con acqua di betonica.
10. Con acqua di betonica, e di eufragia.
11. Con vino mulso, se non haurà febre, con acqua passulata, s' haurà febre.
12. Con due oncie, & vn quarto di aceto scillitico.
13. Con la posca, se'l male è fresco, con acqua piouana, ouero di portulaca, se il male è antico, ouero con acqua di soldanella.
14. Con vn poco di vino, se l' infermo è senza febre, con acqua di acetosa, se haurà la febre.
15. Con brodo, ouero con vino.
16. Sola, ouero con vino.
17. Con acqua di gramigna, ò vino inacquato.
18. Sola, ouero con vino.
19. Con acqua di gramigna, ò vino inacquato.
20. Con brodo simplice.
21. Col brodo del gallo.
22. Con aceto mulso, e col decotto di assaro.
23. Col vino.
24. Col decotto } di Assaro.
25. Col decotto }
26. Con vino mulso, ouero acqua di gramigna, ò di pimpinella.
27. Con vino mollo.
28. Col decotto di apio, ò di petroselino.
29. Col decotto di altea, e di seme di melone.
30. Con vino.
31. Col brodo di cece rosso.
32. Con acqua mulsa, nella qual sia bollito il Dittamo, ouero la Ruta.
33. Col decotto }
34. Col decotto } del Sumac.
35. Col decotto }
36. Con vino, ouero con brodo.
37. Col decotto } d' Iua.
38. Col decotto }
39. 41 42 43 Col vino.

In BOLOGNA, per Giacomo Monti.   1663.   Con licenza de' Superiori.

Fig. 5.6. Le virtù e facoltà Principali della Teriaca di Andromaco Seniore, a theriac *virtue* published in Bologna by Giacomo Monti in 1663.

ASB Studio 251, Archivio di Stato, Bologna.

Sixteenth-century *virtues* explained theriac with reference to the humoral system. A *virtue* from 1574 informed readers that "because it [theriac] has a great temperament, and it is very hot, it is not suitable with every weather and every condition, neither for every age, nor for all ailments." The text also framed conditions in terms of humors: "It [theriac] is valid for falling sickness [epilepsy]; by drying the exceeding humidity of the brain, it frees and facilitates and clarifies the vital spirits."[116] By the eighteenth century these mild cautions and explanations had disappeared. Later exemplars were dry to the bone: "It helps against epilepsy."[117] Finally, abandoning any caution and (almost) any link to Galenic medicine, a *virtue* in English described theriac as a panacea (Figure 5.7): "a medicine which may be taken by People of all kinds, & at all times, and may be adapted to every constitution."[118] More similar to the *virtues* accompanying charlatans' wares, eighteenth-century theriac *virtues* conveyed the view that differences between bodies in terms of age, complexion, season, sex, and ailment were irrelevant when it came to theriac. The more the audience of such leaflets diversified in number and background, the more the instructions for using the medicament became generic. As Theriaca magna became a panacea and a staple of pharmacy, the Galenic humoral system faded away.

In this chapter I have argued that the production of *Theriaca magna Andromachi* grew considerably in the first half of the seventeenth century, especially in Venice. Previously, in the last quarter of the sixteenth century, only "the aristocrats and the wealthy" could obtain "true theriac." While quantities of Theriaca magna increased, the broader concept of theriac caught the imagination of patients. Alongside ever-present fake or adulterated theriacs, a number of by-products became easily available to buyers, such as theriacal salt, vinegar, and water, as well as "theriacs for the poor." Endorsed by public authorities who made sure its price was not excessive, theriac became relatively affordable, allowing even salaried artisans to buy a few doses when needed.

Through public ceremonies and publications, apothecaries distributed theriac across the social spectrum, with the support of political and medical authorities. An extraordinary variety of apothecary materials accompanied theriac's sales and production, a unique case in the pharma-

THERIACA FINA IN VENEZIA.

OF THE USE, VIRTUES ET DOZE

OF THE TREACLE OF ANDROMACHUS THE ELDER,

MADE IN THE APOTHECARY'S SHOP

AT THE SIGN OF THE BLAK EAGLE
IN St. SAVIOUR'S SQUARE, AT VENICE,

In the prefence of the moſt Illuſtrious Magiſtrates of the ancient Juſtice, the Doctors of the College of Phyſicians, Apothecaries & other Deputies.

THe Treacle of Andromachus is a compoſition ſo well regulated in all its parts, & ſo beneficial in the effects it produces, that for the ſe twenty Ages paſt it has excell'd all other medicines, and therefore from its great reputation it may be inferr'd that the uſe of this grand remedy will laſt to the end of the world, provided it be prepar'd with Drugs of the moſt perfect quality, & in the ſome manner as is practis'd at the *Black Eagle*.

It ſerves particularly for the preſervation of health, freeing the human body of all impurities by tranſpiration.

It is a preſervative againſt contagious Diſtempers, & by taking it in ſcordion water, cures the moſt peſtilential Diſeaſes.

It heals ſuch as have been ſtung by Scorpions, bit by Dogs, Vipers, & other venimous animals, by drinking it & applying it to the wound.

A Drachm of it infuſed in wine hinders all ſorts of poiſon from taking effect.

It cures all Kinds of putrid periodical & peſtilential Fevers, by taking it in white wine.

It is very good for the ſtomach-ach, Belly-ach & inteſtine cholick; It Kills worms in Children and forces them out of the body.

It ſtops the ſpitting of blood and acid humors that affect the lungs: Is a cure for the moſt inveterate and violent cough, and facilitates breaching in ſuch as are *aſthmatick*.

It incites women's Terms & Hemorrhoids, and if need be, moderates an overcopiouſneſs of the ſame.

And finally it is a cordial very uſeful in *Syncopes*, palpitations of the heart, quakings, Apoplexies and other nervous diſtempers; and in a word it may be ſaid that this famous antidote cures or extenuates every the moſt dangerous diſeaſe of the human body.

It is a medicine which may be taken by People of all kinds, & at all times, and may be adapted to every conſtitution by rightly proportioning the Doze, which muſt never exceed the weight of half a Drachm.

The Doze is as follows:

2. SCruples to be taken in water, broth, or any other liquid, once a wee k, by young People & of a ſtrong conſtitution to preſerve their health.

Half a drachm to be taken in white wine by old & weak People.

In venimous or peſtilential diſtempers the ordinary Doze muſt be a Drachm in ſpiritu repeating the ſame three times a day till cured.

Fig. 5.7. Eighteenth-century Venetian theriac *virtue* in English titled "THERIACA FINA IN VENEZIA." The handbill survives because it was used as an inside cover for the *Book of Receipts for Cookery and Pastry &c*, suggesting that, at least at the time of binding, such documents were not valued. The text implies little differentiation in doses between patients. Wellcome Collection.

ceutical landscape of early modern medicine. Such publications—all of which came free (were "donated") with their respective remedy—reveal the complex web of social relations demanded and created by theriac. *Virtues* derived directly from Galen's texts, and conveyed abridged scholarly knowledge to patients in the form of handbills and longer pamphlets. Apothecaries' adoption of handbills for theriac implies that charlatans heavily influenced apothecaries' marketing practices.

CHAPTER 6

A Preservative of the Social Order

*E*ARLY MODERN physicians were unrelenting in their pursuit of greater social standing and scientific authority. They had many means to pursue higher status: publications, collections, patronage relations, institutions such as medical colleges, and presenting themselves as useful allies to political authorities. The extent to which physicians actually gained this authority—especially with respect to apothecaries—varied greatly, according to local political economies and the leverage of apothecary guilds compared to that of local medical colleges. Conflicts between these guilds and colleges were commonplace in early modern Europe, where attempts at medical hierarchization, a deliberate process to create a vertical governance among medical actors as well as patients, were the norm rather than the exception.[1]

In this chapter I present two case studies—those of seventeenth-century Bologna and Venice—to explore the relationships between medical colleges, apothecary guilds, and the state; the political economies determining the outcomes of the conflicts among these institutions; and the social role performed by Theriaca magna at this time. We have encountered debates on theriac before. In Chapter 1 we saw how collectors and learned apothecaries used theriac to promote an innovative agenda for scientific research. By contrast, Chapter 3 demonstrated that treatises on theriac published from the 1570s to the end of the century argued for corporatism, control of medical practice, and hierarchization.

This chapter moves away from programmatic and written medical debates to focus on tangible actions in order to gauge the social effectiveness of theriac in the seventeenth century, taking intermittent productions of theriac as a starting point. Interruptions in production disrupted the ordinary medical and economic life of Bologna and Venice. At least three times Bolognese apothecaries were reluctant to make theriac officially, to the point that authorities had to step in. In 1659, 1679, and 1688 the Collegio Medico decreed that apothecaries had to "perform the due and necessary preparations to compose as soon as possible and with the utmost possible accuracy such an important and noble medicament."[2] Similarly, in 1618 Venetian apothecaries abruptly ceased theriac production for three years, running voluntarily at a loss. If Theriaca magna was profitable, why would apothecaries have refused to produce it?

As a state drug, theriac needed to be firmly in the hands of the institutions that best represented the state's interests. In this sense, Bologna and Venice in the seventeenth century offer contrasting scenarios. The honey dispute discussed below exemplifies the inability of the Venetian Collegio Medico to control the city's theriac production and assert its authority over the apothecaries. In Venice the apothecary guild maintained its autonomy, fighting off all attempts by collegiate physicians to restrict its prerogatives. Conversely, in Bologna the preeminence of the Collegio Medico was never substantially questioned. Until the eighteenth century—when the apothecaries reorganized their guild—Theriaca magna productions were major advertising events for the Collegio Medico rather than a regular profitable business for apothecaries.[3]

Despite the two cities' divergent responses to conflict over theriac and pharmacy, this chapter also highlights their similarities. In both cities the local political economy played a fundamental role in shaping the outcomes of controversies. The victor was always the party that could win the support of the state—and the state sided with the institution that best represented its interests, primarily its economic interests in the case of Venice. Physicians in both cities fought aggressively to assert their superiority over apothecaries by establishing their scientific authority and expertise, using their institutional prerogatives, especially medical regulations. For their part, apothecaries defended their intellectual ownership of materia medica, a field that was traditionally theirs, and attempted to contain what they perceived to be physicians' arrogance and intrusiveness into their daily activities. Writing and publishing practices were pivotal in shaping the relationships between the two groups.

Theriaca magna performed a conservative role in society. In the seventeenth century, the battles between apothecaries and physicians over theriac were part of a greater struggle for authority within the established medical hierarchy. Yet these intense conflicts had little impact on understandings of medicine, disease, healing, and bodies, remaining within traditional understandings of natural and human life. Moreover, when performing theriac ceremonies in the *calli* or university courtyard, apothecaries, physicians, and state officials made sure to collaborate for the benefit of those in attendance. By projecting the vision of an orderly medical establishment, theriac productions reinforced and maintained the existing social structure. But out of public view, bitter controversies abounded.

Venice's Bitter Honey

In 1621 in Venice, several state officials drew up a political document that put an end to a harsh dispute between the city's apothecary guild and the Collegio Medico.

> The production of this antidote has always followed the old recipe book that the Medical College gave many years ago to the apothecaries, which is recorded in the Giustizia Vecchia office. Now, it appears that some modern physicians have had a new thought to change the production of theriac; but their opinion has begun a contention, since many think it not convenient to alter what has been done before, celebrated, and used by such great men; nor is it convenient to introduce new non-experimented ways to abandon the old approved ways used continually by many people and experienced for hundreds of years, the same way found in books by famous authors. In conscience, many physicians expressed their

judgment in written statements [*fedi*] and oaths, which is that this novelty will arouse suspicion in the people without bringing any benefit.[4]

This passage contrasted the "old approved ways" of pharmacy with the "new non-experimented ways" of "some modern physicians," framing the state officials' decision in medical terms. However, the document also made explicit that, in Venice, the business of theriac was profitable to both individual actors and the state because of the fees on its trade and the taxes on the tin containers in which it was stored. Furthermore, the production and marketing of theriac generated ancillary commercial traffic, with the activities of buyers and investors triggering import and export duties. The honey dispute that led to this official statement shows that, in Venice, the state's economic interest took precedence over the medical claims of "modern" physicians when they risked damaging state interests.

It all began when an ambitious physician sought to make a name for himself in the medical field. In 1613 Angelo Busti (1582–1615), a Venetian collegiate physician, published a short dissertation in Latin titled *De mellis convenienti atque legitima quantitate ad theriacam componendam* discussing the "convenient and legitimate" quantity of honey in the composition of theriac.[5] A graduate of the University of Padua, Busti had a keen sense of the intellectual world he wished to join. He was already acquainted with such naturalists as Prospero Alpini, and corresponded with Caspar Bahunin (1560–1624).[6] As well as being a hot scholarly topic, a treatise on theriac would give the author visibility beyond the world of academia, since its production was constantly increasing; for example, in the previous year alone Venetian apothecaries had produced 825 kilograms of official theriac.[7] In his text Busti argued that the city's apothecaries should reduce the quantity to bring Venetian theriac in line with that produced in Bologna, Rome, and Florence.[8]

In Galenic pharmacy, honey was commonly mixed with electuaries, including theriac, to stabilize, preserve, and sweeten the mixture. Like wine, honey was also used to dilute or give bulk to medicinal preparations. Ancient and Arab authors already recognized honey's importance as a food and an ingredient in medicines.[9] Renaissance authors discussed honey's medical properties in relation to humoral theory, but all agreed that, in the case of theriac, honey was a pharmacological vehicle useful for binding other ingredients.[10]

Busti argued that the quantity of honey required in theriac depended on the proportion of minced dry spices and other liquid ingredients—juices, oils, and (liquefied) gums. The theriac recipe listed ingredients by weight, but the initial quantities varied as a consequence of the preparation they underwent, such as crushing and mincing. By "long-standing custom," Venetian apothecaries added 1 pound of honey for every 3 ounces of dry spices, for a total of 14.5 pounds of honey per batch.[11] After careful examination of ancient and modern authors, and acknowledging that the weight of minced ingredients varied, Busti concluded that apothecaries should add 1 pound of honey for every 4 ounces and 2 drachms of spices (dry and liquid), for a total of 10 pounds of honey in a single batch. In sum, apothecaries should reduce honey by about 50 percent, instead of 14.5 pounds per batch they should use only 10 pounds.[12] According to Busti, this would prevent Venetian theriac from becoming diluted, too sweet, and less effective.

In theory the Venetian Collegio Medico oversaw the recipe for theriac. But it wielded less authority than the medical colleges tied to prestigious universities such as Padua and Bologna, despite having been established as early as 1316. Moreover, in Venice the production and sale of medicaments involved several institutional actors besides the Collegio Medico: the College of Apothecaries, the Giustizia Vecchia, and the Health Board (*Provveditori di Sanità*). The latter two offices were led by officials who were neither physicians nor apothecaries, and their functions often overlapped, leaving considerable room for negotiation—but also ample opportunity for conflict. For example, the Giustizia Vecchia repeatedly asked the Health Board not to intervene in matters concerning apothecary shops. For a short time in 1590, the Health Board forbade the Giustizia Vecchia from dealing with apothecary matters. But the Giustizia Vecchia was soon able to reaffirm its grip on apothecary goods.[13] Furthermore, while the Giustizia Vecchia's supervision of theriac was centuries old, the Collegio Medico's supervision dated only to 1507.[14] The centuries-long relationship between the Giustizia Vecchia and the apothecary guild meant stronger bonds had been forged between these two institutions than either had with the Collegio Medico. But this did not dissuade the Collegio Medico from pursuing greater prestige and authority, the kind enjoyed by other medical colleges across Europe.

Nevertheless, in the early years of the seventeenth century, just before Busti published his treatise, relationships between the Collegio Medico and College of Apothecaries were as much collaborative as conflicting. For example, in 1601 the Collegio Medico complained that apothecaries were too numerous and yet underqualified: "Recently the number of apothecary shops has greatly grown in this city. Everyone who worked one or two years as an apprentice wants to license his own shop, and it happens that, being them poor, they cannot supply the quantity and quality required for the medicaments necessary to the life of men."[15] Moreover, according to the Collegio Medico, inspections of apothecary shops took place less than once a year, sometimes even just once every other year. By comparison, Bolognese Protomedico inspected apothecary shops four times a year. In addition, Venetian inspectors were selected from the officials of the Giustizia Vecchia. In claiming that the city's inspections were inadequate, the Collegio Medico was attempting to gain more control over apothecaries.

In other areas, such as regulation of exotic materia medica, relationships between the two bodies appeared more cooperative. In 1604, for example, the Venetian Collegio Medico promptly accepted apothecary Francesco (Cechino) Martinelli's findings about amomum, and ruled in favor of its use.[16] Coming from a distinguished family of apothecaries, Martinelli had republished the results of his uncle, who had traveled to the Indies via Crete, Cyprus, and Syria during the 1560s. Martinelli Sr. had sent back rare plants, including two ingredients for theriac: amomum (an unidentified species of the genus *Amomum*) and *Calamus aromaticus* (today known as sweet flag or *Acorus calamus*).[17] On the basis of his uncle's letters, Martinelli Jr. claimed amomum was a grape and *Calamus odoratus* a cane, both from Malacca.[18]

The Venetian Collegio Medico not only demonstrated a degree of receptivity to an apothecary's scholarship, but also championed it in the face of other scholars' objections. In 1605 an anonymous author from Mantua, possibly apothecary Antonio Bertioli, questioned Martinelli's botanical identification, publishing a treatise furnished with detailed engravings.[19] The author criticized Martinelli's understanding of Latin, and added that "it would be better not to introduce new medicaments into apothecary shops [. . . which] stay in the shops for years, impoverishing incautious apothecaries."[20] Notwithstanding the opposition, the Venetian Collegio Medico stood by its decision.

The Collegio Medico also showed flexibility, repeatedly ruling on theriac ingredients and thereby allowing apothecaries to modify the recipe depending on supplies. In 1605 the college ruled that apothecaries could use galangal (then called *Alpinia officinarum*) as a substitute if amomum cost more than 15 ducats per pound or was not available.[21] Similarly, in 1613 the Collegio Medico permitted the substitution of a less pure storax instead of storax in lacrima (*Liquidambar orientalis* Mill.), provided that apothecaries purified it.[22] Again in 1627, the college set a maximum price for storax in lacrima of 50 ducats per pound, above which apothecaries could use a substitute.[23] By recognizing the high cost of theriac's exotic ingredients, the Collegio Medico acknowledged that apothecaries might struggle to procure expensive ingredients for theriac, and gave them some leeway to adapt the approved recipe according to actual prices and the conditions of production.

In 1613, however, Busti's treatise caused a rupture between the apothecary guild and the Collegio Medico. Venetian apothecaries found his book nothing less than outrageous, and the first meeting convened to discuss it was recorded as being an uncharacteristically anxious affair. Several apothecaries complained that collegiate physicians were trying "with all their powers" to modify the recipe of theriac; they wanted to alter the "ancient custom based on reason and experience." Apothecaries firmly believed that "no innovation" was necessary, and they were ready to demonstrate their conviction with "evident reasons." In a petition addressed to the Collegio Medico, they conceded that it was the Collegio Medico's privilege to approve the final recipe, but stressed that physicians should still defer to apothecaries, who were the ones composing the antidote at their own expense.[24]

Interestingly, the apothecaries also complained that Busti had written a book without having informed them. They lamented that rather than having debated the question of the proper quantity of honey with words (*à bocca*), Busti had published a book discussing the matter using "demonstrative words."[25] It is possible that apothecaries had been taken off guard by Busti's dissertation. His treatise threatened them because, as they affirmed, it contradicted both Galenic texts and their experience, which was "the true teacher."²⁶ To Busti, the quantity of honey depended on the interpretation of Galen and other classical texts, but to the apothecaries their best practices were more relevant than any text. Although taken aback, they soon realized they had to compete on the same ground as Busti. Thus they commissioned another collegiate physician, Fabio Olmo, to work on a rebuttal, and asked the Collegio Medico to wait for his treatise before deliberating.²⁷ The commission, as well as the complaint about the subject not having been discussed with words, marked an important—although not definitive—shift regarding the space where and the manner in which controversies should be broached.

The volatile power dynamic between the Collegio Medico and the apothecary guild affected apothecaries' economic interests. More honey meant a slightly sweeter product, but more crucially a higher yield for a smaller investment. By reinterpreting the literature, Busti had placed apothecaries' revenues at risk. Even worse, they feared that changing the recipe would damage the reputation of Venetian theriac and have negative consequences for exports. More fundamentally, a new recipe implied that Venetian theriac, whether past or present, was not perfect.

Money, reputation, and prestige were at stake. Unsurprisingly, the honey dispute escalated, worsening the relationship between the two colleges. It also exposed tensions within the Collegio Medico. The same month that Busti's book was published, the Collegio suspended a production of theriac, as the commission of physicians overseeing its production—including Busti—was split on the quantity of honey to be used. The apothecaries asked the physicians to decide quickly on whether production could proceed; they had already ground the spices and liquefied the gums, so these expensive materials were now at risk of going to waste.²⁸ A consensus was never reached.²⁹ Toward the end of 1613 the Collegio Medico sought to break the deadlock by accepting the offer of apothecary Pompeo Sprechi (or Sprecchi) to make theriac following *two* recipes, with different quantities of honey. After the usual period of fermentation, physicians would verify and compare the results.³⁰ In the meantime all production and distribution of theriac ceased. In 1614, while Sprechi's theriac sat fermenting, Olmo's answer to Busti was published. Over the course of more than one hundred pages in *De mellis opportuna decentiue quantitate pro theriaca, mithridatoque componendis,* he explained the apothecaries' rationale in choosing the appropriate quantity of honey when compounding theriac and mithidate, supporting them with a detailed analysis of classical literature. Olmo's conclusion was that apothecaries should continue with their traditional recipe because, even though the literature was inconsistent on the question of honey, apothecaries' best practices, honed by experience, validated their recipe.[31]

The proposal of a trial came from a learned apothecary, a mediator between the realms of apothecary and physician. Pharmaceutical testing practices followed a hands-on approach to materia medica that was common among medical institutions, physicians, and naturalists, as well as in the household.[32] Pompeo Sprechi, a learned apothecary at the sign of the Two Moors, boasted a scholarly reputation and was well known for his theriac both in Venice and abroad. He corresponded and exchanged specimens with Giovanni Pona (1565–1630), the Campi brothers in Lucca, and Swiss physician Jacob Zwinger (1569–1610).[33] Sprechi had also published his own monograph on a species of yarrow.[34] According to Busti, Olmo did all he could to stop the experiment.[35] Unfortunately, there is no account of how exactly physicians assessed the two compounds. In May 1614 the Collegio Medico inspected Sprechi's two theriacs and voted twenty-five to four to change the recipe according to Busti's proposal.[36]

In the meantime, the honey dispute exposed producers of theriac to attacks by other apothecaries, opening up an internal front. In 1614, apparently unrelated to the honey dispute, Ottavio Campolongo, an apothecary from Parma active in Venice, published a booklet, *Considerationi intorno alla Theriaca*. He claimed Venetian apothecaries used incorrect procedures to liquefy gums, crush herbs, and age theriac; indeed, he denounced practices at the very core of apothecaries' knowledge.[37] An author writing under the pseudonym Asdrubale Mostravero (Shows truth)—probably Martinelli Jr.—immediately published a rebuttal.[38] Mostravero defended Venetian apothecaries and criticized the timing of Campolongo, whose publication appeared right when the Collegio Medico was debating the recipe of theriac.[39]

With the apothecaries under attack on multiple fronts, the Collegio Medico began a final opportunistic offensive. In 1615 it first appointed a physician to write an official pharmacopoeia, which Venice still lacked. Then the Collegio Medico officially changed the recipe of theriac, modifying the quantity of honey.[40] Two years later, two publications reinforced the message: a new *Pharmacopaea* by physician Curzio Marinelli, and

Busti's now posthumous rebuttal to Olmo.⁴¹ Marinelli's *Pharmacopaea* openly advocated for physicians' authority over apothecaries, who protested that the text was "full of insults and slander against all apothecaries."⁴² Historian Sabrina Minuzzi has shown that Marinelli "structured his work around apothecaries' errors."⁴³ For his part, Busti concluded that, on the matter of honey, the apothecaries' custom was wrong. Traditions, he argued, could and must change once they are recognized as inappropriate or harmful.⁴⁴

Up to this point apothecaries had fought their battle by commissioning Olmo's rebuttal to Busti and petitioning the Collegio Medico. But then they changed their strategy, focusing instead on local institutions and pressure groups. A month after the publication of the pharmacopoeia, apothecaries pushed Avogaria di Comun—a board of magistrates charged with protecting the interests of Venetian communal institutions—to withdraw *Pharmacopaea* and prohibit its sale.⁴⁵ Not until 1790 would physicians try again—and fail again—to impose a pharmacopoeia.⁴⁶ The swift intervention of Avogaria di Comun, a state office, shows that apothecaries were both well organized and experienced in dealing with the Venetian administration.

Even though the battle against the pharmacopoeia was easily won, the battle over the quantity of honey proved much more arduous, taking many years before the apothecaries ultimately emerged victorious. At first they ceased all production of theriac, which adversely affected not only the makers of theriac, but also retailers, merchants, physicians, patients, and of course the guild. The apothecaries who made theriac were the same who took administrative roles in governing the guild. Several physicians and druggists lent support to apothecaries, demonstrating that an entire economy hinged on theriac. Possibly solicited by the apothecaries, a group of twenty-five physicians presented a petition to the Giustizia Vecchia, swearing that changing the recipe of Venetian theriac would foment suspicion among consumers and bring "notable damages to both public and private interests."⁴⁷ A similar petition was presented by several druggists, who could sell but not produce theriac, affirming that, for several years now, they had "not seen the same number of merchants from foreign nations" as before. According to druggists, when foreign merchants came to Venice to buy theriac, they bought other goods as well.⁴⁸ Without theriac, Venice would lack an important economic engine.

Such hyperbolic statements were typical of petitions. However, along with apothecaries, druggists, and physicians, the Giustizia Vecchia was also concerned that interrupting the production of theriac might diminish the city's commercial reputation. By 1621, fearing damage to the prestige of Venetian theriac abroad, the Giustizia Vecchia asked several ambassadors and consuls to report on the matter. The Venetian consuls in the Low Countries sent testimony of the importance of Venetian theriac and mithridate: "People in these countries consider the usual theriac made in this city [Venice] as a highly precious treasure for human health; it is extolled as the most perfect of all others, and for this reason they import great quantities of it."[49] The British and French ambassadors and two consuls from the "German Nation" sent similar statements. Venetian theriac still had high prestige in these nations, but a gap in the production of theriac risked its standing.[50]

The dispute came to an end in 1621, when apothecaries were able to gain consensus from a vast swath of state offices: the College of Apothecaries, Giustizia Vecchia, Provveditori of Giustizia Vecchia (a board of magistrates with appeal powers over cases concerning the Giustizia Vecchia), and Savi alla Mercantia (an influential organ of the state with jurisdiction over foreign commerce as well as custom duties). Representatives from these institutions drew up a definitive document that brought theriac back into the hands of apothecaries. The first part outlined explicitly the importance of theriac to the Venetian state:

> Venetian theriac is very popular and has a great reputation because renowned physicians approve of it, many authors celebrate it, and many nations frequently use it and import it [... and] ultramontane nations always desire theriac. Hence, for many years a lot of theriac has been sold, and the Signoria [the Republic of Venice] acquires profit from duties on both import and export derived from theriac itself and from the tin receptacles in which it is stored. Moreover, those who come to buy theriac directly on such occasions invest big sums in other merchandise as well, which all together are contributions to the benefit of the duties.[51]

The document noted another reason the Signoria (the government of the Republic) incurred "notable damage" when theriac production ceased:

other producers were stepping in and stealing the market. The Signoria therefore allowed apothecaries to make theriac according to the Venetian custom, provided they did so in the presence and to the approval of the collegiate physicians. Expecting opposition from collegiate physicians, the Signoria set a considerable fine of 500 ducats on any physician who refused to fulfill his duty.[52]

As we saw at the beginning of this section, the document also elucidated the place of medical knowledge—especially new medical knowledge—in relation to the economic interests of the Venetian state. Considering that these were at stake, the state took sides in the medical dispute, backing the "old approved ways," suspicious of what they called "non-experimented ways." In the end they deemed that the innovations of "modern physicians" should not harm the health of state coffers. By suspending their most lucrative production for several years, apothecaries won the battle against physicians with the help of an alliance of numerous state offices. Apothecaries gained leverage from the revenues theriac generated for the Venetian state, and they also gained strength from their substantial connections. Seventeenth-century Venice had little room for new interpretations of ancient texts or botanical matters when they collided with the economic interests of the state.

"Shoemaker, Not Beyond the Shoe": Apothecaries and Theriac in the Bolognese Medical System

In the seventeenth century, the place of apothecaries and theriac in the Bolognese medical system differed greatly from that of Venice. Naturalist Ulisse Aldrovandi researched theriac for several decades, bringing prestige to Bologna's production across Italy, despite there being no mention of its exports beyond the city. Unlike in Venice, the apothecary guild in Bologna joined forces to make Theriaca magna in the university courtyard in a single great ceremony, under the watchful eyes of collegiate physicians.

According to available sources, apothecaries in seventeenth-century Bologna produced theriac only about ten times, a poor result.[53] Furthermore, they kept only modest quantities of theriac in their shops, no more than 300 Bolognese pounds (98 kilograms) at any given time (Table 6.1). Even the single greatest Bolognese theriac production of 305 pounds

Table 6.1 Quantities of theriac, vipers, and mithridate in Bolognese apothecary shops (1601–1656) in Bolognese pounds (= 325.665 grams).

Year	Theriac	Vipers	Mithridate
1601	235		
1604	140		
1648	305		
1656	285	567	50
Undated 17th cent.	304		58

Source: ASB, Studio 213.

could not compare to the quantities produced in Venice, whose annual average was more than three times greater between 1605 and 1618.[54]

Evidently irritated by apothecaries' reluctance to make theriac, the Bolognese Collegio Medico issued *bandi* (decrees) at least three times (in 1659, 1679, and 1688) ordering apothecaries to produce theriac according to the local pharmacopoeia. In addition, the cardinal legate and the Senate prohibited anyone from exporting or buying vipers, dead or alive, which were to be reserved only for making theriac, "considering how necessary is theriac to the health of people and that it is not possible to make without a great quantity of vipers."[55]

The arm wrestling over theriac between the Collegio Medico and apothecary guild exemplifies the uneasy relationship between these two institutions in the seventeenth century. One of the main areas of conflict regarded the sale of medicaments, which both institutions agreed was disorderly. But while the Collegio Medico attributed responsibility to the apothecary guild, its members and other sellers' unruliness for this state of affairs, the guild blamed the confusion on the Collegio's intrusion into their sphere, their uneven enforcing of restrictions, and the fact they were not doing enough to protect regular apothecaries from the competition of religious apothecary shops. Furthermore, unlike their Venetian counterparts, and despite several attempts, no Bolognese apothecary ever became recognized as a learned apothecary in the Republic of Letters. In Bologna, collegiate physicians maintained authority over knowledge of materia medica and medicines. Until the very end of the seventeenth century, when apothecaries reformed the structure of their guild, apothecary actions often manifested only as a passive resistance.

A rich city with a thriving silk-weaving thread industry, Bologna also boasted a well-established university of considerable prestige throughout Europe. The city had belonged to the Papal States since 1506 and was administered by a so-called mixed government (*governo misto*) made up of local institutions, such as the Senate (comprising forty senators from the aristocracy) and the cardinal legate, the papal representative. In Bologna, the state favored the Collegio Medico and actively endorsed the separation of responsibilities in the medical professions; in the Middle Ages the blurring of those lines had been damaging to patients.

Gianna Pomata has illustrated that the elitism of the Collegio Medico increased during the sixteenth and seventeenth centuries, as did the hierarchization of the medical professions over which it presided.[56] The Collegio was a fundamental component of the university, an oligarchy of select physicians with the mandate to organize and control medical life.[57] It faced especially stiff opposition from the apothecary guild, which was one the richest and most influential guilds, integral to an institutional and productive system at the core of Bologna's social and economic life.[58] The relationship between the physicians and apothecaries was "marked by constant tension."[59] The primary means by which the Collegio Medico and the Protomedicato (a board of collegiate physicians) wielded control over apothecaries were licensing examinations, the official pharmacopoeia, inspections of their shops, and overseeing both the opening of new shops and the making of theriac.[60]

The loss of the guild's archives during the Napoleonic Wars prejudices our understanding of apothecaries' perspective on their relationship with the Collegio Medico.[61] However, we do know that from the early sixteenth century, apothecaries resented their formal subordination to the Collegio. In 1518 they tried to avoid presenting their customary Christmas gifts to the Collegio Medico. The attempt failed, and the college swiftly punished its instigator, apothecary Domenico Aligine, by prohibiting physicians from ordering medicines from his shop.[62] This episode was a harbinger of both the apothecaries' growing resentment and how the Collegio Medico's control over apothecaries would expand in the following decades.

In the second half of the sixteenth century, the apothecary guild faced a wave of provisions strengthening physicians' control over its activities and prerogatives. Aldrovandi loomed large behind these regulations, his stated objective being to actualize a subordination that had been hitherto more symbolic than real. In 1551, right after the publication of its statutes (today lost), the apothecary guild "willingly" submitted itself to the Collegio Medico with an official document.[63] In 1557 the Collegio Medico revised the prices of all simples and medicinal compositions.[64] In 1567 the Collegio issued a regulation on apothecaries, titled *Moderatione,* then expanded and revised it in 1581, 1594, and 1600.[65] In 1568 the responsibility to set official prices passed from the apothecary guild to the Protomedicato.[66] In 1574 the Senate commissioned Aldrovandi to publish Bologna's first official pharmacopoeia, the *Antidotarium,* which bound apothecaries' preparations to its formulas. The *Antidotarium* quickly became a point of reference for physicians and apothecaries not just in Bologna but beyond the city, too.[67] Yet its popularity belied the controversies preceding its publication, which showed that most collegiate physicians resented Aldrovandi's energetic initiative, his ties to the Senate, and the Senate's pressure on the Collegio.[68]

Growing resentment finally exploded in 1575 with an acrimonious dispute over theriac that shook long-standing ties between apothecaries and collegiate physicians.[69] In the years prior, Bolognese apothecaries had failed to stand out in the quest for "true theriac." Visiting the city in 1554 "to see those apothecaries making theriac," apothecary Calestani from Parma was especially unimpressed with the production, which lacked many ingredients.[70] He toured Italy to learn from other apothecaries, and defined Bolognese theriac as "extravagant"—which was not a compliment. Begrudging Aldrovandi's grandiose theriac making at the San Salvatore convent in 1574, Bologna's apothecaries set out to make their own in 1575. In June, Protomedici Aldrovandi and Antonio Maria Alberghini were called to approve of the cutting of the vipers. They refused, claiming the snakes had been caught at the wrong time of year and in the wrong places, and that some were even pregnant. The infuriated apothecaries protested, backed up by the majority of collegiate physicians. That year marked the first time a Bolognese apothecary published a plea to the Senate, expressing his concern for apothecaries' situation in the city and defending their reputation.[71] Aldrovandi took the dispute beyond the realm of the Collegio Medico when he involved a senator and the papal governor, which led to a brutal rupturing of the college, as its physicians expelled not only him but also Alberghini.

·

Far from giving in, Aldrovandi immediately gathered support for his scientific positions in the Republic of Letters and soon won the backing of Pope Gregory XIII, flipping the situation in his favor. In 1577 the pope not only reinstated Aldrovandi and Alberghini to the Collegio Medico, but also endorsed the separation of physicians and apothecaries. In 1585 new regulations redefined the boundaries between the medical professions, once again forbidding partnerships between physicians and apothecaries and reinforcing the hierarchy that governed them. The fine for any association between apothecary and physician was raised to the exorbitant sum of 200 golden scudi.[72]

Relations between the Collegio Medico and apothecary guild remained tense in the last year of the sixteenth century, reflecting half a century of encroaching medical regulation and ever-present hostility. At this time Bologna's population was suffering famine, banditry, and violent conflicts among aristocratic families.[73] Aware of the social discord and professing the will to mitigate it, the cardinal vice-legate, representing the pope, stepped in to mediate the reconfiguration of the relationship between the two institutions. The college and the guild held acrimonious negotiations for at least two years, with recurrent disagreements and complaints.[74] Finally a document signed by the cardinal vice-legate as warrantor called *Conventioni* was published in 1606. The preface of the agreement stressed the interdependence of apothecaries and physicians as well as the hierarchy: "Neither can the Physician accomplish his goal without the ministry of the Apothecary, nor can the Apothecary fruitfully practice his salvific art without the *rule* of the Physician." The document evidenced the importance of hierarchy by affirming that "it is not for one person to both give orders and execute them."[75] To make sure no apothecary could claim ignorance of the agreement, the Protomedicato presented "the new orders" in person to sixty-four apothecaries in Bologna.[76] At the same time the conventions were published, the Senate issued a new edition of the Bolognese *Antidotarium*.[77] Together, the *Conventioni* and the *Antidotarium* marked, once again, the boundaries of the apothecary profession. The vice-legate's involvement represented papal legates' increasing intervention into local affairs to pacify the city toward the end of the pontificate of Pope Clement VIII (1592–1605). The legates' interference undermined local institutions, emboldened single-interest groups, and weakened the formation of a local oligarchy as a single interlocutor of the papal power, all while claiming to protect the mercantile and lower classes from aristocratic abuse and machinations.[78]

Apothecaries were unhappy with the *Conventioni* and did not respect them. They continued to sell medicaments without prescription and give medical advice to patients, just as they had been doing for centuries. In 1617, just over a decade after the agreement, the cardinal legate reissued a medical provision on the grounds that "especially apothecaries and barbers ... sell and give medicines and poisons without prescription, and they themselves want to act as physicians, and the majority among them has not guaranteed that they carry good stuff [*robbe buone*] in their shops."[79] Apothecaries continued to "act as physicians," encroaching on the latter's responsibilities. One apothecary admitted that the "College was full of vicious, very ignorant, and rogue men, who pretend to know medicaments better than apothecaries."[80]

The conflict between apothecaries and physicians unfolded at a time when, as Gianna Pomata has demonstrated, preoccupations about the quality of medical goods and services resonated across social strata and the role of the Protomedicato was widely accepted. The legitimate of the Protomedico came primarily from its role as guardian of medical knowledge, as a body within the Collegio Medico.[81] Throughout the early modern period, people in several capacities actively used the Protomedicato to press charges against physicians, healers, and sellers of medicaments, on the grounds of medical abuses.[82] Apothecaries conformed to such a context, and in their petitions used the same language as patients, pushing the Protomedicato to enforce the rules. Apothecaries stressed that, if they had to follow regulations, others should as well: "If you [the Protomedicato], only punish those who prescribe although they could not, you also have to punish those who give them [medicines] even if they should not because they know nothing of the art."[83] For example, both apothecaries and patients issued complaints against druggist Antonio Cardoni, who sold pills, syrups, decoctions of manna and cassia, and other medicines without permission, and was accused of making many mistakes. Even worse, Cardoni sold these goods to private citizens as well as to traders, such as an agent (*sensale*) working in the public square who resold the medicines, and a "farmer who acts as a physician in the mountain." The plaintiffs suggested that the Protomedico burn Cardoni's merchandise in the public square.[84]

Bolognese apothecaries failed to demonstrate authority in their petitions, and were also unable to build scientific authority and prestige. Throughout these chapters we have encountered many learned apothecaries, not least from Venice, Naples, Lucca, and Mantua, but none was from Bologna. Attempts by Bolognese apothecaries to bolster their status as men of science were scarce, ineffective, or actively stopped by the city's Protomedico and physicians. In 1613 Francesco Sartorio celebrated his production of theriac at the Santa Maria della Morte hospital, and promoted himself as a learned apothecary with a theriac *celebration*.[85] Soon after, the Protomedico issued a restriction (*Editto d'inhibitione*) affirming that Sartorio's booklet contained "many lies," and prohibited its circulation.[86] It is possible that another tentative attempt by apothecaries to establish their scientific authority was their founding of an academy of the *speziali medicinalisti*, those among their number who were approved to make and sell medicines. The academy met at the convent of San Francesco beginning in 1647, focusing on the production of chemical remedies. Unfortunately no further information on the academy has survived.[87]

Among the few publications authored by Bolognese apothecaries are Adriano Riccardi's *Istruttione intorno al comporre la Theriaca d'Andromaco* (1606) and *Venticinque discorsi del modo di preparare i semplici medicinali* (1613). Little is known about Riccardi, other than that he was the benefactor of a well-known comedian, Domenico Bruni.[88] In the latter text, addressed to the "Young scholars of the apothecary art," Riccardi sought to elevate his art, and affirmed that "the Apothecary Art is the first among all the manual arts."[89] According to him, the "nobility" of the apothecary came both from the "quality of the instruments" and the goals of their work. Because apothecaries used all possible materials to preserve human health—"animate, inanimate, sensitive, without sense"—Riccardi placed apothecaries above jewelers, who used only gold and precious stones to adorn. Apothecary art was also "nobilissima" because it derived from the work of a king, Mithradates.[90] By drawing on such traditional arguments, Riccardi insisted that apothecaries were only one small step behind physicians.

Not a word on the nobility of the art, nor a comment on the character of the ideal apothecary, can be found in *Gl'indirizzi dell'arte dello spetiale medicinalista* (1658), a booklet by Ovidio Montalbani published on behalf of the medical college, of which he was a preeminent member.⁹¹ Montalbani was a famous physician, better known for his astrological work. He had also authored a book against innovation using astrology, *Antineotiologia cioé discorso contro le novità co gli astrologici presagij dell'anno 1662*.⁹² Similar to Riccardi's text, Montalbani's booklet was written to "methodically" educate aspiring apothecaries. In contrast to the pompous and hyperbolic prose typical of Montalbani's medical writings, *Gl'indirizzi dell'arte dello spetiale medicinalista* is succinct and direct. The first thirty-two pages present lists of substances—earths, stones, herbs, flowers, seeds, animals, and animal parts—followed by a brief review of the procedures necessary to compound these materials.⁹³ The spirit of this work was summarized in the final Latin motto: *Sutor, ne ultra crepidam*—"Shoemaker, not beyond the shoe." An apothecary should not have ambitions beyond his area of expertise.

The Collegio Medico was the repository of medical knowledge, which was the reason for its responsibility toward the community, which it fulfilled in many ways, such as by controlling the quality of medicaments. In the public discourse, such as in the introductions to public documents, the medical role of the Collegio often intertwined with maintaining the social order and fortifying the social hierarchy. For example, in *Bandi e Provisioni*, a compendium of laws jointly issued by all public authorities in 1617, the discussion of the quality of medical cures and goods was interwoven with that of poverty relief and care for the poor.⁹⁴ *Bandi* presented medical laws as protection for people living in poverty, stating that "especially the poor, who do not know"—who were not able to distinguish between medicaments—"mostly suffered from illicit sales."⁹⁵ Being poor was taken to correlate with greater ignorance, and ignorance increased one's vulnerability to fraud. Following the principle of distributive justice (which maintains that the differences between social groups are "natural"), society's upper echelons tasked themselves with protecting the weakest. Whereas the Collegio Medico occupied an authoritative position in the city, apothecaries were merchants as much as artisans. This liminal social position meant they were caught in a public discourse they did not have the language to oppose.⁹⁶

Furthermore, apothecaries' real thorn in the side were religious apothecary shops. Since the Middle Ages, especially in rural areas, monasteries had been crucial centers for the practice of medicine. Monasteries' production of medicines continued and even increased during the Renaissance. Some monasteries, such as the Aracoeli monastery in Rome and the convent of San Salvatore in Bologna, became renowned hubs of pharmaceutical experimentation. Religious people and their products had two inherent advantages over apothecaries: their symbolic association with divine healing forces, and a certain freedom, because they operated outside the guilds. The sale of remedies was often a major source of income for monasteries, as Sharon Strocchia has shown in the case of Florentine nuns.[97] To compete with religious healers, as I have argued elsewhere, apothecaries claimed that their art was driven by quasi-religious motivations, and that they themselves were merciful caregivers granting assistance to their patients.[98]

Bolognese apothecaries perceived monasteries' production as wrongful competition and lobbied to protect their businesses. In 1574 apothecaries petitioned the city authorities to prevent the "infinite damage" that monastery shops were causing to apothecaries, patients, and even to themselves, since monks and nuns were not supposed to trade (*fare mercantie*). Apothecaries accused monasteries of both smuggling foreign remedies into the city by pretending they were for their personal use, and producing medicines without the supervision of the Protomedico.[99] In 1606 apothecaries managed to have an article added to the *Conventioni* stating that if monasteries were to sell medicaments, they too should follow the *Antidotarium*.[100] Monasteries did not heed this ruling.

One of the many reasons apothecaries resented monastery apothecary shops was that they produced and sold theriac. When the father apothecary at the Certosa, a little convent just outside the city, advertised that he was gathering the ingredients to make many doses of theriac in an "unusual" ceremony, the outraged apothecary guild petitioned the Protomedico against it.[101] As they had before, apothecaries complained in 1677 that both regular and secular convent apothecary shops were selling medicaments publicly and dispensing remedies without recipes. While apothecaries were "forced to make theriac," monastery apothecary shops sold medicines and "especially theriac against the forms, good orders, and conventions, with great damage for the shops that spend so much to make it. And in particular the apothecary shop at the convent of S. Domenico sells medicines and especially theriac in greater quantity than all the apothecaries put together. In the meantime, apothecary father Lodovico prepares the ingredients to make a bigger dose of theriac than the one made officially this year. Since the Protomedico is so zealous, it should take care of this."[102] Bologna's most important conventual center, the apothecary shop of S. Domenico was a major retailer of medicines, and sold more theriac than the apothecaries just meters from the Collegio Medico. In 1678, a year after the apothecaries' petition, the Protomedicato held its first inspection of the hospital of Santa Maria della Morte, which was run by a religious brotherhood.[103] Thus, while the Papal States nominally empowered Protomedico to regulate all pharmaceutical production, boundaries were barely enforced.

Apothecaries' reluctance to make theriac derived not only from their resentment of monasteries' unlawful competition and illegal sellers and smugglers, but also from the lack of control they had over its revenues. Making theriac according to the pharmacopoeia's standards required a number of costly ingredients, an expensive procedure, and the ceremonial apparatus, which religious apothecaries probably did not follow as accurately. Moreover, the retail price of official theriac was set by authorities. In 1607 apothecaries sought permission to sell theriac at 10 soldi per drachm, and lobbied for a three-year ban on imports of foreign theriac. Instead the Collegio Medico and the cardinal legate decided that theriac should be sold at 4 soldi and 16 denari per drachm in order not to "weigh on the population."[104] Over the course of the century, the price of theriac in Bologna oscillated between 4 soldi and 16 denari and 2 soldi and 6 denari per drachm (roughly a dose), in line with other Italian states.[105]

Apothecaries never clearly disclosed how much a production of theriac cost.[106] During a trial in 1754, apothecaries declared three different ways of calculating the final production cost. An anonymous reviewer underlined this opacity: "These are three models, but the truth is one." Again in 1795 the apothecaries offered another example of their murkiness in an almost untranslatable text: "The compound is expected to yield 1,235 pounds, of which we want only 1,200 pounds, from which 50 pounds are removed as a donation, leaving 1,150 pounds, which are also expected to be 1,100 pounds. If 1,100 pounds cost 2,263 lire, each pound will cost 2 ½ lire. Considering it only 1,000 pounds, each pound costs 2 lire, 5 soldi, and 4 denari. The whole thing is a jumble of no account, and if the theriac were only 900 pounds, it would cost 50 bajocchi per pound."[107] In the seventeenth century, the lack of officially produced theriac embarrassed the Collegio Medico and the cardinal legate, so they found alternative solutions. In 1639 the college entrusted a single apothecary, Paolo de Aldrovandis, to make theriac in the university courtyard because the apothecary guild had affirmed its inability to produce it. In 1642 theriac was made in the monastery of the Carthusians.[108] In 1665 Michelangelo Butij, a Roman apothecary nicknamed "the Idiot" (*l'Idiota Spetiale*), made theriac in the apothecary shop of the convent of San Salvatore, with great publicity. Verses were composed for the occasion in both Latin and the vernacular: "Today, for you, Michel, by changing [viper] considerably made it a weapon for life."[109] Theriac may have been a weapon against disease, but in seventeenth-century Bologna it was also a weapon against apothecaries.

Compared to their Venetian colleagues, Bolognese apothecaries were indecisive in their publishing, as well as slow at reforming their guild. The Bolognese apothecary guild did not reform its statutes until 1689, putatively to formalize the order of the guild's management: "In present times, [the guild] is ruled more by the discretion of those who govern it than by laws and statutes."[110] The reform project was meant to bring peace to the guild's administration by creating a structure whereby a small group of people held most of the power. The new statutes promised to rationalize the relationships between the city's apothecaries by relaxing guild membership criteria while tightening access to its governing bodies. This was an elitist project. The first ten of thirty-two articles regulated access to the two governing bodies of the guild, the *Larga* and the *Stretta*. Such division was influenced by the example of lay confraternities that since the fifteenth century had established a *Larga* and a *Stretta* to manage levels of participation.[111] The *Larga* was the assembly of all fee-paying apothecaries enrolled in the guild, while the *Stretta* was a council of twenty-four members. As with the old statutes, membership of the *Stretta* required proof of citizenship dating back at least two generations. The new statutes additionally restricted access to the *Stretta*: members could only pass their privilege to their sons or relatives patrilineally.[112] Only when a family line died could a new family enter the *Stretta*. The *de facto* restriction of guild governance to families already belonging to the *Stretta*, combined with the exclusively patrilineal inheritance of membership, created an elite corps.

The guild and its oligarchy oversaw a larger group of merchants and artisans known as the "observants" (*obbedienti*), who were required to pay an annual fee to the guild to pursue their activities. Among their number was every artisan making remedies, including Galenic, spagyric, and distilled waters; producers of wax, paper (from rags), and sweets and sweet beverages; druggists, perfumers, confectioners, and colorists; and sellers of oil, olives, wafers, and tobacco, be they itinerant or selling in shops or private houses.[113] Observants' annual fees constituted the guild's primary source of income, and was gathered by collectors whose license lasted three years.

The new statutes also reaffirmed the guild's monopoly over theriac and mithridate productions, which had to be made publicly, financed by the guild, and sold to retailers. The statutes declared apothecaries' determination to make theriac and reinstated a prohibition against importing theriac or mithridate, a protectionist measure typical of most apothecaries' statutes.[114] The reformed guild was not only an elitist project based on a limited group of families and patrilineality, but also extractive, with a few families managing all the profits: from the observants, from sales of theriac and mithridate, and from the investments and businesses made in the name of the guild. If anything, the project was *too* exclusive; by 1754 the *Stretta* had a mere six overburdened members, and the entrance fee was lowered considerably to attract new members who had previously refused to enter because of the exorbitant cost of membership.[115] The guild's reform did not put an end to conflict over the price of theriac and its production, but in the eighteenth century the apothecaries were able to better defend their monopoly and profit from sales.[116]

Writing the history of the Venetian Collegio Medico, an eighteenth-century author presented the powerful apothecary guild in diminishing terms, stressing its dependence on the Giustizia Vecchia and apothecaries' low status as mechanical artisans: "At the beginning, [Venetian] apothecaries represented a body of only little reputation, which, like all the other mechanical arts, depended on the magistrates of the Giustizia Vecchia ... Toward the end of the sixteenth century, this body sought nobilitation."[117] These words should be read as an admission of weakness by the Collegio Medico. The college was never able to establish its preeminence over the apothecaries and, aware of its relative weakness, showed animus toward apothecaries well into the eighteenth century. Cognizant of and consistent with their own position within this power dynamic, apothecaries ran profitable businesses and contributed to the state coffers. The case of the honey dispute presented in this chapter shows that the Venetian political authorities prioritized the lucrative business of theriac over the medical innovations of physicians.

The political economies of Venice and Bologna drove the outcome of conflicts between the cities' apothecary guilds and medical colleges. Bologna's apothecary guild was less successful than Venice's at resisting efforts by the Collegio Medico and the political authorities to curb its autonomy, at least until the eighteenth century. Strong state support for the college and the prestige of the city's university meant the authority of collegiate physicians was never seriously challenged in Bologna. The state, the papal administration, and the Senate supported the hierarchical dominance of the Collegio Medico over all medical professions, and justified this position by embracing physicians' claims of medical authority. Apothecaries' attempts to establish their own scientific authority were timid and ineffective. Given theriac's symbolic importance, the Collegio Medico tried to compel apothecaries to make it, but eventually had to rely on monasteries and foreign apothecaries to keep up with demand.

These two case studies have shown that the state was neither the instigator of the contest for pharmacy nor a passive bystander. States favored apothecaries or physicians depending on the local political economy. Venice and Bologna diverged greatly in their economies, forms of government, and international relevance. Yet rather than political differences determining the outcome of conflicts between the two cities' medical professions, the political authorities' interests with respect to pharmacy often proved the deciding factor. Theriac was a state drug in the seventeenth century, and as such it was a preservative of the social hierarchy.

III

Paradoxes of Success

CHAPTER 7

From "Antidote of All Antidotes" to Pharmaceutical Monster

*B*ETWEEN THE 1650s and the 1750s, missionaries, soldiers, and merchants took theriac with them around the world and initiated productions abroad. In the meantime in Europe, apothecaries were producing theriacal spirits, waters, and chemical Celestial theriac alongside Theriaca magna, and exhibits of theriac were becoming ever more elaborate, in a triumph of wealth, medical authority, and commercial wisdom. Local versions of theriac were produced in the Dutch and Portuguese Empires, while theriac exports gained momentum in the Russian and Ottoman Empires. In the 1720s, theriac served as a yardstick for determining suppliers of medicines for the Royal African Company. Even the Chinese imperial court adopted theriac. The global spread of the remedy is in itself testament to the diffusion of Galenic pharmacy around the world.

At the heart of the ever-growing British Empire in 1745, at the peak of theriac's global popularity, English physician William Heberden published *Antitheriaka. Essay on Theriac and Mithridatium* after having taught materia medica at Cambridge for ten years. Heberden found Mithradates's knowledge of simples to be "very inconsiderable"; Pompey, who took care to secure Mithradates's recipes, was "possessed with the vulgar opinion";

the medicine found in Mithradates's cabinet was "a trivial one"; and, in previous eras, "people in the dark" had given too much credit to "ignorant" old physicians. Theriac and mithridate, followed Heberden, were no more than charms and amulets "delivered down to us by witchcraft." Furthermore, he affirmed, the fortunes of theriac among patients were on the wane.[1] Heberden's authoritative verdict influenced the deletion of theriac and mithridate from the 1756 *Edinburgh Pharmacopoeia*, the first such text to expunge the two electuaries. This was especially notable because Edinburgh housed a flourishing and influential medical school at the time. The expunction was a calamitous blow to theriac; historian David Cowen considered it a landmark in the history of pharmacy.[2]

However, the demise of theriac was not a quick, uniform, or straightforward process. In northern Europe, productions ceased a few years after Heberden's *Antitheriaka*—in Nuremberg in 1754 and in Delft in 1763, for example—but most pharmacopoeias were slower than Edinburgh's to expunge theriac. The *London Pharmacopoeia* first simplified the theriac recipe in 1746, but it took until 1788 for the Royal College of Physicians to remove theriac definitively.[3] Simplified versions of the remedy ("reformed theriac") continued to appear in pharmacopoeias across Europe throughout the nineteenth century.[4] Meanwhile in Paris, the Société libre des Pharmaciens de Paris performed the last theriac-making ceremony in 1798.[5] In Bologna and Naples, the arrival of the French army terminated public productions of theriac; they resumed with the Restoration, but by this point they had permanently lost their grandeur. In the Kingdom of Naples, official productions continued until the fall of the Bourbons and the unification of Italy in 1860.

A comprehensive narrative of theriac's global diffusion and final demise in the eighteenth century is beyond the scope of this work, which has been to provide an account of the establishment of early modern theriac as a state drug, with a focus on the Italian peninsula. In this chapter, though, alongside an overview of theriac's trajectory in eighteenth-century Italy, I will survey the expansion of theriac in trans-imperial contexts in the seventeenth and eighteenth centuries. Both aspects of theriac's history are related to theriac's status as state drug. Theriac enjoyed global diffusion and success *because* of its official prestige and primacy in Galenic pharmacy. Within the medical, commercial, and political institutions of the ancien régime, theriac's status as a state drug expedited its geographical expansion and increased production, both locally and worldwide.

At the same time, I will discuss theriac's demise in eighteenth-century Italy by analyzing medical, cultural, and economic sources. As production escalated across most of the eighteenth century, theriac lost favor with a portion of the higher classes and lost prestige, influenced by changing medical ideas and theriac's demise in northern Europe. Physicians were reluctant to express skepticism about theriac, especially when they were part of the medical hierarchy. They supported Galenic pharmacy because it was official pharmacy, and they provided the drug to the many patients who continued to favor it. But socioeconomic groups that were pushing for new political and cultural structures, such as the emerging bourgeoisie, saw theriac and Galenic pharmacy as vestiges of the past, warranting scrutiny. Divergent conceptions of medicine coexisted in the same spaces. The elites of the ancien régime and the bourgeoisie inhabited the same cities, patronized the same apothecary shops, and relied on the same medical institutions. Because Galenic pharmacy was still the official pharmacy of Italy, the overlap of the old and the new science—two orders of knowledge, in Foucauldian terms—led to either embarrassed silences among physicians or choices justified by utilitarian arguments.[6] In this context, only the fall of the ancien régime could ultimately dethrone theriac, by dismantling apothecaries' privileges and reforming the medical system.

This political interpretation of the fall of theriac challenges the claim that the expunction of theriac from pharmacopoeias was a "victory for science."[7] Indeed, such an argument has already been objected to, as Alex Berman argued, if the English rejected theriac before the French, it could not have been because France lacked competent scientists.[8] In Italy, with its own cadre of skilled scientists, the displacement of theriac from its privileged position was much more a political and social affair than a medical or scientific one. Canceling the guild system and proclaiming by law a new order of knowledge swept theriac away as an official drug and a beacon of the state. Nonetheless, many patients continued to use theriac, although it slowly morphed into a relic of yesteryear, favored only by traditionalists.

In the first section of this chapter I explore theriac's various global transformations in the late seventeenth and eighteenth centuries. Sometimes theriac's introduction into non-European cultures was tied to colonization and conquest, as was the case with the Dutch and Portuguese Empires. Elsewhere, in the Russian, Ottoman, and Chinese Empires, which were not subject to European military conquest, either commercial trends or leaders' own political objectives provided fertile soil for theriac's adoption. In these cases, the prestige enjoyed by theriac and Galenic pharmacy in Europe was paramount to facilitating its adoption overseas. Theriac's ever-expanding diversity and metamorphoses around the globe defy any single interpretation, but the geographical diffusion of Galenic pharmacy across the centuries was fostered by its official status.

In the second section I focus on theriac in eighteenth-century Italy. Initially it looked like findings about the social depreciation of theriac contradicted emerging data on its production. Theriac production was increasing, yet its prestige was clearly declining. When we place these findings against the European background of medical and scientific change and the emerging fashion of the bourgeoisie, it becomes evident that there was a shift among consumers. Demand for theriac grew high, especially among the lower classes, those the bourgeoisie called "the vulgar."[9] Following northern European medical and cultural trends, learned society turned away from theriac toward simpler remedies, while also abandoning wonders and the marvelous. Metaphors of theriac evolved in response, and its status dwindled. Actors in popular eighteenth-century plays asserted that old women were "only good to make theriac." With their typical educational and paternalistic approach, end-of-the-century periodicals associated theriac with the lowlier figures of the social hierarchy: women, humble workers, "savages," and animals. Once the drug of Marcus Aurelius and Nero, theriac was now good for cows.

Global Metamorphoses of a State Drug

European colonizers' desire to find new spices, crops, and materia medica was a defining feature of the early modern period. This apparently unquenchable thirst drove much of European exploration, conquest, and exploitation of lands and people. But less well known is that, along with familiar animals, seeds, and plants, Europeans took with them preparations of Galenic pharmacy, including theriac.[10] Having their own medicines and comfort goods helped Europeans settle far from home and retain their identity while sharing their customs with or imposing them on other populations. Theriac was often included in the personal baggage of missionaries and explorers. In 1655 Jean-François Mousnier, minister at the Vincentian mission of Fort Dauphin, Madagascar, wrote to Vincent de Paul (1581–1660), head of the order, to instruct on what new missionaries should pack. Among other things he mentioned theriac and orviétan.[11] Europeans did not always consider their remedies superior to those of indigenous peoples. Describing the antidotes in use among the Illinois nation, explorer Robert de la Salle (1643–1687) wrote that the Illinois "know several herbs which are a quicker and surer remedy against their [serpents'] venom than our treacle and orviétan."[12] De la Salle, however, also administered theriac to the Illinois, who apparently appreciated it.[13] The exchange of remedies was part of this encounter.

New versions of theriac developed in overseas empires when producers of theriac in Asia and South America adapted its recipe to local materia medica. By substituting ingredients, Europeans converted previously unknown local plants into Galenic elements, incorporating the new and blending it with tradition. With its well-documented and far-reaching pharmaceutical activities, the Jesuit order was one of the institutions responsible for popularizing theriac beyond Europe. The Jesuits' involvement in pharmacy encompassed a wide variety of activities: imports and exports of medicaments and materia medica through commercial, charitable, and patronage channels; the writing of pharmacopoeias and studies of natural history and materia medica; the exchange and appropriation of healing practices through intense relationships with local populations; and, of course, bioprospecting.[14] As part of their medical activities in the Portuguese Empire, the Jesuits destined a section of their colleges and of their principal residencies in Brazil to infirmaries, including that in Bahia, established at least as early as 1598. Here they began producing medicaments using materia medica imported from Europe. "Close to it [the infirmary], there was the pharmacy, which also supplied outsiders. And, in cases of epidemic or public calamity, the college's pharmacy was everyone's pharmacy."[15] However, the high costs of importing ingredients, combined with the Jesuits' growing knowledge of local plants and collaboration with native practitioners, gradually led them to modify the recipes.[16] In the eighteenth century (and possibly earlier), the Jesuits developed *Triaga brasilica,* made primarily with local plants. Triaga brasilica was defined as "legendary," and became the Jesuits' most prized compound.[17] It was compared to Theriaca magna from Rome or Venice for its versatility, efficacy, and prestige.[18] Triaga brasilica was prescribed as an antidote against poisons, venoms, and a wide variety of ailments.[19] While in Europe a theriac with too many substitutes was deemed low-quality or even fake, an eighteenth-century author reported, "If it [Triaga brasilica] is not better than theriac from Europe, it is not inferior to it in any respect."[20] Thus, Triaga brasilica was conceived of as a new product built on ancient foundations.

The creation of Triaga brasilica slotted neatly into the Jesuits' wider project of evangelization. They conceptualized pharmacy and healing as tools with which they could gain the confidence of indigenous populations and then conquer them and spread Christianity, while discrediting local healers by proving the worth of Christian pharmacy—that is, Galenic. Local medical knowledge, such as the healing properties of plants and safe dosage, was gained through several practices, including confession.[21] In line with the Jesuits' objectives, in Bahia the recipe of the new Triaga brasilica became a secret, contrasting with the recipe of Theriaca magna in Europe, which was never hidden away from the public eye.[22] Such secrecy enhanced the Jesuits' authority and boosted the commercial value of the recipe itself. In 1760, when the Jesuits suddenly had to leave the college, one particularly astute officer made sure he got a copy of the recipe before anyone else, hoping to auction it for a considerable sum.[23]

Triaga brasilica enjoyed some circulation in Europe, certainly in Portugal, showcasing how pharmaceutical knowledge and practice could spread globally, adapt locally, then recirculate in their new formulation. The 1697 edition of *Polyanthea medicinal,* a popular medical compendium written by the Portuguese pharmacist João Curvo Semedo (1635–1719), did not mention Triaga brasilica.[24] However, a substantial addition enriched the 1716 edition: a celebration of the numerous simples and compounds that "from East India, America, and other parts of the world come to our kingdom to heal many illnesses," which instructed how and when to use these remedies. The text presented Triaga brasilica as an antidote especially effective against venomous animals, made in Brazil with local ingredients. It is not clear from the document whether Portuguese patients or physicians could actually buy the compound.[25] The Jesuit headquarters in Rome received ample information on Triaga brasilica, and a few samples, too.[26]

Similarly, in the Dutch Empire the recipe of theriac changed to include local ingredients. Within their fortified outposts, the Dutch built several hospitals with apothecary shops for soldiers, state officials, civilians, and travelers. There is no evidence that the local population was granted access to these medical facilities.[27] Rather than establishing a connection with the indigenous populations through medicine and pharmacy in the manner of the Portuguese, the Dutch of the United East India Company (VOC) relied on a familiar array of remedies.[28] This does not mean that the Dutch were indifferent to local materia medica. In fact, beginning in the mid-1660s the VOC hired physicians and chemists to learn about local medicinal plants and find substitutes for medicines imported from the Netherlands. VOC officials sought to save on the cost of exporting materia medica from Europe and Batavia (now Jakarta), and to provide specimens for wealthy Dutch collectors, the main beneficiaries of Dutch bioprospecting.[29] Eventually Dutch physicians and chemists discovered suitable substitutes. They also made a commerce of theriac in the area. According to Swedish naturalist Carl Peter Thunberg (1743–1828), Dutchmen from Batavia trading in Japan on behalf of the VOC in the seventeenth century brought theriac to sell to the Japanese, but it is uncertain where it came from.[30]

Between 1656 and 1796, the Dutch ruled Sri Lanka, where they founded several hospitals. Working for several years in the Colombo hospital was Swedish physician Hermanus Nicolaas Grimm (1641–1711). He authored *Insulae Ceyloniae thesaurus medicus laboratorim* (1679), which listed recipes for pharmaceutical preparations made with local ingredients and used by the physicians and local population of Sri Lanka. The book also included recipes for Theriaca magna, mithridate, and a *Theriaca ceylonica*, all made with local ingredients. Grimm extolled the virtues of Theriaca ceylonica, which did not induce sleep, and claimed that one scruple worked better than a pound of any "deceitful theriac." He went further still, asserting that the products purveyed by "sellers of theriac roaming throughout the entire world" should be prohibited.[31] The earliest official Dutch pharmacopoeia recorded in Sri Lanka, from 1757, listed both a Theriac of Andromachus and a Theriacal spirit, a distillation of theriac, but there was no mention of Theriaca ceylonica.[32] However, the recipe for Theriac of Andromachus included ingredients such as cubeba, a particular kind of pepper; calumba (*Jateorhiza palmata*), a plant from East Africa; and ekaweriya (*Rauwolfia serpentina*), a local plant used in Ayurvedic medicine.[33] In the Dutch empire as well as among the Jesuits in the Portuguese Empire, theriac retained its therapeutic connotations of antidote against venoms, poisons, and diseases, even though apothecaries had transformed its recipe with local ingredients.

Theriac was also employed in the British Empire. Unlike the Dutch and the Portuguese, British physicians and surgeons never initiated local productions; instead, in Africa and North America they relied on theriac imported from England or Europe, and often prescribed it as an antidote.[34] In 1733 Joseph Moseley, a surgeon at a holding facility for enslaved people in the Gambia region prescribed theriac (along with Peruvian bark) to treat fever.[35] According to John Atkins's 1742 edition of *The Navy-Surgeon*, theriac was one of the nine medicines navy surgeons were expected to carry with them.[36]

Theriac also appears in a cautionary tale of the dangers the English might encounter in Africa, narrated by physician Robert Boyle: "In another part of *Africa*, a famous Knight, who commanded the *English* there, and lately died a ship-board in his way home, was so poysoned at a parting Treat, by a young *Negro* Woman of Quality, whom he had enjoy'd and declin'd to take with him, according to his promise, into *Europe*. And though my Relator early gave him notice of what he suspected to be the cause of this Indisposition, and engag'd him thereupon to take Antidotes, and Cordials, as Treacle, *&c.* yet his languishing distemper still increased, till it kill'd him."[37] In retelling this episode, Boyle was warning his countrymen to be careful when entertaining relationships with African women, to not overestimate their naivety or underestimate their presumed propensity toward poison. Neither theriac nor other medicines (civilizing objects) could be of help if they disregarded the danger of misleading locals with false promises.

It is unsurprising that Englishmen occupied in running an empire would carry theriac. More unexpected is the fact that the Royal African Company used theriac as a yardstick in the Atlantic commerce of humans. In 1720 the Royal African Company decided to reconsider the drug supply contract for the slave trade; supplying such drugs was a highly lucrative business run by a select few apothecaries. During tendering, the Company asked London apothecary James Goodwin to produce theriac in a bid against the two apothecaries who held the contract. Goodwin produced theriac at a lower price and soon supplanted the two apothecaries as sole supplier of drugs for the slave ships.[38] As previously mentioned, no single approach to theriac is detectable in imperial settings. The British brought theriac along for medical purposes, and the Royal African Company used it to determine commercial partners in the slave trade. They neither used theriac as a means to acquire prestige and credibility among indigenous populations, like the Jesuits with Triaga brasilica, nor transformed it, like the Dutch in their official pharmacopoeia in Sri Lanka.

The Chinese and Russians also differed in their adoption of theriac, depending on local circumstances. These regions embraced Theriaca magna only when doing so became politically favorable, mainly for internal reasons. In China, theriac arrived repeatedly across the centuries. Its initial introduction came in the Low Middle Age, when a Byzantine embassy brought it along the Silk Road as a gift to the emperor.[39] Then during the Yuan (1271-1368), Ming (1368-1644), and Qing (1644-1912) dynasties, theriac was included in several medical commentaries, transliterated as *deliyage* or *diyejia*.[40] The author of the *Bencao gangmu*, a sixteenth-century encyclopedia of Chinese materia medica, misread or misrendered a character, labeling the compound "pig gall bladder."[41] As Carla Nappi has argued, this represented a normalization of Galenic pharmacy: from a complex compound, theriac was translated into a simple ingredient in the Chinese medical framework.[42] Something similar happened in Tibet. An eighth-century Tibetan text introduced the word *daryakan*, whose origin has been traced to the Persian word *taryak*, a dark-red remedy for snakebite. Over time, *daryakan* became *daryakan smugpo*, "treacle berries," a dark-red berry used in medical preparations.[43] These two examples show that an artifact—however complex—arriving from a foreign culture might lose its meaning and be normalized through known terms.

Ultimately, despite repeated introductions into China over the course of many centuries, theriac failed to generate enough momentum to be integrated into the Chinese medical framework. Only in the late seventeenth century did the Qing court appropriated and attempted to indigenize theriac. Jesuit missionaries had brought it to China both as a gift to the emperor and for their own use.[44] Philippe Couplet (1623?-1693) brought theriac from Goa to Macau along with icons and glasses.[45] As described in the Introduction, theriac was used in the imperial court of Emperor Kangxi. When the physician of the Chinese court diagnosed a Jesuit's illness in Chinese medical terms, he nonetheless prescribed theriac, thereby incorporating it into his practice.

As part of his policy, Emperor Kangxi welcomed Jesuits and their knowledge at court. Because the Qing dynasty had originated in Manchuria, outside of China, he chose to promote a multicultural identity within his court, one more open to foreign cultures than traditional Han culture. Thus, the emperor's interest in theriac was as much political as medical, perhaps even more so. The symbolic values attached to theriac in Europe facilitated its acceptance at the Qing court. For an emperor eager to receive foreign suggestions that aligned with his wider political objectives, theriac was an excellent instrument.[46] At the Chinese court, theriac retained the social meaning it had enjoyed in sixteenth- and seventeenth-century Europe, if not its medical meaning—which further research could clarify.

Theriac in Russia was also tied to imperial objectives, which shows that religious rules and cultural values could either hamper or facilitate the adoption of foreign medicines. Traditionally the Russian Orthodox Church was reluctant to embrace medicines compounded with animal or human flesh, such as theriac and *mumia,* allegedly made with resinous exudate scraped out from embalmed Egyptian mummies. These medicines violated religious rules on the consumption of poisonous creatures and the proper treatment of dead bodies. This reluctance manifested in outright bans in 1620, when theriac was prohibited. Therefore, in Russia during the first half of the seventeenth century, theriac was neither imported nor prescribed.

However, starting in the 1660s (before the birth of Peter the Great) and throughout the early eighteenth century, theriac came into use in Russia. As Claire Griffin has argued, this was the outcome of religious, cultural, and political changes tied to the politics of Westernization. In this context, the czar Peter the Great (1672–1725) pushed to shift attitudes regarding animal flesh and dead bodies, such as by opening a museum displaying anatomical specimens. Furthermore, the Russian Orthodox Church changed the cult regarding the bodies of dead saints; indeed, one of the czar's advisors even used theriac as a positive metaphor in his sermons, as it was usual in Western Europe. During the 1730s to 1750s, as a consequence of this politics, theriac was listed in the Russian tariff, and the Medical Chancery made regular use of both Theriaca magna and Theriaca coelestis, even sending them to the army.[47]

Unlike all abovementioned cases, the success of Venetian theriac in the eighteenth-century Eastern Mediterranean was unrelated to colonization, conquest, and internal political objectives. Populations in the Ottoman Empire, such as Turks, Egyptians, Greeks, and Arabs, needed no introduction to theriac: Galenic pharmacy was an integral element of their medical culture. In fact, until the late sixteenth century Egyptian theriac enjoyed great prestige in Italy, and Turkish theriac figured as a valuable gift to Christian princes, dukes, and ambassadors. Although it still needs further investigation, Venetian theriac's popularity in the eighteenth-century Ottoman Empire should be understood as part of a widespread appreciation for Western consumption goods, including colonial goods, such as sugar and cheap coffee from the Antilles, and European manufactures, such as textiles, porcelain, and timepieces.[48]

Local production of theriac endured in Egypt and Turkey well into the seventeenth century. Ottoman traveler Derviş Mehmed Zillî, known as Evliya Çelebi (1611–1682), left a detailed account of the grandiosity of the productions (*Tiryaki Faruk*) performed in the Qualaáun hospital in Cairo. The elaborate manufacturing process involved the harvesting and subsequent killing of thousands of extremely venomous snakes. Çelebi reported that the Egyptians exported their theriac to Anatolia, Persia, Arabia, and Europe, and also sent it as a gift to the "king of Dunkarkiz" (Dunkirk).[49] Similarly, in his first visit to Istanbul in the 1630s, French merchant and traveler Jean-Baptiste Tavernier (1605–1689) reported that, at the imperial palace, it was "in the Cup-bearer's Apartment that the Treacle is made, which the Turks call Tiriak-Faruk, and there is a great quantity of it made, because they use it as a Universal remedy, and charitably bestow it on all sorts of people, as well in City as Country."[50]

Toward the end of the seventeenth century, the medical marketplace of Istanbul became oriented more toward medicines than services, and expensive drugs became increasingly fashionable.[51] When Tavernier left for his journey in the 1660s, heading to Persia through Turkey, he took twenty-four vases of theriac. (None survived the trip: the theriac fermented because of the heat, and every vase broke over the course of the journey.)[52]

Why would Tavernier have taken theriac to Turkey, where it was plentiful and of good quality? Perhaps because it was a gift he had received from the Grand Duke of Tuscany, or because, by this time, the balance of prestige between Venetian and Eastern Mediterranean theriac had started to shift. Thus, when the English ambassador arrived in Istanbul in 1687, among the presents he brought for the Ottoman court was Venetian theriac. Accounting for the importance of gifts at the court, a historian noted, "One could say that the world of William Trumbull was held together by Venetian theriac."[53] Several accounts from the Venetian ambassadors (*baili*) in Istanbul reported that Ottoman officials valued Venetian theriac highly. Venetian officials brought theriac, along with velvet and mirrors, to lubricate their relationships with their Ottoman counterparts and obtain favors. In 1719 *bailo* Emo brought six vases of theriac.[54]

By the mid-eighteenth century, though, Venetians were exporting theriac as a good rather than as a gift. Especially after the treaty of Passarowitz in 1718, which favored the Austrians, the Venetians and Ottomans were both weakened militarily and had to reorganize. The French, English, and Dutch supplanted Venice as privileged commercial partners of the Ottoman Empire, and negotiated better tariff payments in the process. At the same time, other Adriatic ports became more competitive, such as Ancona and Trieste.[55] Although *bailo* Foscari lamented the declining appreciation of Venetian goods in Turkey in 1757, Venice remained an important commercial partner of the Ottoman Empire. However, Foscari also affirmed that theriac "was a singularity of Venetian production" because the remedy was "greatly valued here [Istanbul], beyond all belief."[56] Exports of Venetian theriac to Istanbul, Aleppo, Smyrna, Alexandria, Thessaloniki, and Larnaca (Cyprus) continued until at least the end of the century.[57] Between 1754 and the 1790s, Venetian merchants usually sent one or two trunks of theriac to their correspondents.[58] Venetian apothecaries, like the brothers Robustelli, apothecaries at the sign of the Silver Apple, advertised their products in Arabic to potential clients in the Ottoman Empire, informing them that their network reached as far as India.[59]

As in the past, commerce in "true" theriac was closely intertwined with commerce in "fake." To protect its theriac, the Venetian state used its leverage at the Ottoman court to prohibit imports from Trieste, whose apothecary shops had the same names as those in Venice.[60] To prevent forgeries, Venetian theriac was labeled and accompanied on its travels by documents from the Venetian Health Board. When he noticed discrepancies in its accompanying documents in 1793, Pietro Choch, Venetian consul in Thessaloniki, rejected an entire shipment of theriac, judging it to be "fake and foreign."[61] A process held in Venice in 1777 sheds light on the commerce and production of counterfeit theriac in the eighteenth-century Adriatic Sea. Such theriac was produced in Trieste in the Habsburg Empire, by Succi, a former laborer of a renowned Venetian apothecary shop. Once in Trieste, Succi worked as a nurse at the local hospital by day and produced theriac by night, packaging it with fake seals, labels, and virtues, identical to those of the most renowned Venetian producer of the time, the apothecary shop at the sign of the Golden Head. Succi's production lasted at least twenty-five years, and employed his son as well as several printers in Ferrara and Gorizia. Production was directed to commercial partners on the Dalmatian coast and in Puglia in southern Italy—and to the Ottoman Empire, where theriac was sold at 4-5 kuruş apiece, rather than the 7 kuruş apiece commanded by "true" Venetian theriac—but the two products were virtually undistinguishable to customers.[62] Even though the quantities of exported theriac the Venetians recorded in the account books were not impressive, the emphasis of *bailo* Foscari and the presence of frauds suggest that in the Ottoman Empire, Venetian theriac—both official and forged—was a profitable business. Demand remained lively until the end of the century.

The Persistence of Theriac in Italy

As it traveled around the world, theriac remained a topic of scientific investigation, albeit in diverse scenarios. Between the 1490s and 1650s, the most influential studies of and innovations surrounding theriac took place in the Italian states, but thereafter the center of gravity moved. In the field of medicine, the evolution of physiology and pathology in the seventeenth century cultivated ideas regarding the effects of materia medica on the body. Theoretical medical systems—iatrochemistry, iatrophysics, animism, vitalism—competed, compelling physicians to either confirm or refuse the use of traditional drugs, such as opium, and to advocate new specific drugs, such as Peruvian bark. Consequently experimentation on drugs became more and more relevant, to the point that Andreas-Holger Maehle has placed the origin of experimental pharmacology in the eighteenth century.[63] At the time, Italian universities were struggling to maintain their prestige in the face of rising European academies and scientific institutions, where new theories and experimentation abounded. Students were increasingly flocking to Leiden and Edinburgh over Bologna and Padua. Meanwhile, apothecaries were experimenting freely with chemical procedures, and exotica arrived by the boatload in Atlantic ports from all over the world.

By the eighteenth century, theriac was so entrenched in Italy's medical institutions as to seem immovable. However, medical ideas coming from abroad influenced both patients and medical practitioners. The response of Italian physicians to new medical approaches that discredited theriac was ambiguous: they continued prescribing it, albeit in moderation, and did not write against it—but between the lines appears growing skepticism about the remedy's efficacy and workings. This caused the slow but certain decline of theriac's prestige, and by the end of the century theriac had lost its status. This decline, though, was not reflected by a downscaling in production. Quite the contrary: production in Bologna and Venice consistently increased over the century. Theriac's appeal continued unabated, especially among the elites attached to the values of the ancien régime and the lower strata of the population.

Medical approaches toward theriac varied greatly. As we saw with the dispute between Francesco Redi and Moyse Charas, experiments and reflections on poisons and antidotes were popular in the seventeenth century. Several physicians tried to explain the contradictions of theriac *within* the Galenic framework. In 1700 Friedrich Hoffmann (1660–1742) and Jacques Descazals (fl. 1700) argued that in traditional complex compounds such as theriac, substances with different properties acted together to mitigate the effects of opium, thus justifying its numerous ingredients.[64] In doing this, Hoffmann and Descazals joined a long line of physicians, including Marco Oddo, physician at the University of Padua, who in 1583 published a table to systematize theriac's ingredients according to their humoral qualities and how they balanced one another.[65] Other physicians such as Charas did not even try to make such an argument, discarding it on the grounds that theriac was simply well known for being efficacious.[66]

Especially in the seventeenth century, French and English physicians condemned theriac and thought about writing against it, but refrained from publishing their ideas. In 1648 French physician Guy Patin (1601–1672) privately wrote a merciless attack on theriac, which remained only in manuscript form.[67] Later, in a private letter to Heinrich Meibomius (1638–1700), Patin requested a copy of Meibomius's father's treatise on theriac, published in Nuremberg in 1652, but nonetheless admitted that he looked upon theriac "with a twisted eye." Patin affirmed his plan to pen a treatise titled *Ergo nulli bono teriaca* (Thus theriac is no good to anyone), but this never came to fruition.[68] English physician Robert Boyle (1627–1691) held a milder position than Patin—that theriac was more useful than noxious, and that in theory "mixture gives the electuary a higher virtue."[69] Boyle was also of the mind to further investigate "this difficulty of discerning, what Ingredient it is of a very compounded Medicine, that helps or hurts the Patient," believing that only a few of the components were active. In Boyle's drawer were several drafts on this topic, but he ultimately chose not to enter such an insidious arena: "I had once thoughts of drawing up a discourse of the Difficulties of the Medicinal Art; and had [diverse] materials by me for such a work, which afterwards I laid aside, for fear it should be misimploy'd to the prejudice of worthy Physicians."[70] Openly criticizing the medical science they followed could put practicing physicians in a difficult position with their patients.

Boyle's and Patin's hesitation to express doubts about theriac and Galenic polypharmacy was shared by Nicolas Lémery (1645–1715), a leading French chemist and member of the French Academy of Science. In his *Pharmacopée Universelle,* first published in 1697, Lémery claimed, "Theriac is an assemblage of a great number of ingredients of different kind and virtues; even if they seem badly assorted, nonetheless they produce a good effect on many ailments; still it would be appropriate to cut from its description many drugs which are either harmful or useless." Although Lémery believed a better antidote could be made with fewer drugs and a simpler process, he included in his treatise the two main staples of polypharmacy, mithridate and theriac, and advocated for the use of fresh theriac over the extract thereof, whose preparation "loses what is more volatile and essential in this composition."[71] Famous for their clarity, Lémery's manuals of pharmacy and chemistry became a point of reference for generations of apothecaries and physicians.

North of the Alps the debate on theriac became harsher in the eighteenth century. Probably the most impressive countermelody to Heberden's attack on theriac was that of French physician Théofile Bordeu (1722–1776), a vitalist and collaborator of the *Encyclopédie*. In 1764, in a book on the advantages of empirical medicine and inoculation, Bordeu stated, "[Andromachus made a] composition which endures, and will always endure; which will be the pitfall of all reasoning, of all systems, and it will be never banned; theriac, so to speak, follows the heart, follows the instinct, or follows everybody's taste." In his invective, Bordeu called theriac "the masterpiece of empiricism."[72] Theriac had centuries of popularity and medical experts' approval on its side, and he was unimpressed by Edinburgh Medical College, which had recently expunged theriac from its official pharmacopoeia. According to Bordeu, doctors who criticized theriac lacked common sense and did not know the rules of good pharmacy. Combining theriac and inoculation under the concept of "empiricism" in the manner of Bordeu opens up fascinating speculations. Both forms of therapeutic placed a small portion of the "evil"—be it the smallpox pus or the poison or viper—at the core of the healing process. As theriac began to wane, vaccination began to rise.

In 1768, a few years after Bordeu published his book, chemist Gabriel-François Venel (1723–1775) responded to him in the *Encyclopédie*.[73] The tone of Venel's entry recalls Heberden's. According to Venel—a convinced supporter of chemical pharmacy—even those who advocated for simplified versions of theriac showed a "blind and superstitious respect for celebrity." Theriac was a "pharmaceutical monster," and the best reform was to pull it from both pharmacopoeias and apothecary shops. The *Encyclopédie* recognized no virtue at all in theriac; in all cases it could be replaced with simpler and more effective medicines.[74] Untouched by disbelief and critique, French apothecaries continued to publicly produce theriac in the traditional way until 1798, and patients continued to buy it. It was 1908 before the official French pharmacopoeia expunged the last theriac.[75]

Changing pharmaceutical trends and attitudes toward theriac first manifested in Italy in the form of private letters and personal communications. In 1671 Redi and Fiorentini had already been privately sharing their incredulity that theriac could respond well to testing.[76] In 1751, however, the news reached Italy that theriac had been expunged in England.

Johan Gassel, a German living in Venice, anonymously published *Lettere famigliari sopra le novelle letterarie oltramontane*, (letters with news from Western Europe) dedicating one of the letters to an apothecary.[77] Gassel informed readers that the 1746 *London Pharmacopoeia* "lightened up" the recipe of theriac and reduced the overall number of medicaments. Since Venice still lacked an official pharmacopoeia, the letter explained to Venetian readers that the *London pharmacopoeia* was "different from other pharmacopoeias because it is a solemn law and a universal rule." According to the author, apothecaries should rejoice over this new pharmaceutical trend, which relieved them of the burden of keeping in stock "hundreds of useless syrups and waters."[78]

Gassel's letter proposing the simplification of remedies clearly nodded to the *vix medicatrix naturae*, the healing power of nature. The organism's ability to heal itself when left alone was a neo-Hippocratic concept that grew in popularity among both physicians and the bourgeoisie. Giambattista Paitoni (1703-1778), a Venetian Protomedico and member of the Royal Society, was an ardent supporter of simplicity and began refusing licenses for charlatans' remedies whose purported effects could be derived from simpler medicines.[79] As ideas of simplification took hold, Galenic polypharmacy, the baroque fortress of the entrenched medical establishment, went out of fashion among the bourgeoisie. Furthermore, as Elena Brambilla has argued, for the bourgeoisie new ideas of simpler medicines came together with pressing demands to open up the ranks of the medical profession. Some thought it was time to reward physicians for the merits acquired in the field, rather than for privileges acquired by birth.[80]

If most Italian physicians held views against theriac, however, they were not forthcoming in expressing them, and they continued prescribing theriac throughout the eighteenth century, albeit in moderation. Clinician and experimenter Francesco Torti (1658-1741) usually prescribed theriac only in combination with other drugs, or as an ingredient for other compositions: "If Signora Benedetta's fever continues and cannot be kept under control, I would finally approve the use of China mixed in equal amount with powder of lesser centaury and theriac."[81] Similarly, Bolognese physician Giuseppe Azzoguidi (1700-1767) in his medical consultations prescribed theriacal water for a variety of ailments, such as rheumatism, hypochondria, gout, abdomen pains, and cramping.[82] In his treatise on professional diseases Bernardino Ramazzini (1633-1714) prescribed theriac and theriacal vinegar only twice, as antidotes for rag and scrap merchants, and for factory workers handling metals.[83] More than anything, physicians remained silent on theriac.

Anatomist Germano Azzoguidi (1740–1814) exemplified the ambiguity of Italian physicians toward theriac. Author of successful booklet *La spezieria domestica,* first published in 1782 and running for several editions, Azzoguidi included theriac among the thirty substances "that on the most frequent occasions can be needed and profitably employed" in the household.[84] Nonetheless, Azzoguidi affirmed that he would say little about theriac for fear of being lumped in with those "vulgar people" who spoke highly of it. Except for "transient migraines," theriac was useless. Azzolini would even "not be opposed" to expunging it from the apothecary chest entirely. Yet, he added, "I would be sorry if that happened only because of my advice: . . . if ever the lack of theriac were to cause some disgrace . . . , the loss of profit theriac might bring could not be reduced to my oversight."[85] Unwilling to be associated with the "vulgar people" yet reluctant to disavow theriac, Azzoguidi seemed ultimately unable to take a definitive stance on the matter.

Late eighteenth-century physicians' rationale for retaining theriac as part of their medical practice is also clarified by an episode involving foremost physician Luigi Galvani (1737–1798), famous for his research on bioelectricity. Galvani made explicit the favor in which patients still held theriac, as well as physicians' reliance on what today we call the "placebo effect." In 1792 the Bolognese Senate asked the Protomedico to appraise a rabies remedy developed by Baron Anton von Störck (1731–1803) that was outlined in a treatise translated into Italian in 1784.[86] The new remedy's primary ingredient was *meloè,* a beetle from the genus *Meloe*—and the secondary ingredient was theriac. In response to the Senate, Luigi Galvani and two other physicians wrote a wide-ranging and informative report on von Störck's electuary, contextualized within a broader exploration of the contemporary bounds of medical knowledge:

> This [rabies] is one of those many fatal illnesses for which we still desire new light. Many of the most knowledgeable and expert masters are working to find a lead, both for prevention of those who are under menace, and to cure those who unfortunately catch the disease. The infinite remedies proposed and

> praised as specifics since the earliest times of medicine, as well as the new methods of cure that every day are created and published in both medical journals and erudite publications, are quite convincing proofs of the uselessness of human intelligence and medical industriousness.[87]

Physicians felt hopeless against rabies. Given the limited efficacy of the remedies at their disposal, the three physicians considered the best course of action to be to treat the wounds—mostly dog bites—with traditional methods. They also believed it would be better for a physician "to be considered too timid than not enough cautious or prudent." Finally, they added: "[To] soothe any concerns in the soul of the injured, and to free them from the perpetual fear that accompanies them, a fear that experience has unfortunately shown to aggravate the development of the hidden poison, it is of great benefit that there be some remedy, whose reputation awakes in the injured confidence and supports hope." Galvani and his colleagues believed that the emotional state of the injured affected the efficacy of the cure. Consequently, they favored the use of "ineffective" remedies as long as the patient had faith in them. Their concluding advice to the Senate was to ask apothecaries to prepare von Störck's electuary against rabies for the following year.[88]

The incident shows the awareness of Bolognese Collegio Medico physicians of the effectiveness of the medicaments at their disposal to treat such diseases as rabies—which was always fatal before a vaccine was developed at the end of the nineteenth century—as well as of the limits of human intelligence. It also demonstrates end-of-eighteenth-century physicians' approach to patients' well-being, which was considered more a responsibility of the higher classes and those in charge than an individual responsibility. Galvani and his colleagues' declaration only partly confirms several historians' interpretation of eighteenth-century pharmaceutical practices. According to this view, because physicians lacked both effective medicines and new medical theories, they continued using many traditional remedies, including Galenic ones, so as to not lose their authority.[89] In fact, Galvani's psychological justification for keeping ineffective remedies leveraged his clinical experience while considering the mental well-being of the patient. Rather than offering no hope or administering ineffective remedies, physicians instead did what they thought best for the patient. In accepting Galvani's advice, however, the Senate adopted a patronizing approach: they took responsibility for their patients, while keeping them in the dark and denying them a choice. This is an ethical dilemma that every era approaches according to its current values.

Physicians' ambiguity toward theriac altered the social prestige of theriac, as did changing medical and scientific ideas. During the late sixteenth and seventeenth centuries Theriaca magna regained ground lost in previous centuries, when theriac had often been associated with deception and fraud, but medieval associations with treachery were now resurfacing in the eighteenth century. A Dutch etching from the 1720s depicted John Law (1671–1729), a Scottish economist associated with financial collapse and deceit, celebrating the carnival in Venice, dealing in theriac, mirrors, and rose-tinted spectacles.[90] In Italy the plays of Carlo Goldoni (1707–1793), son of a physician, were a harbinger of theriac's changing status, especially in Venice. A defining feature of his plays was their uncanny portrayal of the mid-rank society of contemporary Venice. Goldoni can hardly be considered a champion of women's emancipation, but many of his female characters were strong, witty, independent, and capable of navigating complex situations. However, in two of his plays published in the late 1750s, theriac was associated with women in derogatory terms:

> Men, even when old, are worth something: but you women, when you are old, you are only good to make theriac.[91]

> The proud woman wants to contradict everything. I would like to have a hundred of these women, and grind them in a mortar like theriac.[92]

In these crude lines, theriac is made by grinding stale and wasteful ingredients. Theriac's association with old women contrasts starkly with its origin stories, inhabited as they were with emperors, kings, and indeed Christ, and clearly marked its declining status.

Negative views of theriac grew further in late eighteenth-century newspapers, one of the primary means through which the emerging commercial class could both express and dictate its new ideas to society. Antonio Piazza's *Gazzetta Urbana Veneta* melded commercial information and leisure; his stated intention was "to please every kind of people, educated, noble, boorish, and communal alike."[93] A few pieces in the *Gazzetta*

Urbana Veneta indirectly discredited theriac by associating it with the lower classes, people from other continents, and animals. In one article, two "rude mountain dwellers . . . resembling savages from Canada" spent a leisure day in Venice. A cunning thief tricked them by making them believe they had gained a gold coin and doubled their money, when in fact they had just lost it all. The two simpletons then entered an apothecary shop to buy some theriac.[94] In this story, the equation was straightforward: vulgar = savage = theriac. In another tale, in an emergency an honorable woman ventured out of her home without a chaperone. While crossing the bridge where apothecary laborers were making theriac, the woman fainted for shame as the theriac grinders expressed their appreciation for her beauty with outrageous words.[95] Again, theriac was associated with low-class workers and women who were fainting, feeble, or inattentive. Both articles presented theriac as a medicine for ignorant, incompetent, and backward individuals. Moreover, during the same years, books for breeders and journals presented theriac as a remedy suitable for animals. In 1760 the *La Gazzetta Veneta* reported that English breeders were adding Venetian theriac to bovine remedies.[96] In the social hierarchy, women, "the vulgar," "savages," and animals scored quite low—and now so did theriac.

By the 1780s, however, the bourgeoisie neither constituted the majority of society nor yet ruled it. Apothecaries persevered in their business, and patients, with their autonomy and own medicinal preferences, still sought theriac. Public theriac productions became so excessive that their grandiosity became proverbial, reflected in other festivities, such as the Festival of Chinea held in Rome in 1773 (Figure 7.1). Data on productions in Venice and Bologna shows that production increased compared to previous centuries. Bolognese archives have a remarkably complete record of theriac quantities held in apothecary shops for most of the eighteenth century, thanks to the quarterly inspections that took place for more than 200 years. This bequeathal illuminates the city's special reputation among contemporaries for the attention its Protomedici paid to the quality of medicaments.[97]

The structure of inspection reports inevitably changed several times over such a period. In the sixteenth century, possibly under the influence of Aldrovandi, reports were many pages long, and featured long lists of the medicaments available at each shop.[98] But over time they shortened, perhaps because keeping such detailed records was simply unsustainable.[99]

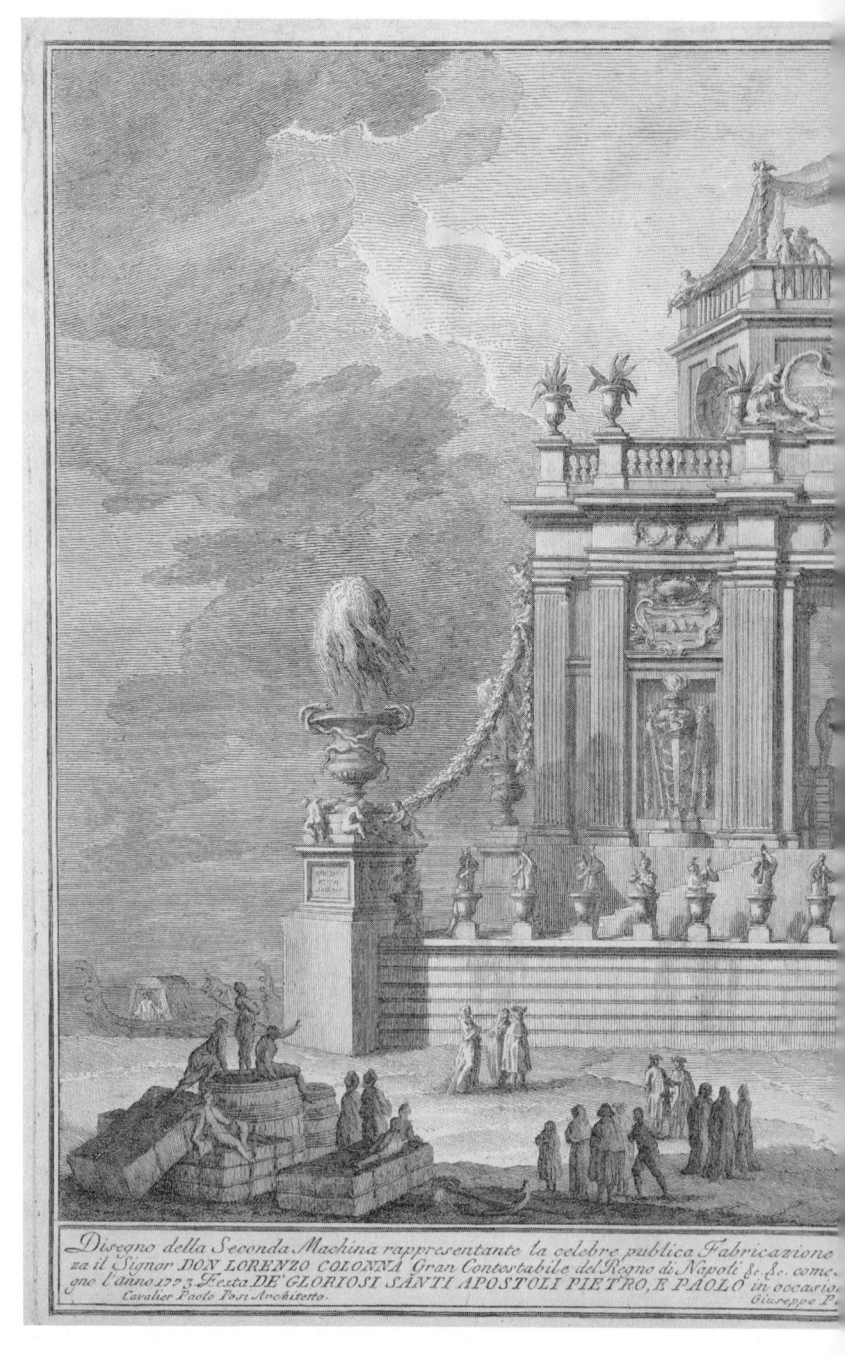

Disegno della Seconda Machina rappresentante la celebre publica Fabricazione za il Signor DON LORENZO COLONNA Gran Contestabile del Regno di Napoli &c. &c. come. gne l'anno 1773 Festa DE GLORIOSI SANTI APOSTOLI PIETRO, E PAOLO in occasio Cavalier Paolo Posi Architetto. Giuseppe P.

Fig. 7.1. The public preparation of theriac in Venice became such a renowned event that its representation, designed by the architect Paolo Posi, featured in the Chinea festival. Every year on June 29, the day of Saints Peter and Paul, the king of Naples (or his representative) would pay a tribute to the pope, consisting of a considerable sum and a horse (called *Chinea*

FROM "ANTIDOTE" TO PHARMACEUTICAL MONSTER 223

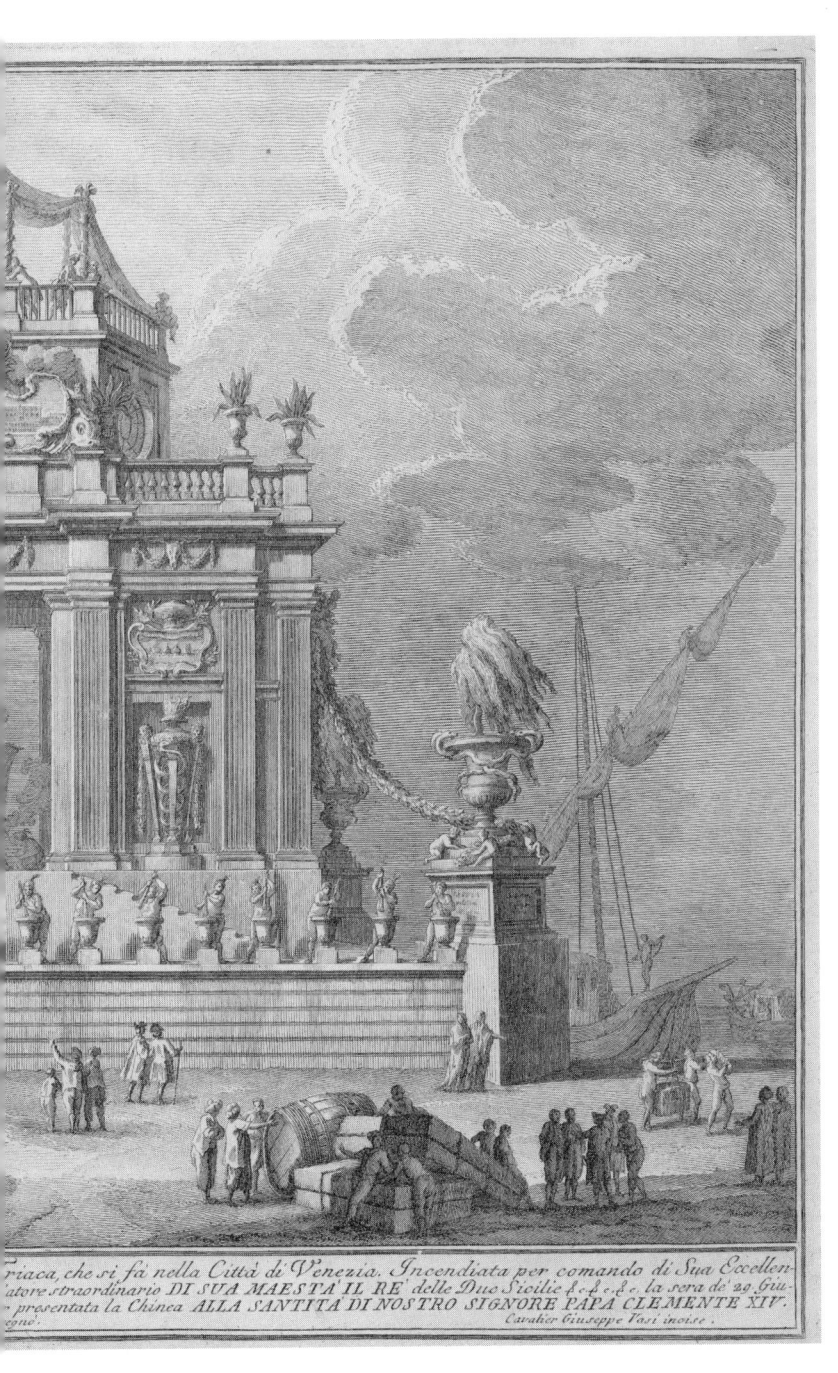

riaca, che si fà nella Città di Venezia. Incendiata per comando di Sua Eccellen- atore straordinario DI SUA MAESTÀ IL RE delle Due Sicilie &c. &c. &c. la sera de' 29 Giu- presentata la Chinea ALLA SANTITÀ DI NOSTRO SIGNORE PAPA CLEMENTE XIV.
Cavalier Giuseppe Vasi incise.

from the Hackney breed). For the celebrations, the king commissioned grand temporary structures that were burned down at the acme of the festival, as happened with this one in 1773. Drawing of Giuseppe Palazzi, engraving by Giuseppe Vasi.

National Gallery of Art, Washington.

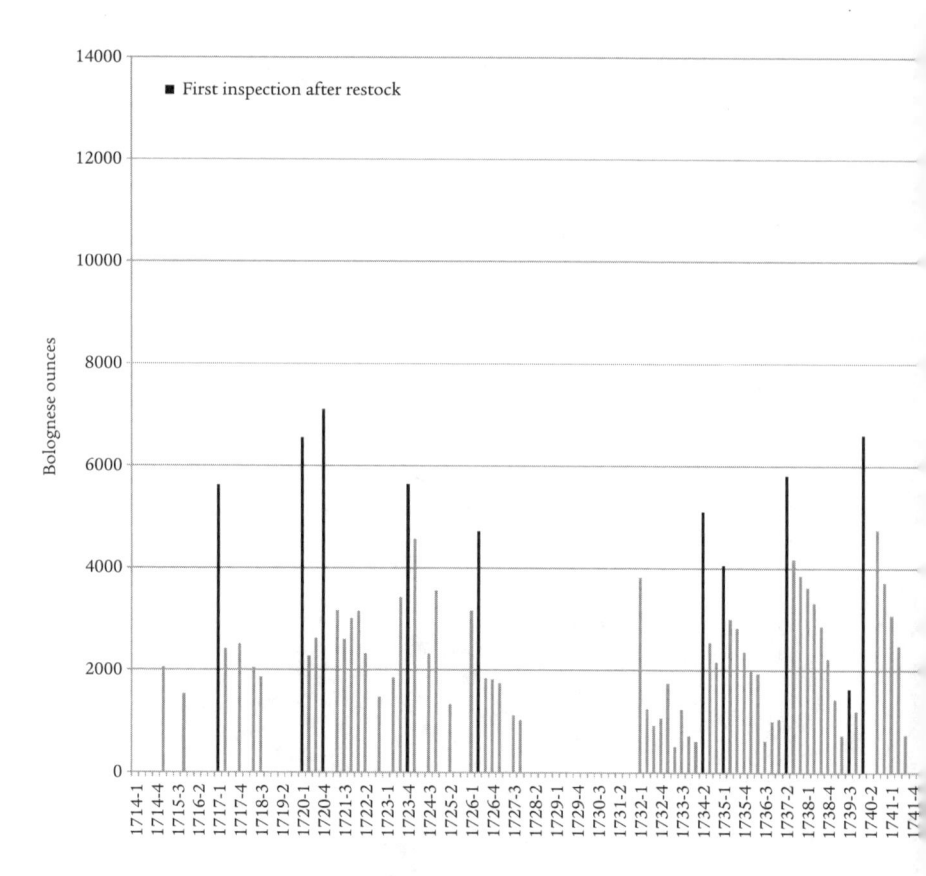

Fig. 7.2. Quantities of theriac in Bolognese ounces held in Bolognese apothecary shops between 1714 and 1776, according to the Protomedicato's inspection records. Each year were carried out four inspections.

(*Data source:* ASB, Studio 326, 327, 329.)

Beginning in 1704, inspection reports concentrated exclusively on how much theriac was being kept in each apothecary shop, leaving aside any other observation. In 1717 this practice was institutionalized, with the Collegio Medico stating that, to verify that apothecaries were not holding any unlawful theriac, only those quantities present in the shop should be noted during inspection. Unlike during the previous century, in the eighteenth century the now-reformed apothecary guild made an official theriac every three years, let it rest for a year, then distributed it among the *obbedienti* (obedient ones) and those apothecaries involved in its production. Each apothecary would receive an amount proportional to what they

FROM "ANTIDOTE" TO PHARMACEUTICAL MONSTER 225

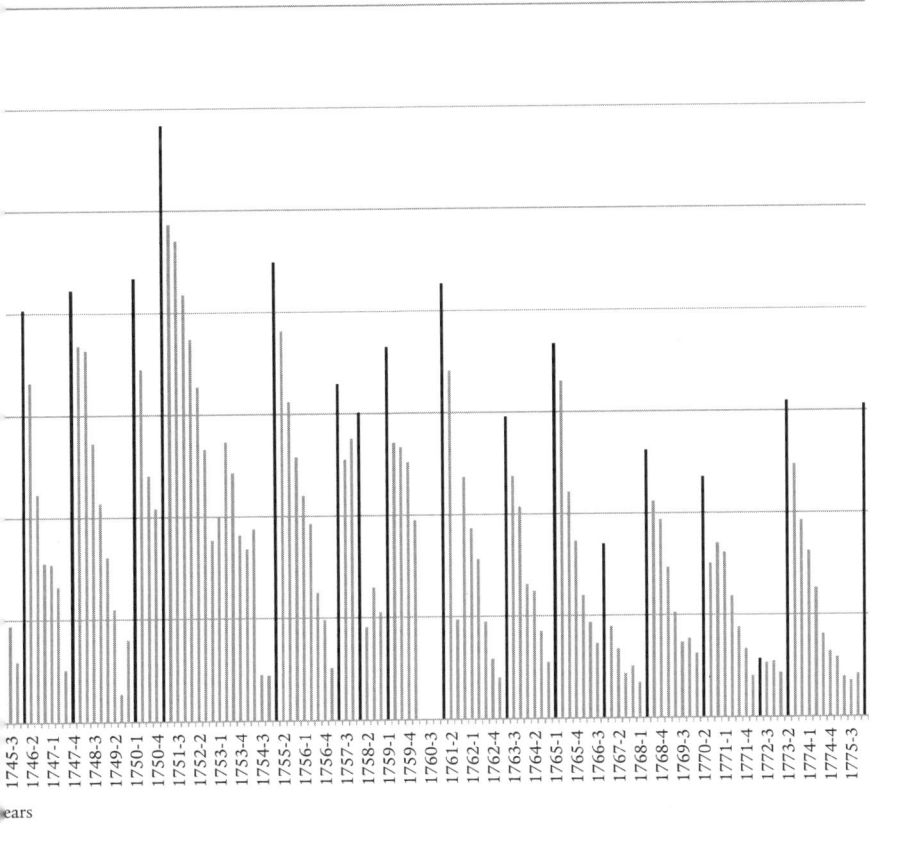

had invested in the production or how much they were able to buy. Thus, the sum of all quantities of theriac should not have exceeded that of the previous year (or should not have exceeded that of the total production). The same regulation stated that theriac old and new should be stored separately, since "signori Medici" prescribed theriac for different occurrences.[100] The reason Protomedici began paying attention only to theriac was never clearly expressed. Because it was nearly impossible to check every product listed in the pharmacopoeia, perhaps they decided to focus only on the most consequential one. Whatever the reason, theriac was still a focal point in the relationship between the Collegio Medico and the apothecary guild in the eighteenth century.

Figure 7.2 shows the quantities of theriac held in apothecary shops between 1714 and 1776. Theriac was distributed every three years, then sold until the next distribution. Theriac distribution in Bologna reached its maximum quantity in the 1750s: 11,500 Bolognese ounces (316 kilograms). Quantities decreased over the following decades; in 1776, for example, only 165 kilograms were distributed. Toward the end of the century, however, quantities increased again: 1,220 Bolognese pounds in 1791; 1,104 in 1793; and 1,139 in 1795 (respectively, 396, 358, and 370 kilograms).[101] In terms of quantity, even at its highest, Bolognese theriac production never competed with that of Venice, which by the early seventeenth century had reached 453 kilograms per year. Nonetheless, Bologna was a significant producer of theriac, especially considering the fact it was made mostly for local use.

Theriac production also increased in eighteenth-century Venice, although no records exist similar to those of Bologna, and sources are patchy. In the 1740s physician Giuseppe Bolis, then prior of the Venetian Collegio Medico, expressed his concern about the near impossibility of checking the quality of the vipers employed in the production, because of their constantly growing population. As discussed in Chapter 2, by 1747 the plans for Venetian production involved killing 2,800 vipers (although apothecaries were able to process only 2,200—the rest were dead on arrival).[102] In 1799 a single apothecary killed 3,000 vipers for his production.[103] Making multiple batches of theriac was a quasi-industrial undertaking in terms of investment and organization. Theriac production remained an artisanal procedure that a well-organized apothecary, such as Vincenzo Varè at the sign of the Doge, could undertake six times between 1786 and 1805.[104] Varè left carefully annotated records of costs and quantities, and even created drawings of his exhibits.[105] Ultimately production was limited by the inherent complexity of its constituent processes.

In the late eighteenth century, increased production exacerbated authorities' challenges with substitutes and counterfeiting. In 1769 the age-old problem of substitutes resurfaced in the Collegio Medico's books. Unlike in the past, however, this time collegiate physicians appeared open to using specific substitutes, even when the original ingredient was available. Nutmeg oil gave theriac "an aromatic and pleasant scent" and was preferred to opobalsamum, of which apothecaries had finally secured a steady supply from the Eastern Mediterranean.[106] But the sale of illegal theriacs was far from having been resolved. In 1700 and again in 1758, the Giustizia Vecchia issued new regulations for handling theriac. The description of the procedure became extremely convoluted, more closely resembling a ceremonial handbook than a practical routine. For example, once "seen, identified, and weighed," ingredients should be kept in a trunk. During their grinding, which took several days, the trunk was to be locked every evening. Once the compound was ready, a sample of 3 ounces was to be placed in a vase, sealed and signed by the producer, who also signed an oath regarding the quantity produced. This sample was kept in case a comparison became necessary. The bulk of the compound was to be sealed in jars locked with two keys, one kept by the prior of physicians, the other by the prior of apothecaries. The sheer number of certifications, seals, signatures, special cases for comparison, keys, cupboards, and officials involved is testament to the inadequacy of these measures.[107] After all, in the end these precautions did little to prevent apothecaries and forgers from pursuing their illicit activities; they could still falsify theriac and also the very containers, seals, and certifications that were supposed to guarantee legitimacy. Venetian authorities also threatened ship captains with exorbitant fines and the loss of patents if they transported forgeries.[108] Yet regardless of physicians' skepticism and theriac's depreciated social prestige, forgeries and increased production confirm that patients' demand for theriac endured in the eighteenth century. Patients—and not necessarily only those of a lesser rank, as the gazettes would have had us believe—remained faithful to a remedy they appreciated, although as time passed they might have felt more compelled to justify their choice. The learned society, attached to the past, was still relying on theriac, as were the defenders of the traditional ways. In 1787 the abbot Ludovico Preti (1727–1810) wrote to his friend in Venice, the later Bishop of Montepulciano:

> I cannot avoid to pray you, kind Count, leave a little corner of your trunk for my needs. A little jar of the famous theriac from the apothecary shop at the Madonna, and a box of Zanichelli pills, called Santa Fosca pills. Do theriac and pills appear to you as commission for an apostolic man, a proven preacher? And why not? If theriac is a fruitful remedy for so many diseases, and the pills a light medicine for the vices of the stomach, is it not all but appropriate that you bring the one and the other to a friend who has cured with the sanctity and efficacy of his words so many vices of the human heart?[109]

Despite being in Bologna, Preti asked for a special theriac in Venice. He felt he had to justify his choice, presuming resistance from his friend: "Theriac?" "And why not?"

Patients' affection for theriac was so entrenched that political and medical establishments continued leveraging it during the nineteenth century to shore up their power. The Venetian Republic fell in 1797, concluding a glorious history. In 1803 Ferdinand von Bissingen (1749–1831), governor of the newly formed Austrian-Venetian provinces, issued an order to establish the first official pharmacopoeia for Venice. The new pharmacopoeia was intended to introduce gradual innovation, by retaining weights and measures, accompanying the old medicaments' names with "modern chemistry," and "disregard[ing] the absurdity of paltry recipes" made with a "barbaric multiplicity of ingredients, purging them with severity, as reason demands." At the same time, the new pharmacopoeia was to keep those "medicaments protected by the blind faith of the plebs."[110] According to the Austrian governor, even though "reason demanded" specific actions, the state should not cause unnecessary frustration to its subjects. The new pharmacopoeia was to respect the common people's attachment to medicaments, lest the social peace be disrupted. The pharmacopoeia did, however, prohibit public ceremonies of theriac.[111] Von Bissingen's view of the people oscillated: on the one hand, they were "men of good faith," not to be grieved; but on the other hand, they were "vulgar plebs" who must be guided. This perspective was simultaneously aristocratic and enlightened, echoing contemporary statements regarding colonial subjects in other continents. Von Bissingen's project for an official Venetian pharmacopoeia ultimately failed, and Venice never got its own pharmacopoeia.[112] A few years later the Austrian government of Venice adopted the *Pharmacopoea Austriaco-Provincialis Emendata*, which included a reformed theriac purged of vipers.[113]

The Kingdom of Naples was theriac's last stronghold as a state drug, and remained so for most of the nineteenth century.[114] Here the state attempted to exploit patients' inclination toward theriac, hoping to gain some economic advantage from its monopoly. In 1781 the king of Naples granted the monopoly over theriac to the newly formed Academy of Sciences and Fine Letters. Founded in 1778, the Academy was to serve as a ministry of culture and education: its president had to manage several affairs, such as the renovation of the museum for antiquities and the distribution of scholarships to promising artists.¹¹⁵ Together with the monopoly over theriac, the king gave the Academy other sources of funding, which, like theriac, were unable to provide a constant flow of money into the Academy's coffers.¹¹⁶ Until that moment, theriac produced locally was expensive and of bad quality. The Eights (*gli Otto*), a small elective body within the apothecary guild, held the privilege of making theriac, and they did so out of the public eye. To avoid buying theriac from the Eights, most apothecaries imported it from Rome and Venice, or produced their own fake theriac of even lower quality. So in 1779 the king ruled that the Academy should produce theriac in public, following the example of other "wise [*culte*] nations," and its price was lowered. These decisions were explicit attempts at modernization. The production of theriac in Naples took place in both the "chemical laboratory" and the backyard of the Academy—today the Museo Archeologico Nazionale—where only authorities could attend the event.¹¹⁷

Selling theriac was irksome for the Academy. Considerable quantities of its theriac were distributed to public hospitals, such as the Royal Hospital in Aquila, which consumed more than 50 pounds of theriac in 1790 alone. Overall, however, the Academy was unsatisfied with sales of theriac. The kingdom's apothecaries considered it expensive and refused to buy it, instead continuing to either make their own or import it from Venice.¹¹⁸ Indeed, the Academy sold theriac at 18 carlini per pound, yet apothecaries could buy it at just 12 carlini per pound.¹¹⁹ At the time, the law required apothecaries to have official theriac in store when inspected, so they circumvented the law by buying small quantities just before inspections. In 1795 the correspondent of the Academy from Salerno noted, "It is not easy to sell theriac here, the apothecaries of the surrounding areas only buy one pound or half a pound when the time of the Protomedico inspection comes close."¹²⁰ Even when the Academy was able to sell theriac, it was not easy to collect payments, as apothecaries kept the containers sealed and often returned them as unsold.¹²¹ In 1791, 30 pounds of unsold theriac was returned to Naples from Acri.¹²²

Regardless of insufficient profits, in 1806, during the Napoleonic period, the newly formed Royal Society for the Promotion of the Natural Sciences (Istituto di Incoraggiamento) inherited the monopoly over theriac from the former Academy. In what might seem like a paradox, the institute for the advancement of science and technology was to be funded through the sales of that most ancient of medicaments: theriac. The institute survived the Bourbon Restoration, and the official production of theriac continued in the kingdom until Italian Unification in 1860, although profits never met expectations.

The global expansion of theriac and its trajectory in eighteenth-century Italy can be understood in the light of theriac's status as state drug. The greatest diffusion of theriac worldwide took place between the 1650s and 1750s, as part of a more general diffusion of Galenic pharmacy (and European colonization), because of the prestige theriac enjoyed in Europe and despite the complexity of its recipe and production. The diversity of theriac's transformations around the world precludes a single interpretation. The authority it wielded was vital to its adoption, as is most evident in the case of China and Russia, where it was certainly not imposed.

Theriac's prestige waned in the eighteenth century, especially in England and northern Europe, where its institutional character was perhaps less established. Meanwhile in the Mediterranean countries, theriac's use continued unabated, and even increased. Comparing and contrasting sources regarding medical theory, practice, and pharmaceutical production, and the perception of medicaments in literary sources, we are left with a complex picture of theriac's standing in eighteenth-century Italy. Medical beliefs are a cornerstone of medical practice, but so are institutional setups and pharmaceutical fashions; after all, medicines are not only commercial products but also objects charged with political meaning. Whatever eighteenth-century Italian physicians thought of theriac's efficacy, they chose not to directly undermine their patients' propensities. This was for several reasons, including their therapeutic sensibility, and the institutional standing theriac held until the fall of the ancien régime. Theriac consumption continued in the nineteenth century, although it remained a state drug in only a handful of states, including the Kingdom of Naples.

Conclusion

*I*N 1835, while the Austrian Empire ruled over northern Italy, Defendente Sacchi (1796–1840), a Lombard journalist of anti-Austrian sentiments, wrote of theriac: "For a long time, [through ceremonies] Venetian theriac upheld its market reputation as the best, and it truly was; some may laugh at the ceremonial production of a medicine. However, I believe the Venetian government showed great wisdom. With rigor, Venice was able to establish and maintain a near-exclusive trade in theriac. In 1804 a statistical table showed that theriac yielded the state about 120,000 silver ducats, or half a million francs . . . The Venetian Republic fell, but theriac is still there."[1] By reminding his readers of the state's sponsorship of theriac, Sacchi highlighted the savvy of the Venetian Republic's administration. He also expressed hope that Italian traditions would outlast the Austrian occupation—and theriac did indeed outlast both the Venetian Republic and the Austro-Hungarian Empire. In the 1930s nostalgic patients could still buy theriac at the apothecary shop Santa Maria alla Scala of the Discalced Carmelites in Trastevere in Rome, although it lacked viper, as the last *viperaio* had died around 1910.[2] If you happen to visit the Santa Maria alla Scala pharmacy, look for the large jar in a niche—it still contains theriac. If you ask the friar-guide, he might let you smell it. In 1966 one could still purchase a remedy called "theriac" in the Venetian apothecary shop at the sign of the Golden Head, right off the Rialto Bridge.[3] Today, above the river of rapt tourists and hasty passersby, the sign of the Golden Head remains—pay attention not to miss it—but the shop now sells garments. These are the last remnants of a medical tradition that persisted for almost two millennia.

"Some may laugh," wrote Sacchi in his article, referring to the irony that ceremonies of theriac production aroused in some readers in the 1830s. Between the eighteenth and nineteenth centuries, theriac was labeled both a "pharmaceutical monster" and a "universal panacea." In the twentieth century, historian Erwin Ackerknecht called it a "hellish brew."[4] These epithets signify that theriac had become an embarrassing symbol of what medicine should never have been, in contrast with modern biomedicine, the rational medicine of modernity. Nineteenth- and twentieth-century physicians were eager to distance themselves from the medicine of yesteryear, which they judged ineffective and scientifically unsound. Eventually theriac slipped into oblivion. Few today know what theriac was; at best you may find it flaunted as a curio, for the amusement of tourists, sitting in display cases alongside medieval torture devices and magical potions. Ultimately, while I myself did start this research fueled by curiosity, more than anything I began with the presumption that theriac deserved serious historical consideration, and that its longevity and prestige should surely render its history a useful window into the early modern history of pharmacy and medicine, if not more. I did not expect this to become primarily a history of the early modern political use of pharmacy.

By delving into the social significance of theriac in the early modern Italian states, it swiftly became apparent that theriac was multifaceted: it was at once a medicine, an object of scientific inquiry, a market commodity, a subject of medical regulation, and a metaphor. A comprehensive understanding of this phenomenon emerged only by integrating the diverse social dimensions of theriac. This necessitated uncovering the interconnections between the actions and statements of the various social actors involved with the drug, including apothecaries, remedy sellers, physicians, patients, state officials, rulers, medical regulators, and health practitioners. To achieve this, I employed an integrated approach, combining micro- and macro-analysis, and utilizing both quantitative and qualitative methods. The investigation would go on to span the history of science, medicine, institutions, consumption, commerce, and culture. My analysis concentrated on three key themes: the political, examining how state authorities demonstrated their concern for public health; the social, exploring how public provision fostered social cohesion; and the medicinal, investigating the persistence of classical pharmacy into the early modern period.

I have argued that, in the early modern period, theriac transitioned from renowned antidote of the Galenic tradition with a declining reputation to a symbol of medical and state authority. Theriac became a state drug, intimately tied as it was to the objectives of the early modern Italian states. Theriac was intrinsically interwoven with the ancien régime. Unlike most early modern drugs, its relationship with the state was therefore unique, embodied in a visible system of certification, managed by medical colleges, apothecary guilds, and state offices. This system began in the Middle Ages, and expanded in size and complexity over the centuries. From the beginning, the certification system was justified by the elaborate process of theriac manufacture, and aimed to grant legitimacy to the remedy's purported extraordinary efficacy. The certification system oversaw the entire life cycle of theriac: the definition of the recipe, production, distribution, sales, and pricing. This system was foundational to theriac's status as state drug—although, of course, neither being certified nor boasting elaborate branding alone sufficed in rendering it such.

Patients primarily associated theriac with Venice, the city that since the Middle Ages had most successfully established a brand for the remedy. Venice maintained its trade and production of theriac for several centuries, exporting it throughout Italy, Europe, and in the eighteenth century even the Eastern Mediterranean, upending the balance of prestige between Venetian and Egyptian theriac. However, the *concept* of theriac was by no means only Venetian or indeed Italian: it was integral to the Galenic tradition. Different states used theriac in different ways, for different purposes, and to different degrees of success. Like the Venetian Republic, the Kingdom of Naples, for example, sponsored theriac to profit from its sales, albeit unsuccessfully. In contrast, most northern Italian cities leveraged theriac primarily to gain prestige and medical authority. Most states used theriac as a measure of public health during outbreaks of disease. The prestige the remedy had acquired in Italy set an example for other European regions, where it also found fertile ground in which to thrive, although the extent to which theriac become a state drug elsewhere needs further investigation.

The medical strata involved with the production, sale, and management of theriac were primarily traditional settings such as guilds, universities, and public health boards, in accordance with its status. However, my investigation confirmed the existence of unlawful or hidden activities performed by apothecaries as well as inadequately documented producers of preposterous or "untrue" theriacs who were sufficiently organized, held international connections, and employed workers in different capacities, such as printers to forge labels. In this respect, theriac was no different from many other products whose success led to rampant forgery and imitation.

While the institutional renown of theriac was not new to historians, a wholly new aspect of the history of theriac that emerged over the course of my research was the extent of the durable, intentional, and strategic connection between this one drug and the state (in its many forms). Although pharmacy was an early modern activity carried out in multiple spaces—households, makeshift and court laboratories, apothecary shops, botanical gardens, religious institutions—it constituted an interest of state institutions. This interest was not limited to pharmacopoeias, patent systems, and apothecary shop inspections, but extended in a way that fostered a shared narrative, which organized and hierarchized products, remedy makers, and practitioners. This narrative aimed to demonstrate the state's commitment to protecting society from disease and building social cohesion. Sometimes there was also an economic advantage for the state, or at least for the people and institutions involved in the trade. The profits theriac yielded did not appear to be outstanding from the perspective of this study, especially compared to those of other early modern productions, but they must have at least appeared significant to the Neapolitan officials who thought it wise to fund an Academy of Science with theriac sales.

Pharmacy remains an understudied subject in relation to medical practice, regulation, and the market. Pharmacopoeias are yet to be investigated thoroughly, as are tariffs, hidden within which is much detail regarding when and which medical matter entered into practice. It would

CONCLUSION

be especially fruitful to cross-check this information with account books and inventories. The actual use of exotica, for example, might further illuminate links between empires, commerce, and medicine. The relationship between apothecary guilds and those religious institutions that produced medicaments has also been studied only episodically; indeed, it emerged only toward the end of my study, upon my researching production in Bologna, when apothecaries refused to make theriac and monasteries did so in their place. How states managed—or rather left unmanaged—the balance between lay and religious apothecary shops remains understudied.

The trajectory of theriac as a state drug has been delineated throughout these chapters. By virtue of its economic standing, theriac already held a special status in fifteenth-century Venice. In the sixteenth century, the connection between the remedy and the state intensified and extended to other regions of Italy, as a consequence of the reformation of theriac into "true theriac," a process initiated by a dispute in 1490s Venice. I have demonstrated that the "reinvention of theriac" spanned seven decades, undergoing phases of disbelief, skepticism, excitement, and disappointment—but ultimately generating a consensus that "true theriac" was in fact achievable. Most importantly, whereas the reinvention of theriac was previously understood primarily as an intellectual and medical endeavor, I have shown that the reinvention of theriac also involved courts, commercial entities, and administrative institutions, all of which played key roles in its transformation. Especially in a city such as Venice, whose theriac trade was well rooted, decisions regarding its recipe were not solely medical in nature, but instead were influenced by numerous social forces. In the highly regulated medical market of early modern Italy, medicines were outcomes of multiple interdependent social dynamics.

Renaissance rulers understood the importance of pharmacy as a political enterprise, and possessing "true theriac" became a mark of distinction. Within courtly culture, the origin tale of theriac, involving kings, generals, and emperors, was pivotal in positioning the drug as a desirable option for rulers and the medical elite. In an era when authority and trust were rooted deeply in a classical past, theriac's pedigree was a foundation upon which physicians could build incrementally. The emphasis physicians placed on theriac when discussing the organization of the pharmaceutical field was a reminder of the remedy's symbolic significance within the medical community. While rulers' interest in pharmacy predates the early modern period, the Renaissance fervor forged the systematization of the field, which in turn was part of early modern state building.

In this process, the plague of 1575–1577 played a pivotal role in further establishing theriac as a state drug. Theriac's notable connection with the state was reinforced by its use as a measure of public health in times of plague, first in the 1570s when at least some of the medical community reached a consensus that "true theriac" was attainable. This period was one of heightened hopes, although the product itself was not yet widely available. Theriac came to prominence as a public health measure during certain periods, notably in the last decades of the sixteenth century; during other infectious outbreaks in lazarettos and hospitals; and especially during the plague of 1630. This was evident in provisions of theriac made to protect cities, bans on exporting theriac, and rulers' interrogations of physicians regarding its use and adequacy during epidemics.

In the seventeenth century, the medical community's perception of theriac began to diverge, reflecting a growing tension between orders of knowledge. The plague of 1630 also came about at a time when more observationally inclined physicians, such as Francesco Maria Fiorentini, noted that theriac was not having the expected results. However, more numerous and renowned physicians, such as Ludovico Settala, continued to publish works presenting theriac as the primary resource against the plague. Until the end of the seventeenth century, only authors who were more critical of (or less integrated into) the intellectual and medical system, such as Leonardo Fioravanti and Bernard Palissy, were willing to openly voice their doubts about theriac. They did so despite knowing that critiquing theriac and mithridate would "attract the hate of many," especially of "notable physicians."[5] Most conspicuous among those who kept their doubts concealed were Robert Boyle and Guy Patin. The contemporary presence and absence of knowledge in different sectors of society about specific facts that may appear evident—such as "Does theriac cure plague or does it not?"—is an intriguing avenue to keep exploring. After all, even today questions of trust, authority, and observation may be less settled and more dependent on context than we would like to think.

In addition to theriac being used as a public health measure, the certification process was augmented by the transformation of public pro-

CONCLUSION   237

ductions into solemn ceremonies, displays of medical skillfulness and knowledge, visual affirmations of the state's promise of health and protection. Theriac-making ceremonies were initially a commercial response to a medicine market that by the mid-sixteenth century was bursting with new products, exotic medicaments coming from all manner of places and directed to all manner of pockets. Insofar as they were official providers of medicines, apothecaries could not claim divine healing powers; this advantage was enjoyed only by religious producers of medicaments. Nonetheless, apothecaries could and did respond to the popular performances of charlatans with theriac-making ceremonies, supplemented by a flurry of publications exclusive to theriac and no other medicament: *virtues, formulas,* and *celebrations.* By publicizing their official standing through theriac and theriac-making ceremonies, apothecaries clearly marked their role in society, while disseminating medical knowledge among patients and reinforcing their own position in the market.

By the mid-seventeenth century, theriac had recaptured the imagination of rulers, patients, and administrators alike, and constituted a solid trade for apothecaries. Across early modern Italy, state officials controlled the price of theriac, ensuring that it remained affordable to the public. The price of medicines, then as now, is as much an economic question as a political and social one. In the Italian states, the price of medicines, like the price of most basic goods, was not left to the market to determine. Yet ultimately theriac could never be inexpensive if its purveyors wished to maintain its prestige; cheapness would of course have marked it as being of little value. However, theriac was not expensive to the point that a salaried worker could not afford a few doses in the case of extreme illness. Furthermore, the poor could receive theriac as a treatment at the hospital, like the peasant bitten by a snake and cured by Johannes Faber in Rome. Moreover, one could choose from several by-products of theriac, which some patients may have felt granted them access to the heavenly and earthly powers contained within, even if they could not afford the remedy itself.

The history of theriac in eighteenth-century Italy presents a complex picture. On the one hand, I have shown that production increased consistently over the course of the century in response to patient demand. On the other hand, theriac's prestige progressively waned, culminating in its becoming a remedy for the lower classes and the more traditionally minded patients. For their part, physicians remained largely ambiguous about theriac, caught between new medical theories and subject to changing therapeutic sensibilities, and at the mercy of the lack of effective remedies and the need to protect their authority. A new class separation opened up at this time. In the sixteenth and seventeenth centuries, the gap between remedies for the rich and remedies for the poor widened as a result of the preciousness of the former's ingredients, as well as the presumed differences in the constitution of the respective classes' bodies. The rich were considered more delicate, and thus in need of rarer and more expensive ingredients for their medicines. However, the pharmaceutical framework remained the same for both classes. In the eighteenth century the bourgeoisie demarcated itself from the lower classes in terms of both consumption and the medical theories it adhered to, moving toward simpler remedies and away from polypharmacy.

Meanwhile the apotheosis of theriac ceremonies cohabited with the decreasing status of the drug. For some, theriac was now only the symbol of a bygone era from which they wished to dissociate themselves. Different classes no longer shared the same medical points of reference, sources of authority, or indeed political symbols. Thus, while certain performative political aspects more common in the sixteenth and seventeenth centuries continued being enacted through the eighteenth century, they were actually meaningful only to certain sectors of society. Rather than interpreting this in terms of delay or tardiness, which might imply a "right" time for developments or a set schedule for modernization, I prefer to describe this in terms of continuities and discontinuities. Interestingly, those who are considered to have been enlightened men of science, such as Luigi Galvani, existed at the border of these shifting paradigms, and did their best to negotiate between their official roles, scientific ideas, and medical ethics. Institutionally, the fall of the ancien régime ended the public productions of theriac, but its consumption continued well into the nineteenth century, supported by states such as the Kingdom of Naples.

I have also argued in this book that theriac's effectiveness extended beyond its purported biological efficacy, which still needs to be either confirmed or disproved by current standards. Other than serving as a politically potent tool, theriac's effectiveness was both economic and social. For centuries the Venetian state coffers benefited from its commerce. Theriac was a source of revenues for not only the apothecaries who officially produced it, but also for the numerous remedy sellers who created theriacal by-products, as well as those who forged it, those who sold it (legally or otherwise), and those producing the numerous publications related to theriac, which no other remedy could match in either number or variety. When considering the social effectiveness of medicines, the business they generate cannot be underestimated.

Regarding its social efficacy, theriac long served as a beacon of stability for apothecaries, patients, physicians, and officials. It was something to hold on to as a resource, an anchorage. Initially, albeit briefly and for a restricted group of historical actors, theriac enhanced the social standing of learned apothecaries, who based their authority on the quality of their "true theriac," their superior knowledge—for example, as authors of manuals and monographs—and their morals, which granted them distance from mercantile reproaches to their profession. Moreover, the history of theriac reminds us that "apothecary" is a category in need of specification. An apothecary could be a learned individual, a successful merchant, a skillful artisan, a shrewd administrator—but not necessarily all at once. For example, seventeenth-century Bolognese apothecaries lacked a shared language they could use to define some of their fundamental procedures and their understanding of their own compounds. This suggests that, while artisanal knowledge was embodied, not all artisans were interested in or able to carry this knowledge further and conceptualize it more concretely. This might have lent credence to the claim of "learned apothecaries" that they were distinct from their peers. Examining the production of theriac also hints at an economy of laborers, sellers, remedy makers, snake hunters, and physicians providing certifications and authorizations, which has been only partially investigated. Finally, this research shed only *some* light on the internal dynamics of apothecaries, showing that, at least in Bologna, there was a process of hierarchization within the guild in the seventeenth and especially the eighteenth century.

Each Italian city has its own political and institutional history, and this is true also of medical institutions. Theriac production was central to several disputes between medical colleges and apothecary guilds throughout the seventeenth century, resulting from the social dynamics and power struggles among institutions in both Venice and Bologna. The different political economies and the influence of state interventions shaped these controversies' outcomes, as well as the social meaning of theriac. In Venice, where state interests aligned with the economic interests of the apothecary guild, theriac remained in the hands of apothecaries. But in Bologna theriac stayed under the control of the medical college, which was more authoritative than that of Venice. Through the analysis of treatises and disputes, patterns emerged in the relationships between apothecary guilds and medical colleges. Such patterns might be dependent, for example, on the presence of a prestigious university, and might be further investigated. Regardless of the context, however, once established as a state drug, theriac mainly helped preserve the social order, functioning as a symbol of stability and protection rather than an agent of innovation.

The history of theriac tells much—but it hides much, too. Despite its moniker "the queen of medicaments," theriac was associated both practically and symbolically almost entirely with men. These were men who held decisional power in medical and pharmaceutical matters, and masculine figures symbolizing medical authority and political power. The narrative of theriac aimed to build cohesion and trust in institutions. However, regardless of how compelling a symbol is, it does not necessarily reflect the reality of early modern healing. In early modern Europe, women were the main health care practitioners. The sheer overabundance of early modern institutional documents regarding theriac and its production obscures the much greater presence of homemade remedies and the daily labor and resourcefulness of female healers. In theory, the noble antidotes theriac and mithridate were part of the same medical framework as the health care and medicines provided by women and shaped around diet and botanicals, a framework to which most secrets concocted by patented remedy sellers also belonged. What set theriac apart from other medicines was its elevation above all other drugs by the medical and state systems. In a culture such as that of early modern Italy, in which everything was hierarchized by value—stones, flowers, animals, foods—medicines too were ordered strictly according to prestige and effectiveness. For those prone to follow and trust authority, theriac's prestige was a strong incentive to use it. Theriac's visibility, however, is testament to its institutional character. Especially in the sixteenth and early seventeenth centuries, such visibility was not in itself proof of theriac's widespread use among patients, although its use certainly increased from the mid-seventeenth century.

CONCLUSION

Theriac's material composition was of paramount importance to its history. It was a point of reference for patients, who knew what to expect; for apothecaries, who built their careers and reputations on it; and, for a long time, also for physicians, who relied on it even as they started doubting its efficacy. Examining theriac's sensory characteristics—its taste, smell, and consistency—yields a deeper understanding of the remedy as being more than just a medicinal substance. Apothecaries could base their authority on theriac because of the complexity of its recipe, which entailed the precise measuring and handling of dozens of disparate ingredients. Making theriac demanded expertise, knowledge, skills, and means. As production grew consistently throughout the eighteenth century, the complexity of the procedure prohibited its being scaled up into an industrial process. The mechanics of theriac production were constraining in different ways from those of the chemical remedies studied by Zachary Dorner, for example, which were easily turned into full-scale industrial productions. Furthermore, demand for specific ingredients, especially vipers, led to the development of organized hunting, whose significant environmental impact in the Colli Euganei resonated for centuries thereafter. This should make us suspicious of romantic ideals of artisanal productions as being naturally harmonious. The scale of an artisanal production can render it simply unsustainable. By virtue of its sensory characteristics, theriac represented an experience not only for the apothecaries who crafted it but also for the patients who consumed it. The experience was intangible as well as material, as embedded within theriac were spiritual meanings derived from medieval legends that associated the sacrifice of Christ on the cross with the viper's flesh it contained. This points to an emotional side of the consumption of medicines, which also warrants further investigation.

While it is not my intention to overstate the importance of theriac in Italian or European state building, I do suggest that pharmacy is a significant perspective to add when investigating this phenomenon. Theriac's political significance grew at a time when Galenic pharmacy—which since antiquity had constituted Europe's primary learned pharmaceutical tradition—was gaining more weight as the official pharmacy. The establishment of Galenic pharmacy as the official pharmacy across early modern Europe has not been adequately considered to date, and it is not evident whether this process followed similar patterns across Europe. I have argued that the official status of Galenic pharmacy played a significant role in keeping it so persistent over time. The proximity of Galenic pharmacy to the early modern state suggests that pharmacy was critical to the creation of colonial empires. The success and prestige theriac acquired both in the Italian states and across Europe would eventually extend to other continents, beginning with the European expansion. Despite the complexity of its recipe and manufacture, colonizers and missionaries implanted theriac productions in colonial empires, and theriac exports also gained traction in the Ottoman and Russian Empires. The metamorphoses of theriac reflect the diversity of the contexts in which it was received—although its prestige remained ever its defining mark. By following multiple versions of theriac across four continents, I have merely hinted at the flexibility of Galenic pharmacy in different environments, the continued commercial and political relevance of the Galenic framework, and Europeans' demonstrable attachment to it. The ways health practitioners and patients negotiated, accepted, transformed, and rejected remedies once in contact with different cultures and natural environments also awaits further investigation.

Finally, I have demonstrated that theriac was not just an improbable curiosity, and I have addressed my initial question about why a Chinese physician at the court of Emperor Kangxi would prescribe theriac to one of his patients. The history of early modern theriac holds contemporary relevance: the persistence of a pharmaceutical tradition, the interplay between medicine and state authority, and the social and cultural significance of pharmaceuticals are themes that resonate beyond the specific context of theriac. The ways early modern states used theriac to assert authority and maintain social order, and the drug's interconnections with commercial revenues, can inform discussions on the role of government in health care, the importance of state intervention in public health, and the social and political dimensions of pharmaceuticals. The state drug reminds us that connections between health, authority, and society have deeper roots than biomedicine does.

ABBREVIATIONS

NOTES

BIBLIOGRAPHY

ACKNOWLEDGMENTS

INDEX

ABBREVIATIONS

AOIF	Archivio dell'Ospedale degli Innocenti, Florence
AOSMM	Archivi Storici Diocesani di Udine, Archivio dell'Ospedale S. Maria Della Misericordia
ASAN	Archivio Storico della Sovrintendenza di Napoli
ASB	Archivio di Stato di Bologna
ASF	Archivio di Stato di Firenze
ASN	Archivio di Stato di Napoli
ASV	Archivio di Stato di Venezia
BCAB	Biblioteca Comunale dell'Archiginnasio, Bologna
BMC	Biblioteca del Museo Correr, Venice
BNCF	Biblioteca Nazionale Centrale, Florence
BNM	Biblioteca Nazionale Marciana, Venice
BUB	Biblioteca Universitaria, Bologna
VBA	Veneranda Biblioteca Ambrosiana, Milan
DBI	Dizionario Biografico degli Italiani, https://www.treccani.it/biografico/
KJV	King James Version
MAP	Medici Archive Project, bia.medici.org

NOTES

INTRODUCTION

1. First Historical Archive, *Complete Translation;* 1445, 629; also in Puente-Ballestreros, "Antoine Thomas Si," 229.
2. *Lettres édifiantes et curieuses,* 19:318; also in Puente-Ballestreros, "Antoine Thomas Si," 240.
3. Given its diffusion and long history, theriac has been the subject of numerous studies. However, only a handful of book-length histories of theriac exist. The most recent and reliable is certainly Boudon-Millot and Micheau, *La Thériaque* (2020); see also Watson, *Theriac and Mithridatium* (1966); and Holste, *Der Theriakkrämer* (1976). For theriac in antiquity, see especially Stein, "La Thériaque chez Galen"; Totelin, "Mithradates' Antidote." See also Knoefel and Covi, *A Hellenistic Treatise;* Martin, "De theriaca." For theriac in the Middle Ages, see especially Nockels Fabbri, "Treating Medieval Plague"; McVaugh, "Theriac at Montpellier"; Granel, "La thériaque de Montpellier"; Ricordel, "Le traité sur la thériaque"; Ricordel, "Ibn Djuljul"; Gibbs, "Specific Form and Poisonous Properties"; Rubin, "Use of the 'Jericho Tyrus.'"
4. Therefore, here and throughout, I mostly refer to theriac alone, pointing out differences with mithridate only when necessary.
5. Heberden, *Antitheriaka,* 10.
6. Studies on theriac in the early modern period are plentiful, and the following references are only a selection: see Olmi, "Farmacopea antica"; Findlen, *Possessing Nature,* esp. chap. 6; Stossl, *Lo spettacolo della triaca;* Palmer, "Pharmacy"; Laughran, "Medicating"; Rankin, *The Poison Trials,* esp. chap. 1; Pugliano, "Pharmacy, Testing"; Bernhard, *Les médicaments oubliés;* Dian, *Cenni;* Benedicenti, *Malati, medici e farmacisti,* 2:1017–1030; Pazzini, *La triaca in Roma;* Berman, "Persistence of Theriac"; Mongelli, "Diffusione di un medicamento"; Maggioni, "La teriaca 'farmaco di Stato'"; Rosa, "La teriaca a Bologna"; Cowen, "Expunctum est Mithridatium"; Flahaut, "La thériaque diatessaron"; Griffin, "Venetian Treacle."
7. Whyte et al., *Social Lives of Medicines;* Sismondo and Greene, *The Pharmaceutical Studies Reader.*

8. Dorner, *Merchants of Medicines*.
9. Breen, *The Age of Intoxication*.
10. B.D.B., *Theriaque et anthidot prepare*.
11. Gestrich, "The Social Order," 295.
12. For an overview of these complex processes, see Lindemann, *Medicine and Society*, chap. 6. Among many others, see Cipolla, *Public Health*; Cipolla, *Miasmas and Disease*; Park, *Doctors and Medicine*; Cook, *The Decline*; Pelling and White, *Medical Conflicts*; Gentilcore, "'All That Pertains to Medicine'"; Brockliss and Jones, *The Medical World*; Pomata, *Contracting a Cure*.
13. Breen, *The Age of Intoxication*, 131–132.
14. Palmer, "Pharmacy."
15. On Camilla Erculiani, see Carinci, "Una 'speziala' padovana"; Erculiani, *Letters on Natural Philosophy*. On Erculiani and theriac, see Erculiani, *Letters on Natural Philosophy*, 125; Findlen, "Foreword" to Erculiani, *Letters on Natural Philosophy*, 12–15.
16. BNM, Collegio Medico, IT.VII, 2366 (= 9737), Ferdinand von Bissingen to Antonio C. Michelburg, August 19, 1803.
17. Ackerknecht, *Therapeutics*.
18. Rosenberg, "The Therapeutic Revolution," 4.
19. This was the case for heroic medicine in nineteenth-century America; see Warner, *The Therapeutic Perspective*.
20. Breen, *The Age of Intoxication*, 228.
21. See, among others, Bénézet and Flahaut, *Pharmacie et médicament*, 673–677; Mozzato, "Oppio, triaca," 172–173. On opium and theriac, see also Scarborough, "The Opium Poppy." Researchers have analyzed old samples of theriac found in historical hospitals and pharmacies in 1928 (Genua), 1962 (Florence), and 2021 (Rome). Experiments were conducted in vitro and in vivo in the first two cases, and the samples were considered pharmacologically active, with both sedative and stimulant action. See Garello, "Sopra un vecchio campione di triaca"; Piccinini et al., "Una ulteriore luce." For a molecular analysis, see Mattoli et al., "Mass Spectrometry Studies."
22. Stein, "La Thériaque chez Galen," 205.
23. Nockels Fabbri, "Treating Medieval Plague," 280.
24. Maranta, *Della theriaca et del mithridato*, 150–152.
25. Della Peruta, "Infanzia e famiglia," 486.
26. In theriac recipes, the quantity of opium was about 1/80th of the total weight of raw ingredients (in Venice, 24/1892 drachms, or approximately 93 grams over a total of 7.4 kilograms). It is possible that the quantity of opium contained in one dose of theriac—approximately 0.05 grams of opium in a dose of 3–4 grams—was sufficient to act as a painkiller or sedative. These quantities varied because the weight in grams of a drachm depended on the system used; for example, a drachm equaled 3.9 grams in Venice, but 3.39 grams in Bologna. See also Raj et al., "The Real Theriac."

27. On this point, see especially Ahnfelt et al., "Making and Taking Theriac."
28. See, for example, Pisanelli, *Discorso sopra la peste*, 51; Houel, *Traité de la Thériaque et Mithridat*, 11v.
29. Bénézet and Flahaut, *Pharmacie et médicament*, 673.
30. Maranta, *Della theriaca et del mithridato*, 150–152.
31. Three teams of scholars have already attempted to reconstruct theriac. For the reconstruction at the University of Uppsala, see Ahnfelt and Fors, "Making Early Modern Medicine"; and Ahnfelt et al., "Making and Taking Theriac." For the reconstruction undertaken at the Pharmaziemuseum at the University of Basel, see Kluge, "Das Theriak-Experiment," J9, according to which theriac would have had no antimicrobial effects. For the reconstruction at the University of Wrocław, see Raj et al., "The Real Theriac"; and https://projekty.ncn.gov.pl/en/index.php?projekt_id=385062. For biologists' experiments on historical remedies, see, for example, Kadam et al., "From Treatise to Test"; Anonye et al., "The Safety Profile"; and Furner-Pardoe et al., "Anti-Biofilm Efficacy."
32. On the Galenic medical tradition in general, see Temkin, *Galenism*; García Ballester, *Galen and Galenism*; and Hankinson, *Cambridge Companion to Galen*.
33. De Vos, *Compound Remedies*; Debru, *Galen on Pharmacology*; Vogt, "Drugs and Pharmacology."
34. On early modern bioprospecting, commerce, and science, see especially Cook, *Matters of Exchange*; Schiebinger and Swan, *Colonial Botany*; Schiebinger, *Plants and Empire*; and Smith and Findlen, *Merchants and Marvels*.
35. For specific remedies, see Cook, "Markets and Cultures."
36. Grafton et al., *New World, Ancient Texts*; see chap. 1, n6, on Renaissance botany and medicine.
37. McVaugh, "Chemical Medicine"; Moran, *Chemical Pharmacy*; Moran, "Survey of Chemical Medicine"; Urdang, "How Chemicals Entered"; De Vos, *Compounds Remedies*, esp. chap. 5.
38. On the disputes, see, for example, Debus, *The French Paracelsians*. See also Murphy, *New Order of Medicine*, 112.
39. Gentilcore, *Medical Charlatanism*.
40. For the relationship between chemistry and its impact on medical theories in Italy, see Clericuzio, "Chemical Medicine"; Galluzzi, "Motivi paracelsiani"; and Brambilla, "Dagli antidoti."
41. Temkin, *Galenism*, 117.
42. See Youyou Tu, "Discovery of Artemisinin"; Anonye et al., "The Safety Profile"; and Furner-Pardoe et al., "Anti-Biofilm Efficacy." See also the Institute for the Preservation of Medical Traditions (medicaltraditions.org). On using ancient texts for bioprospecting, see Totelin, "Technologies of Knowledge."
43. De Vos, *Compound Remedies*, 5.

44. On substitutes in Galenic pharmacy, see Touwaide, "Quid pro Quo"; and Boumediene and Pugliano, "La route des succédanés."
45. Murphy, *New Order of Medicine.*
46. See, for example, De Vos, *Compound Remedies;* and Newson, *Making Medicines.*

1. THE REINVENTION OF THERIAC

1. Calestani, *Delle osservationi,* 84. Unless otherwise noted, all translations, here and throughout, are mine
2. BUB, Ald. Ms. 21, III, 134r.
3. Watson, *Theriac and Mithridatium,* 12.
4. On the word *theriac,* see Rousseau, "Des Thériaques."
5. For theriac in antiquity, see the Introduction.
6. On Renaissance botany and medicine, see, among others, Stannard et al., *Herbs and Herbalism;* Palmer, "Medical Botany"; Reeds, *Botany;* Findlen, *Possessing Nature;* Ogilvie, *The Science of Describing;* Jardine et al., *Cultures of Natural History.*
7. For theriac as a symbolic enterprise at the core of rethinking materia medica, see Palmer, "Pharmacy," 108–110; Findlen, *Possessing Nature,* 272–277; Olmi, "Farmacopea antica."
8. Findlen, *Possessing Nature,* chap. 6
9. See especially Olmi "Farmacopea antica"; Laughran, "Medicating," 102–104; Griffin, "Venetian Treacle"; Pugliano, "Pharmacy, Testing."
10. The reinvention of theriac has some similarity with, but does not fit precisely the paradigm of, the "invention of tradition." Theriac was only *reinvented,* not invented from scratch; see Hobsbawm and Ranger, *The Invention of Tradition.*
11. A reference to theriac peddlers (or *triacleurs*) can be found in a 1508 French ordinance; see Bernhard, *Les médicaments oubliés,* 90.
12. Bénézet and Flahaut, *Pharmacie et médicament,* 189; Silini, *Umori e farmaci,* 207.
13. Ait, *Tra scienza e mercato,* 89, n35.
14. De Manliis et al., *Luminare maggiore,* 80; Bénézet and Flahaut, *Pharmacie et médicament,* 680. In the late 1470s the Paston family in East Anglia was anxious to receive theriac from Genoa; see Davis, *Paston Letters and Papers,* vol. 1, no. 313.
15. Bénézet and Flahaut, *Pharmacie et médicament,* 127–128, 140, 680.
16. On apothecaries, see Gentilcore, "World of the Italian Apothecary"; Collard and Samama, *Pharmacopoles et Apothicaires;* Halikowski-Smith, "The Physician's Hand"; Palmer, "Pharmacy"; Laughran, "Medicating"; Di Gennaro Splendore, "Craft, Money and Mercy"; Pugliano, "Pharmacy, Testing." On apothecaries and the market, see Shaw and Welch, *Making and*

Marketing Medicine; Welch, *Shopping in the Renaissance,* 151–158; Welch, "Space and Spectacle"; Wallis, "Consumption, Retailing, and Medicine"; DeLancey, "Dragonblood and Ultramarine"; Strocchia, "The Nun Apothecaries"; Strocchia, *Forgotten Healers,* esp. chap. 3 and 4.
17. Mozzato, "Uno speziale aretino."
18. Shaw and Welch, *Making and Marketing Medicine,* 249; Tognetti, "Prezzi e salari."
19. In Venice between 1460 and 1470, theriac in bulk cost 0.18 ducats per pound; see Mozzato, "Oppio, triaca," 172–173.
20. AOSMM, 1064, *Index pretia continens omnium rerum medicinalium simplicium* (1636).
21. Jacquart, "La thériaque," 338.
22. Pulci, *Morgante,* Cantare 25, 112.
23. Rabelais, *Gargantua and Pantagruel,* xlvi, 1041.
24. Pazzini, *La triaca in Roma,* 21.
25. Sanudo, *Le vite dei Dogi* (1423–1474), 1:370.
26. Rossi, "La Sultana Nūr Bānū"; Dian, *Cenni,* 41.
27. Pagano and Postel, *True Description of Cairo,* 22. The caption likely referred to an unidentified square close to the thirteenth-century Qalawun complex, which included a hospital.
28. Dian, *Cenni,* 38.
29. Gentz, "Theriaca," 77; also in Stossl, "Lo spettacolo della teriaca."
30. Adorno, *Itineraire d'Anselme Adorno,* 213.
31. Alpini, *De medicina Aegyptiorum,* 133v.
32. BUB, Ald. Ms. 38, II, v. I cc. 135r–136v (Guilandino to Aldrovandi June 9, 1559).
33. On Melchior Wieland (Guilandinus), see Gillispie, *Complete Dictionary,* 14:335–336.
34. Alpini, *De medicina Aegyptiorum,* 133v.
35. In England, regulation started in 1540; see Griffin, "Venetian Treacle."
36. Until the sixteenth century there were few local differences between apothecary statutes; see Corradi, "Gli antichi statuti," 177.
37. ASB, *Statuto dell'Arte degli speziali,* 1303.
38. Monticolo, *I capitolari,* 159, 163; also in Dian, *Cenni,* 38.
39. Arte degli speziali di Pisa and Vigo, *Statuto inedito,* 15–17. For a critical appraisal of this publication and a general discussion on apothecary guilds' statutes, see Corradi, "Gli antichi statuti," 153–213.
40. Vigo, *Statuto inedito,* 61.
41. On the origin of the Giustizia Vecchia, see Deputazione Veneta di Storia Patria, *L'ufficio della Giustizia Vecchia.*
42. Laws on theriac were issued at least in 1410, 1432, 1437, 1441, 1442, and 1480. ASV, Compilazione delle Leggi Prima serie, 277; Compilazione delle Leggi Seconda Serie, fasc. 31 n. 6. This last is also in Dian, *Cenni,* 39.

43. ASV, Compilazione delle Leggi Seconda Serie, fasc. 231 n. 6; also in Dian, *Cenni*, 39. Electuaries were pharmaceutical preparations comprising pulverized medication mixed with honey.
44. ASV, Compilazione delle Leggi Prima serie, 277, 890.
45. ASV, Compilazione delle Leggi Seconda Serie, fasc. 231 n. 6. See also Dian, *Cenni*, 40. To the best of my knowledge, there is no extant "Libro delle Triache" in Venice.
46. On the Venetian Collegio Medico, see Palmer, *The Studio of Venice*; Bernardi, *Prospetto storico-critico*, also reprinted in Vanzan Marchin, *Dalla scienza medica*.
47. Dian, *Cenni*, 42.
48. Palmer, "Physicians and the State," 57.
49. For the Bolognese Collegio Medico, see Pomata, *Contracting a Cure*, 1–24. For Florence, see Ciuti, "Il Collegio dei fisici." For Rome, see Elisa Andretta, *Roma Medica*, 47–186.
50. Vanzan Marchin, "Medici ebrei," 148–150; Stevens Crawshaw, *Plague Hospitals*, 156.
51. ASV, Compilazione delle Leggi. Prima Serie 277, 805, July 10, 1480.
52. ASV, Compilazione delle Leggi. Prima Serie 277, 88, October 6, 1441.
53. Minard, *La fortune du colbertisme*.
54. De Blainville, *Travels Through Holland*, 79.
55. The most comprehensive study to date on the textual transmission of theriac's recipe is Boudon-Millot and Micheau, *La Thériaque*; see also Watson, *Theriac and Mithridatium*.
56. These works became available in Europe in the fourteenth century. It is debated whether Galen wrote a specific treatise on theriac—the only compound remedy in the Galenic corpus with dedicated specific treatises—because, although he did refer to a treatise on theriac, scholars have not definitively identified it with *De Antidotis*; see Boudon-Millot, "Anecdote et antidote," n.5, 46.

    For *De theriaca ad Pamphilianum*, see Coturri, "Perché." For *De theriaca ad Pisonem*, see Boudon-Millot, *Claudius Galenus, Œuvres*, and Leigh, *On Theriac to Piso*. Both authors and Nathalie Rousseau agree that *De theriaca ad Pisonem* was not written by Galen. In the sixteenth century, physician Giulio Alessandrini was one of the first to doubt the authenticity of *De theriaca ad Pisonem*, as confirmed by a letter from Girolamo Mercuriale to Pietro Andrea Mattioli; see VBA, D198 inf, 78r–79v. Popular books for apothecaries raised doubts on the authenticity of *De theriaca ad Pisonem*; see, for example, Calestani and Bertucci, *Osservationi*, which had fourteen editions.
57. For the use of the anachronism "pharmacology" in this context, see Vogt, "Drugs and Pharmacology," 305. Galen had a complex theory on the ways drugs affected the human body, and pharmacology investigates just that, albeit with different methods.

58. On Galen and pharmacology, see Vogt, "Drugs and Pharmacology"; Debru, *Galen on Pharmacology*; De Vos, *Compound Remedies*.
59. Stein, "La thériaque chez Galen," 206–207.
60. Vogt, "Drugs and Pharmacology," 314.
61. Nockels Fabbri, "Treating Medieval Plague," 266. This was a common theory in the Renaissance; see, among others, Maranta, *Della theriaca et del mithridato*, 10.
62. Leigh, *On Theriac to Piso*, 85.
63. Arnaldus and McVaugh, *Arnaldi de Villanova*, 57; Ricordel, "Variations sur le thème."
64. Avicenna et al., *Libri in re medica omnes*, 1:255, A49–53.
65. On specific form, see Gibbs, *Poison, Medicine, and Disease*, 25–26; and Gibbs, "Specific Form," 19–46.
66. Daston and Park, *Wonders*, 127.
67. Siraisi, *Avicenna in Renaissance Italy*.
68. On the debate on theriac in Montpellier, see McVaugh, "Theriac at Montpellier"; Arnaldus and McVaugh, *Epistola de Dosi Tyriacalium*, 58–59. On Ibn Rushd's treatise *De tyriaca*, see Ricordel, "Le traité"; and Ricordel, "Ibn Djuljul"; Ricordel, "Variations sur le thème," 291. On the circulation of the manuscript, see Hasse, *Success and Suppression*, 345 n. 156.
69. Arnaldus and McVaugh, *Epistola de Dosi Tyriacalium*, 68–69. This was in line with the general framing of the medical discussion on poison; see Gibbs, *Poison, Medicine, and Disease*.
70. Nockels Fabbri, "Treating Medieval Plague," 247–283, 262.
71. On medical theories about poison, see Gibbs, *Poison, Medicine, and Disease*; Wexler, *Toxicology*; Voinier and Winter, *Poison et Antidote*; Grell et al., *"It All Depends on the Dose."*
72. Chase, "Fevers, Poisons and Apostemes," 157. On plague and poison, see also Carmichael, "Contagion Theory," 223–224; Gibbs, *Poison, Medicine, and Disease*, 116–150.
73. Chase, "Fevers, Poisons and Apostemes," 158, 161.
74. Arduino, *Opus de venenis*, 83–93.
75. Ficino, *De vita libri tres*, 28–29.
76. Beecher, "Ficino, Theriaca," 243. Beecher affirmed that theriac at the time was a "drug under empirical siege," but the siege started later on.
77. Ficino, *Consiglio contro la pestilenza*, 1r–1v.
78. Ficino, *Consiglio contro la pestilenza*, 12r.
79. Paracelsus, *Paracelsus*, 149–151.
80. Daston and Park, *Wonders*, 88–90.
81. Calvet, "À la recherche."
82. Panciroli, *Rerum memorabilium*. See also Keller, "Accounting for Invention."
83. On the concept of lost knowledge, see Olshin, *Lost Knowledge*; on lost objects as scientific objects, see Keller, "Storied Objects, Scientific Objects."

On the importance of the concept of lost knowledge for artisans in the seventeenth and eighteenth centuries, see Bertucci, *Artisanal Enlightenment*, chap. 1.
84. Fracastoro, *Hieronymi Fracastorii*, 65.
85. Pugliano, "Pharmacy, Testing," 256.
86. Arduino, *Opus de venenis*, 21, 83, 92, 165.
87. ASV, Compilazione delle Leggi Prima serie, 277, 889.
88. Cordus, *Von Der Vielfaltigen*.
89. Bruno, *De la causa principio*, Dialogo 5, 17.
90. Citation in Harley, "Medical Metaphors," 423 n140.
91. Calzolari, *Lettera*, nn., "et massimamente trovandosi che fra noi si potevano aver le vere serpi né occorreva andar in Levante a trovar le false."
92. Maranta, *Della theriaca et del mithridato*, 44.
93. Leoniceno, *De tiro seu vipera* in *Opuscula*, 108v.
94. Rubin, "Use of the 'Jericho Tyrus,'" 239.
95. Rubin, "Use of the 'Jericho Tyrus,'" 242.
96. Ramusio, *Navigazioni e Viaggi*, 5:286–287. Gonzalo Fernando de Oviedo reports of a deadly serpent tyrus in Tierra Firme, between today's Columbia and Nicaragua; Rubin, "Use of the 'Jericho Tyrus,'" 252 n53, 54.
97. Leoniceno, *De tiro seu vipera* in *Opuscula*, 108v. For this debate, see also Rubin, "Use of the 'Jericho Tyrus,'" 245–248.
98. Rubin, "Use of the 'Jericho Tyrus,'" 253 n71, 72.
99. On Niccolò Leoniceno (Niccolò da Lonigo), see DBI, Paolo Pellegrini, *ad vocem*.
100. Leoniceno, *De tiro seu vipera* in *Opuscula*, 109r. For Leoniceno on Ibn Sīnā, see also Siraisi, *Avicenna in Renaissance Italy*, 68–69. Leoniceno wrote other texts about snakes: *De vipera libellus* (1506), *De dipseade et pluribus aliis serpentibus* (1518, 1532).
101. Leoniceno, *De tiro seu vipera* in *Opuscula*, 109r.
102. Leoniceno, *De tiro seu vipera* in *Opuscula*, 109v. On viper's *trociscus*, see Oszajca, "Trocisci viperini."
103. Dian, *Cenni*, 42.
104. On Venetian apothecaries, see Palmer, "Pharmacy," esp. 106–107; Pugliano, "Botanical Artisans"; see also Palmer, *The Studio of Venice*, 105.
105. Sanudo, *Diarii*, vol. 55, 3 January 1531, 310.
106. Sanudo, *Diarii*, vol. 55, 3 January 1531, 310.
107. Sanudo, *Diarii*, vol. 55, 2 January 1531, 308.
108. Galenus, *Galeni librorum pars prima-quinta* (Venice: in aedibus Aldi et Andrea soceri, 1525). This was a sole edition; see Mani, "Die griechischte Editio."
109. Sanudo, *Diarii*, vol. 55, 2 January 1531, 308.
110. Siraisi, *Avicenna in Renaissance Italy*.
111. Musatti, *La teriaca e il mitridato*.
112. ASV, Giustizia Vecchia 211.

113. Dian, *Cenni*, 43–44.
114. BUB, Ald. Ms. 21, III, 134r.
115. Champier, *Appothiquaires et Pharmacopoles*, 27.
116. Teodosio, *Medicinales epistolae*, 41. On Teodosio, see Manzi, "Un maestro dello studio bolognese."
117. Teodosio, *Medicinales epistolae*, 47.
118. Cordus, *Von Der Vielfaltigen*.
119. Maranta, *Della theriaca et del mithridato*, 44. On the popularity of Dioscorides in the sixteenth century, see Stannard, *Herbs and Herbalism*.
120. Mattioli, *Di Pedacio Dioscoride Anazarbeo*.
121. On Dioscorides's sixth book on antidotes, see Fausti, "Su alcune traduzioni cinquecentesche."
122. Mattioli, *Il Dioscoride* (1548), bk. VI, 7.
123. On Mattioli's scorpion oil and skepticism, see also Findlen, *Possessing Nature*, 269n101.
124. On the importance of Greek texts to the scientific debate, see Nutton, "Greek Science," 16–17.
125. Galenus, *De anatomicis administrationibus*; Galen, *De theriaca ad Pisonem liber*.
126. Camerarius, *De theriacis et methridateis*. On this text, see Stannard, *Herbs and Herbalism*, 152–153.
127. For Nicander in the early modern period, see Radici, *Nicandro di Colofone*.
128. Findlen, *Possessing Nature*, 53–54.
129. Palmer, "Pharmacy," acknowledged the importance of Venetian apothecaries to the development of botany. On apothecaries' contribution to the Scientific Revolution, see Smith, *Body of the Artisan*; Harkness, *The Jewel House*; Egmond, "Apothecaries as Experts"; Anagnostou et al., *A Passion for Plants*.
130. Calestani, *Delle osservationi*, 83–86.
131. Calestani, *Delle osservationi*, 83.
132. Bartolomeo da Orvieto and Paglia, *In antidotarium Joannis filii Mesue*; De Ninno, *Memorie storiche*, 106; Massa Ducale, *Dilucidazione fitologica*, 31.
133. Vallieri, "Le 22 lettere," 211, Maranta to Aldrovandi January 23, 1558.
134. Vallieri, "Le 22 lettere," 203, Maranta to Aldrovandi March 6, 1558.
135. Lavoranti, *Lode della theriaca*.
136. BUB, Ald. Ms. 382, III, cc. 26r–26v (Calzolari to Aldrovandi, July 25, 1554); c. 33r. (Calzolari to Aldrovandi November 5, 1555); c. 39r. (Calzolari to Aldrovandi, September 5, 1558).
137. Maranta, *Della theriaca et del mithridato*, 35.
138. Calzolari, *Lettera*, nn.
139. Mattioli, *I discorsi di M. Pietro Andrea Matthioli* (1563), 743.
140. Mattioli, *I discorsi di M. Pietro Andrea Matthioli* (1563), 743–744.
141. Mattioli, *Il Dioscoride* (1573), 955.
142. Mattioli, *Il Dioscoride* (1573), 780.

143. BUB, Ald. Ms. 21, III, 134v.
144. On Evangelista Quattrami, see De Toni, "Notizie bio-bibliografiche"; Dallasta, "Novità." On Ferrante Imperato, see Stendardo, *Ferrante Imperato*; Findlen, "Why Put a Museum in a Book?" On Antonio Bertioli, see Galassi, "Antonio Bertioli"; Grandi, "La scienza medica."
145. Carinci, "Una 'speziala' padovana," n67.
146. Calestani, *Delle osservationi*, 83–86.
147. Calestani, *Delle osservationi*, 250; BUB, Ald. Ms. 91, 50r, 108v; ASB, Studio 217.
148. On apothecaries publishing on pharmacy, see also Pugliano, "Pharmacy, Testing."
149. Minuzzi, *Sul filo dei segreti*, 116.
150. Palmer, "Pharmacy," 109.
151. Calzolari, *Lettera*, nn.
152. Calestani, *Delle osservationi*, 248.
153. See, for example, Maranta, *Della theriaca et del mithridato*, 52–53.
154. Calestani, *Delle osservationi*, 250; BUB, Ald. Ms. 91, 50r, 108v; ASB, Studio 217.
155. Melich, *Avvertimenti*, 42v.
156. Stieb, "Drug Adulteration." For anxieties attached to snake handlers and itinerant healers, see, for example, Park, "Country Medicine."
157. I discussed the position of apothecaries in Di Gennaro Splendore, "Craft, Money and Mercy."
158. Garzoni, *La piazza universale*, 662, 550.
159. Pastarino, *Ragionamento*, 12.
160. Mattioli, *Il Dioscoride* (1573), 780.
161. BUB, Ald. Ms. 91, 503–559, 532r; *Discorso Naturale*. A full transcription of *Discorso Naturale* is in Tugnoli Pattaro, *Metodo e sistema delle scienze*. For Aldrovandi's opinion on apothecaries, see Di Gennaro Splendore, "Craft, Money and Mercy," 98.

2. THE EXPERIENCE OF THERIAC

1. Bartoli, *Lettere a Lorenzo Giacomini*, 149, December 24, 1574.
2. Whyte et al., *Social Lives of Medicines*.
3. Bynum and Porter, *Medicine and the Five Senses*.
4. ASB, Studio 213.
5. Baley, *A discourse*, nn. It is not certain if the author of this treatise is English physician Walter Bayley (1529–1593).
6. ASB, Studio 213, 29r–30v.
7. Ficino, *Consiglio contro la pestilenza*, 10r.
8. Maranta, *Della theriaca et del mithidato*, 143.
9. Piccinini et al., *Una ulteriore luce*, 36.

10. Ahnfelt et al., "Making and Taking Theriac," 50.
11. Ahnfelt and Fors, "Making Early Modern Medicine"; Ahnfelt, Fors, and Wendin, "Making and Taking Theriac," 57, 60.
12. Larry Principe, personal communication, March 17, 2024.
13. ASB, Studio 213, 14r, 29r–30v.
14. Von Eschenbach, *Parzival*.
15. Palmer, "In Bad Odour," 61.
16. Piccinini et al., *Una ulteriore luce*, 35–39.
17. ASB, Studio 213, 29r–30v.
18. Galasso, *Trattato molto vtile*, 4.
19. Cook, *Matters of Exchange*, 91.
20. "Literary Notes," 420.
21. Fioravanti, *Del reggimento della peste*, 22.
22. Moratti, *Racconto de gli ordini*, 59; Wear, *Knowledge and Practice*, 68; Crawshaw, *Plague Hospitals*, 128.
23. *Lettere edificanti*, 147, Father Fontaney to Reverend Della Chaise, January 17, 1704.
24. Sassetti, *Lettere edite e inedite*, 353, Filippo Sassetti to Bernardo Davanzati, January 23, 1586.
25. ASF, Mediceo del Principato 2944, fol. 371r, October 1607, Francesco Ormanni to unidentified addressee (MAP Doc ID# 5078).
26. AOIF, Filza di ricevute riguardanti la spezieria del conservadorio 1705–1743.
27. AOIF, Giornale della spezieria dal 1729 al 1767, 124r, 133r. Apparently, nuns paid different prices for similar quantities of theriac.
28. Guarguanti, *Della theriaca*, 21.
29. *Il giornale dei letterati d'Italia*, vol. 33, pt. 1, 63.
30. Sterlich, *Lettere a G. Bianchi*, 172.
31. See, for example, Zanella, *Della triaca*; these doses are usual in medical literature.
32. ASB Studio 248, Draft of the 1727 Conventions, art. 12.
33. For similar conclusions drawn from other sources, see Cavallo, "Secrets to Healthy Living"; Cavallo and Storey, *Healthy Living*, 221.
34. Hoffmann, *Botanotheca Lauremergiana*, sig. [A3]r, in Cooper, *Inventing the Indigenous*, 69.
35. Maranta, *Della theriaca e del mithridato*, 164.
36. Voiture, *Les oeuvres*, 22.
37. Dian, *Cenni*, 37.
38. Metastasio, *Lettere*, vol. 5, 203.
39. ASB, Assunteria di Studio 87, March 17, 1687.
40. Ahnfelt et al., "Making and Taking Theriac," 43; Kluge, "Das Theriak-Experiment."
41. Collegio dei Medici di Roma, *Antidotario romano* (1624) 37.

42. Melich, *Avertimenti nelle compositioni* (1575), 42–43.
43. On artisanal awareness, see Smith, *Body of the Artisan*.
44. See also Rosa, "La panacea dell'antichità," 334.
45. ASN, Badia di Mileto 268, 33r; vitriol was part of an apothecary's list of missing ingredients for making theriac.
46. BUB, Ald. Ms. 21, IV, 127v.
47. De Sgobbis, *Universale theatro farmaceutico*, folding sheet at 424–425.
48. Just like ingredients, parts may vary depending on the recipe and interpretation; these are according to Maranta, *Della theriaca e del mithridato*.
49. Maranta, *Della theriaca e del mithridato*, 50–52.
50. Riccardi, *Istruttione*, 4.
51. Strocchia, *Forgotten Healers*, 260 n62.
52. Collegio dei Medici di Roma, *Antidotario romano* (1612), 37.
53. BUB, Ald. Ms. 70, 36v, 37r, 45v.
54. Danuta Raj, personal communication on December 6, 2022.
55. Riccardi, *Istruttione*, 4.
56. Bertioli, *Breue auuiso*.
57. This practice remains understudied. On substitutes in Galenic pharmacy, see Touwaide, "Quid pro Quo"; and Boumediene and Pugliano, "La route des succédanés."
58. Maranta, *Della theriaca e del mithridato*, 33–34.
59. Pomata, "Practicing," 121.
60. BCAB, Ms. B2468.
61. Maranta, *Della theriaca et del mithridato*, 147; Sartorio, *Discorso*, 45–47.
62. Riccardi, *Istruttione*, 8.
63. BUB, Ald. Ms. 136, XI, 127v.
64. Costa, *Discorsi sopra le composizioni*, 46r.
65. BMC, Grevembroch, *Gli abiti de Veneziani*, 120–121.
66. Castiglione, *Prospectus pharmaceutici*, 32. See, for example, Maranta, *Della theriaca et del mithridato*, 33–34; Cardullo, *Teriaca d'Andromaco*.
67. Candrini, *Teriaca*.
68. Openness was associated with trust until the late nineteenth century; see Gabriel, *Medical Monopoly*.
69. For the textual transmission of theriac's recipe, see Boudon-Millot and Micheau, *La Thériaque*; see also Watson, *Theriac and Mithridatium*.
70. Prévost, *Dispensarium Magistri Nicolai*. Widely accepted as a standard dispensatory as early as the thirteenth century, the *Dispensarium* was attributed to Nicolaus Salernitanus, a twelfth-century physician, and had been incorporated into the Paris medical curriculum by 1270. At least ten different manuscripts and several printed editions of the *Dispensarium* survive. See Zamuner, "Un volgarizzamento fiorentino."
71. See, for example, Collegio dei Medici di Roma, *Antidotarium Romanum*, 22v–23r.

72. Galenus, *L'antidotario di Claudio Galeno;* Arte de' medici e speziali di Firenze, *Ricettario utilissimo* (or *Ricettario Fiorentino,* 1556); Maranta, *Della theriaca et del mithridato;* Arte de' medici e speziali di Firenze, *Il ricettario medicinale;* Collegio degli speziali di Napoli et al., *Antidotario napolitano;* Capello and Capello, *Lessico Farmaceutico-Chimico;* Sartorio, *Discorso;* Riccardi, *Istruttione.*
73. Leigh, *On Theriac to Piso,* XII, 127.
74. BMC, Mariegola 209, 31. Also in Dian, *Cenni,* 74.
75. BNM, *Theriaca Andromachi senioris* (Venice: Joanne Baptista Albricci, 1756).
76. Part of the discussion on theriac formulas builds on Di Gennaro Splendore, "The Triumph of Theriac."
77. BMC, Mariegola 209, 31. Also in Dian, *Cenni,* 74.
78. On recipes as a medical genre, see Pomata, "The Recipe and the Case." For recipes in the early modern context, see Leong, *Recipes and Everyday Knowledge;* Leong and Rankin, *Secrets and Knowledge;* and Eamon, *Science and the Secrets.*
79. BMC, Mariegola 209, 31. Also in Dian, *Cenni,* 74.
80. For charlatans' publications, see Gentilcore, *Medical Charlatanism,* chap. 10, 337–358. For printed recipes of secrets, see Minuzzi, *Sul filo dei segreti,* 222–243.
81. Wallis and Wright Smith, "Evidence, Artisan Experience," 152.
82. In Bologna, the Protomedicato tribunal consisted of two Protomedici elected every three months by the members of the medical college. The tribunal conducted inspections specifically on physicians and apothecaries. On Protomedicato in Italy, see Gentilcore, "All That Pertains." On Bolognese Protomedicato, see Rosa, "La panacea dell'antichità"; Pomata, *Contracting a Cure,* esp. chap. 1.
83. ASB, Studio 213 1r–6v.
84. Roberts, "Death of the Sensuous Chemist."
85. Wallis and Wright Smith, "Evidence, Artisan Experience," 141–142.
86. Greene, *Generic,* 2.
87. Shapin, "The Sciences of Subjectivity"; Shapin, "The Tastes of Wine."
88. ASB, Studio 213, n.15.
89. ASB, Studio 213, 29r–30v.
90. Smith, *Body of the Artisan.*
91. On Mesue, see De Vos, "The 'Prince of Medicine'"; Ventura, "Les mélanges de médecine."
92. On this text, see Martelli et al., "Galen's Treatise."
93. ASB, Studio 213, 14r–16r.
94. ASB, Studio 213, 7v.
95. ASB, Studio 213, 27r–29r.
96. ASB, Studio 213, 9r.
97. ASB, Studio 213, 10v.
98. ASB, Studio 213, 9v.

99. ASB, Studio 213, 25r–26v.
100. ASB, Studio 213, 27r–29r.
101. Smith, *Body of the Artisan.*
102. See Quattrami, *Tractatus perutilis,* 77.
103. The Wikipedia page "Rod of Asclepius," http://en.wikipedia.org/wiki/Rod_of_Asclepius, lists more than eighty medical institutions that bear the snake in their symbol, but this number is an underestimation. Several medical organizations use the caduceus of Mercurius as their symbol, which may be more of a Freudian slip than an unintentional mistake.
104. Schickore, *About Method.*
105. Abati, *De admirabili viperae nature;* on this text, see Knoefel, "Abati's Work."
106. Panicelli, *Trattato.*
107. BUB, Giornale di Hercole Dal Buono, 8v.
108. De Beauvais, *Speculum naturale,* bk. XX XLVI, 250.
109. Terrusi, "Guittone," 50; Terrusi, *Secondo che Galieno pone.* On the relation between Beauvais and Cantimpré, see also Roy, "La trente-sixieme main."
110. McDonald, "The Serpent as Healer," 21.
111. Charlesworth, *Good and Evil Serpent,* 161–166.
112. John 3:14–15 (KJV). "Sicut Moses exaltavit serpentem in deserto, ita esaltari oportet filius hominis."
113. Neckam, *De Naturis Rerum,* II CIX192. Partially cited in Collard, *The Crime of Poison,* 70.
114. Calvet, "À la recherche," 196.
115. Calvinus, *Commentaries on John* (John 3:14–15), "https://ccel.org/ccel/calvin/calcom34/calcom34.ix.iii.html?highlight=serpent&queryID=37281311&resultID=119828%22" \l "highlight".
116. For the medals, see Holzmair, *Katalog der Sammlung.*
117. Picinelli, *Mondo simbolico,* 360; in Stossl, *Spettacolo di teriaca,* 26.
118. Biller and Ziegler, *Religion and Medicine,* 4; Gentilcore, *Healers and Healing,* 1–28.
119. Krafft and von Christa, *Christus ruft in die Himmelsapotheke;* Hein, *Christus als Apotheker.*
120. Maranta, *Della theriaca et del mithridato,* 46.
121. BUB, Ald. Ms. 100; for the approvals by the Collegio Medico of Rome, Naples, and Florence, see BUB, Ald. Ms. 21/4 cc. 349r–355r.
122. ASF, Arte Medici e Speziali, 269 Registro di Provvisioni e Ricordi detto C.
123. Bernhard, *Les médicaments oubliés,* 62–63.
124. ASB, Studio 233, *Bando sopra le Vipere,* April 20, 1606 (also in BCAB); April 20, 1663; March 31, 1666. BCAB, Raccolta Bandi Merlani, *Bando sopra le Vipere,* March 24, 1683.
125. Gentilcore, *Medical Charlatanism,* 174–180; Park, "Country Medicine."
126. BUB, Ald. Ms. 79.
127. Redi, *Osservazioni intorno alle vipere,* 13–14.

128. ASN, Badia di Mileto 279; Santolillo was paid 5 carlini for his service, while 260 vipers cost 61 ducats and 94 grana; at the time, 1 ducat = 10 carlini; 1 carlino = 10 grana.
129. BNM, Collegio Medico, IT.VII, 2340 (= 9672) holds several such *fedi.*
130. Schott, *Italy,* 37.
131. BNM, Collegio Medico IT.VII, 2340 (= 9672), 185r, 185v.
132. BNM, Collegio Medico IT.VII, 2340 (= 9672), 185v, 187v.
133. Sartorio, *Discorso,* 17.
134. BUB, Ms. 408, I: 159r–159v. A viper cost 13–25 soldi.
135. BNM, Collegio Medico IT.VII, 2342 (= 9695), 121r. Document partially cited in Dian, *Cenni,* 42. ASV, Giustizia Vecchia, 211. Also in Eamon, *Professor of Secrets,* 164.
136. For this information, I would like to thank Daniele Di Rosa, president of the APAE (Associazione Padovana Acquatologica Erpetologica), and Dr. Matteo di Nicola.

3. IMPERIAL ANTIDOTES FOR RENAISSANCE RULERS

1. Bremer-David et al., *Decorative Arts,* 211, no. 367.
2. On Mithradates, see Mayor, *The Poison King.* Attempts to find the original recipe for mithridate have not met with success. Watson, in *Theriac and Mithridatium,* 44, named it a "will-o'-the-wisp"; Totelin, in "Mithradates' Antidote," called it a "pharmacological ghost." Medical treatises by Mithradates himself, the Roman physician Asklepiades (fl. ca. 95 BCE), and Lenaeus (ca. 95–25 BCE), which could have shed some light on the very first theriacs, are now lost.
3. Knoefel and Covi, *A Hellenistic Treatise;* Krumholz McDonald, "The Serpent as Healer."
4. Pliny the Elder, *Naturalis Historia,* xxv, 3, 5–7; also in Totelin, "Mithradates' Antidote," 3–4.
5. Olmi, "Farmacopea antica"; Findlen, *Possessing Nature,* chap. 6.
6. For an overview of publications on theriac between 1465 and 1800, see Di Gennaro Splendore, "The Triumph of Theriac," 445–448.
7. Leigh, *On Theriac to Piso,* 89.
8. Leigh, *On Theriac to Piso,* 73.
9. Totelin, "Mithradates' Antidote," 2–14.
10. Menegacci, *La theriaca et il mithridato,* B3v.
11. Although rational, physicians fully shared the values of a deeply religious society. For example, for centuries they participated in the canonization of saints and evaluations of miracles. Among others, see Pomata, "Malpighi and the Holy Body."
12. Maranta, *Della theriaca,* 1.
13. Chittolini et al., *Origini dello stato;* Reinhard, *Power Elites.*

14. Blockmans et al., *Empowering Interactions*.
15. For the importance of symbolism in politics, see Kertzer, *Ritual, Politics, and Power*.
16. Biagioli, *Galileo, Courtier*, 4, 13. For scientific patronage, see also Biagioli, "Galileo's System of Patronage"; Findlen, *Possessing Nature*, 346–376.
17. For the long-standing relation between politics and poison, see especially Collard, *The Crime of Poison*; Collard, *Pouvoir et Poison*; Rankin, *The Poison Trials*.
18. Rankin, "On Anecdotes and Antidotes," 277; Rankin, *The Poison Trials*; Corradi, "Degli esperimenti tossicologici."
19. Bloch, *The Royal Touch*, chap. 5.
20. Alberi, *Relazioni degli ambasciatori veneti*, ser. 2, 1:356.
21. Bellorini, *The World of Plants*. The first official pharmacopoeia was issued in Florence fifty years before other Italian cities followed suit, showing that an early interest in pharmaceutical matters was alive in Florence. Possibly following this trend, the Medici precociously entered the field of pharmacy.
22. Bellorini, *The World of Plants*, 18–21, 29, 33, 40.
23. In 1530 Emperor Charles V restored the Medici rule in Florence, and in 1532 he bestowed the title duke on Cosimo's predecessor, Alessandro.
24. Strocchia, *Forgotten Healers*, 55–59.
25. Bellorini, *The World of Plants* 29–30; see also Wheeler, *Renaissance Secrets*, 76–77; Alberi, *Relazioni degli ambasciatori veneti*, ser. 2, 1:356.
26. ASF, Mediceo del Principato 241, fol. 84r, 7 January 1573, Cosimo I de' Medici to Francesco I de' Medici (MAP Doc ID# 14353).
27. Bellorini, *The World of Plants*, 23–28.
28. Bellorini, *The World of Plants*, 33. To my surprise, I found only two apothecary publications related to the making of theriac in Florence: a poetic celebration of the compounding of theriac at the Santissima Annunziata monastery in 1748 (Coltellini, *Corona d'applausi poetici*), and a handbill from the end of the eighteenth century related to the theriac made at Santa Maria Novella.
29. Machiavelli, *The Prince*, 9.
30. Leigh, *On Theriac to Piso*, 73.
31. Menegacci, *La theriaca et il mithridato*, nn (13).
32. For the Italian context, see Benzi, *Tra prìncipi e saltimbanchi*.
33. Soll, "Healing the Body Politic."
34. Cohn, *Cultures of Plague*.
35. BUB, Ald. Ms. 70, 63r.
36. Skinner, *Modern Political Thought*, 1:118–119.
37. Houel, *Traité*, 3r, 7r, 11v. On Nicolas Houel, see Warolin, "Nicolas Houel and Michel Dusseau."
38. Calzolari, *Lettera*, nn.

39. Leigh, *On Theriac to Piso*, 73.
40. Grandi, "La scienza medica," 152–158.
41. Tasso, *Lettere*, G1483, March 24, 1595, to Ferdinando de' Medici.
42. ASF, Mediceo del Principato, 2955, fol. nn, 29 January 1621, Duke of Mantua Ferdinando Gonzaga to Grand Duke Cosimo II (MAP Doc ID#5143).
43. Pisanelli, *Discorso sopra la peste*, 49.
44. Lavoranti, *Lode della theriaca*, 6.
45. BUB, Ald. Ms. 70, 26r.
46. Maranta, *Della theriaca et del mithridato*, 3.
47. Overduin, "The Anti-Bucolic World," 626.
48. For Nicander in the early modern period, see Radici, *Nicandro di Colofone*. For an assessment of Nicander from a scientific perspective, see Scarborough, "Nicander's Toxicology."
49. Di Gennaro Splendore, "The Triumph of Theriac," 445.
50. See, for example, Cohn, *Cultures of Plague*, Benzi; *Tra principi e saltimbanchi*; see also Mendelsohn et al., *Civic Medicine*.
51. Settala, *Breve compendio*. On Ludovico Settala, see Rota Ghibaudi, *Ricerche su Ludovico Settala*.
52. Herlihy and Klapisch-Zuber, *Les Toscans*, 299. See also Park, *Doctors and Medicine*, 43n83, for a discussion on the status of physicians and apothecaries.
53. In Florence, apothecaries and physicians belonged to the same guild—the Guild of Doctors, Apothecaries, and Grocers—which was unusual, as these professions were typically separate in most other cities.
54. Halikowski-Smith, "The Physician's Hand," 102–108; Palmer, "Pharmacy," 105–106.
55. Park, *Doctors and Medicine*, 28.
56. Halikowski-Smith, "The Physician's Hand," 102–103.
57. Meneghini, *La farmacia*, 44, esp. n5 and n6.
58. See, for example, Palmer, "Pharmacy," 106.
59. Laughran, "Medicating," 99.
60. Lindemann, *Medicine and Society*, 211.
61. Cook, *The Decline;* Pelling and White, *Medical Conflicts*.
62. Brockliss and Jones, *The Medical World*.
63. Murphy, *New Order of Medicine*.
64. Ghini bequeathed his library to Maranta, Vallieri, "Le 22 lettere," 198. On Ghini, see Findlen, "Death of a Naturalist." On Maranta, see, Micca, "The 'De Theriaca e del Mithridato'"; Tiraboschi et al., *Storia della letteratura italiana*, 556–557.
65. Maranta, *Della theriaca et del mithridato*, Dedicatoria to Imperato.
66. Maranta, *Della theriaca et del mithridato*, Dedicatoria to Imperato.
67. Maranta, *Della theriaca et del mithridato*, 162.

68. Maranta, *Della theriaca et del mithridato*, 7–8.
69. Maranta, *De theriaca et mithridatio*, trans. Camerarius. Joachim Camerarius visited Naples in 1562 and met Maranta personally. See Valtieri, "Le 22 lettere," 203, Maranta to Aldrovandi March 4, 1562.
70. On Bernardino Trevisano, see *Saggi scientifici e letterari*, 1:xxvii–xxviii; De Renzi, *Storia della medicina*, 3:729; on Marco Oddo, see Vedova, *Biografia degli scrittori padovani*, 149–152; on Paolo Crasso, see Vedova, *Biografia degli scrittori padovani*, 301–303; *Saggi scientifici e letterari*, 5:287–278.
71. Crasso et al., *Meditationes doctissimae*.
72. Crasso et al., *Meditationes doctissimae*, 7–8.
73. Crasso et al., *Meditationes doctissimae*, 2, 5.
74. See, for example, Crasso et al., *Meditationes doctissimae*, 286.
75. On this dispute, see Cuna, "Editoria e testi"; Sabbatani, "Di un trattato del Maranta," 240.
76. Stigliola, *Theriace, et mithridatia*.
77. Stigliola, *Theriace, et mithridatia*, 4v–5r.
78. Cuna, "Editoria e testi," 75–76.
79. Gentilcore, "'All That Pertains to Medicine'," 123.
80. Musi, "Medicina e sapere medico," 172; on Protomedicato in Naples, see Gentilcore, "Il Regio Protomedicato."
81. Musi, "Medicina e sapere medico," 170.
82. On sixteenth-century apothecaries in Naples, see Gentilcore, *Healers and Healing*, esp. chaps. 2–5; Russo, *L'arte degli speziali*; Russo, "Contributo alla storia"; Musi, "Medicina e sapere medico," 178. For the rules governing the inspection of apothecary shops, see ASN, Sommaria Arrendamenti Protomedicati 1119, 1217. Few sixteenth-century reports of Neapolitan inspections of apothecary shops are extant in ASN, Sommaria Arrendamenti Protomedicati 1071 relative to the years 1582–1584.
83. On apothecaries in Padua, see Meneghini, *La farmacia*, 72–95.
84. Favaro, *Galileo Galilei*, 2: 86n2. See also Carinci, "Una 'speziala' padovana," 209.
85. Palmer, *The Studio of Venice*, 27–28.
86. Borgarucci, *La fabrica degli spetiali*, nn, Dedicatoria.
87. Borgarucci, *La fabrica degli spetiali*, 490–491.
88. Pezzolo, "The Venetian Economy," 264–265.
89. Laughran, "Medicating," 100.
90. Palmer, "Pharmacy," 104, 106, 107, 109, 116, 117.
91. Melich, *Avertimenti nelle compositioni* (1575) was republished at least in 1596, 1605, 1627, 1648, 1660, 1670, 1678, 1688, and 1720. Georg Melich, *De recta medicamentorum*.
92. Melich, *Avvertimenti nelle compositioni*, a2v.
93. Melich, *Avertimenti nelle compositioni* (1575), 142r; also in Palmer, "Pharmacy," 106 n60.

94. Blair, *Too Much to Know;* on artisanal transmission of knowledge, see also Smith, *From Lived Experience.* On pharmacy, see also Bénézet, *Pharmacie,* 116–121; Pugliano, "Pharmacy, Testing," 238–240.
95. Quattrami, *Tractatus perutilis.*
96. Quattrami, *Tractatus perutilis,* 1–3.
97. BUB, Ald. Ms. 136, XXVI, 98r Evangelista Quattrami to Sigismondo Dondini in Cento, July 18, 1597.
98. Dallasta, "Novità sul semplicista," 167, Quattrami to Ranuccio I Farnese, not dated (between 1597 and 1606).
99. For theriac, Aldrovandi, and medical regulation, see especially Olmi, "Farmacopea antica e medicina moderna"; Findlen, *Possessing Nature,* chap. 6; Di Gennaro Splendore, "Aldrovandi's *Farmaceptica.*"
100. Di Gennaro Splendore, "Craft, Money and Mercy," 101–102.
101. BUB, Ald. Ms. 70, *Avertimenti sopra la Teriaca et Mithridato,* should be dated after 1597 and was never published. On this text, see also Di Gennaro Splendore, "Aldrovandi's *Farmaceptica.*"
102. For the theriac dispute, see Chapter 6.
103. BUB, Ald. Ms. 70, 9v–10r.
104. BUB, Ald. Ms. 70, 16r, 16v.
105. BUB, Ald. Ms. 21 IV, 55r.
106. BUB, Ald. Ms. 70, 27r.
107. BUB, Ald. Ms. 21 IV, 39r, see also 44v.
108. BUB, Ald. Ms. 91, 529v. See also BUB, Ald. Ms. 70, 14r.
109. BUB, Ald. Ms. 91, 529v.

4. A PUBLIC HEALTH MEASURE AGAINST POISON AND PLAGUE

1. Pisanelli, *Discorso sopra la peste,* 50.
2. Del Panta, *Le epidemie,* 170; Alfani, *Il Grand Tour;* Corradi, *Annali delle epidemie,* 2:219–265; Beloch, *Storia della popolazione d'Italia,* 48.
3. Heberden, *Antitheriaka,* 4.
4. Watson, *Theriac and Mithridatium,* 103.
5. Collard, *The Crime of Poison;* Pastore, *Veleno,* 17, 24–25 has argued that this conviction owed much to Heinrich Burkhardt (1861–1914), German historian of the Renaissance; see also Pastore, "Poisoning as Politics."
6. Gentilcore, *Medical Charlatanism,* 203–204.
7. Minuzzi, *Sul filo dei segreti,* 33, 316.
8. Pomata, *Contracting a Cure,* 91–92, 178.
9. ASF, Mediceo del Principato 649, fol. 70r, September 14, 1576, Gian Luigi Vitelli to Cosimo I de' Medici (MAP Doc ID# 22539).
10. I found forty-five nonmedical texts published across Europe between 1490 and 1799 that used theriac as a metaphor in the title. For example: De Lebrija, *La Triaca del alma;* Turner, *A Preservative, or Triacle, Agaynst the Poyson of*

Pelagius; Draconi and Zanni, *Theriaca fina contra il pestifero veleno;* Zalman Zevi, *Theriaca Judaica;* Mather, *A Treacle Fetch'd Out of a Viper: A Brief Essay upon Falls into Sins;* Pascual, *Sueños ay, que verdad son, y punto en contra de los astrologos: triaca magna contra el veleno de la astrologia judiciaria.*

11. It is worth noting that theriac was not referred to as a panacea in sixteenth- and seventeenth-century Italy. We lack a history of the early modern use of the term *panacea*, which derives from the name of the Greek goddess of healing and was later applied to any herb able to cure all diseases. The word *panacea* meaning "a medicine to cure all ailments" probably first appeared in print in Germany in 1581, associated with the supposed healing properties of tobacco. On the term *panacea*, see Rankin, *The Poison Trials*, 210. According to the *Encyclopédie*, the term *panacea* was mostly applied to chemical remedies. See "Panacée" in Diderot and d'Alembert, *Encyclopédie*, http://encyclopedie.uchicago.edu/. When the demand for antidotes and wonder cures increased, the semantic lines between *antidote, cure-all,* and *panacea* may have blurred. In the nineteenth century, *panacea* became a derogatory term when applied to previous remedies. However, when theriac was refashioned into "true theriac," it was not yet considered a panacea but rather still an antidote, to be used against poisons and an almost endless list of ailments, including plague.
12. On fear in the early modern Western world, see Delumeau, *La peur en Occident*, 98–143; Naphy and Roberts, *Fear in Early Modern Society.*
13. BUB, Ald. Ms. 21, III, 134v.
14. Ginzburg, *Paura Reverenza Terrore*, 53–71.
15. Jones, "Plague and Its Metaphors," 108–109.
16. Palmer, "La Gran Moría,"; Cipolla, "Origine e sviluppo"; Cipolla, *Public Health.*
17. Jones, "Plague and Its Metaphors," 111.
18. See, for example, Calvi, *Histories of a Plague Year*, esp. chap. 4; for the plague of 1575–1577, see also Cohn, *Cultures of Plague*, chap. 9.
19. Fioravanti, *Del reggimento della peste*, 37r–37v.
20. Cohn, *Cultures of Plague.*
21. Palmer, "Girolamo Mercuriale"; Cohn, *Cultures of Plague*, chap. 6.
22. Donzellini, *Discorso nobilissimo*, n.p. On Girolamo Donzellini, see DBI, Anne Jacobson Schutte, *ad vocem.*
23. ASB, Studio 217, 142v; also in Olmi, "Farmacopea antica e medicina moderna," 201.
24. BUB, Ald. Ms. 69 I, Aldrovandi to his nephew in Rome, September 13, 1576.
25. BUB, Ald. Ms. 21, III, 134r. *La città felice* (The happy city) was the title of a political treatise by Francesco Patrizio, published in Venice in 1553 by Giovan Griffio.
26. BUB, Ald. Ms. 21, III, 133v–134r.
27. Preto, *Peste e società a Venezia*, 90–97.

28. Rambaldi, *Speranze e crisi*, 24–26.
29. BUB, Ald. Ms. 21 IV, 221v, Andrea Bacci to Aldrovandi, February 6, 1578.
30. Corradi, *Annali*, 2:199–200.
31. Valdagni, *De theriacae*. For this medical dispute, see Redmond, "Girolamo Donzellino," 54–123; Cohn, *Cultures of Plague*, 161–162.
32. Valdagni, *De theriacae usu*, 7r; also in Redmond, "Girolamo Donzellino," 64.
33. Donzellini, *De natura, causis*, 14.
34. Calzaveglia, *De theriacae abusu*.
35. Calogera, *Nuova Raccolta*, 41–54.
36. Alessandrini, *Galeni praecipua scripta annotationes*, 859–888.
37. Alessandrini, *Galeni praecipua scripta annotationes*, 888.
38. Sassonia, *Disputatio de phoenigmorum*. On Ercole Sassonia, see Ongaro and Martellozzo Fiorin, "Girolamo Mercuriale e lo studio di Padova," 38–39, n67.
39. Massaria, *De abusu medicamentorum vesicantium*.
40. Settala, *Preservatione dalla peste*, 36–37.
41. Settala, *Preservatione dalla peste*, 7.
42. Del Panta, *Le epidemie*, 182–185.
43. According to Crawshaw, *Plague Hospitals*, 169, few records about therapeutics used in Venetian lazarettos have survived, and those that have stipulate that theriac and sweets should be given only to those who need them.
44. Cantini, *Legislazione*, 16:89–90; also in Henderson, *Florence Under Siege*, 114.
45. Henderson, *Florence Under Siege*, 201–204, 216.
46. Moratti, *Racconto de gli ordinii*, 121–123.
47. Legates *a latere* were cardinals who received the time-limited right to represent the pope as if they were the pope in person. Brighetti, *Bologna e la peste*, 158.
48. Brighetti, *Bologna e la peste*, 136.
49. Sforza, *F.M. Fiorentini*, 69, 148.
50. Cinelli Calvoli, *Biblioteca volante*, 1:2.
51. Baldi, *Del vero opobalsamo orientale*, 7.
52. On the history of balsam, see Milwright, "Balsam in the Mediaeval Mediterranean"; Milwright, "The Balsam of Maṭariyya"; Di Gennaro Splendore, "Mediterranean Botany."
53. For example, see de Gasparis, *Liquoris artificialis*; Baldi, *Del vero opobalsamo*; Donzelli, *Additio apologetica ad suam*.
54. Redi, *Osservazioni intorno alle vipere*. On Redi's experiments on vipers, see Knoefel, *Francesco Redi on Vipers*; Tribby, "Cooking (with) Clio and Cleo"; Findlen, "Controlling the Experiment"; Schickore, "Trying Again and Again"; Schickore, *About Method*, chap. 3.
55. Tribby, "Cooking (with) Clio and Cleo."
56. Severino, *Vipera Pythia*, 416–437.
57. Severino, *Vipera Pythia*, 434.

58. Redi, *Osservazioni intorno alle vipere,* 6; also in Schickore, "Trying Again and Again," 581.
59. Schickore, *About Method,* chap. 3.
60. Schickore, *About Method,* 34.
61. Schickore, "Trying Again and Again," 590.
62. Redi, *Lettera sopra alcune opposizioni,* 30–31. On this dispute, see Catellani and Console, "Moyse Charas, Francesco Redi, the Viper."
63. Redi, *Consulti medici,* 57; Knoefel, *Francesco Redi,* XIV.
64. Schickore, *About Method,* 31.
65. Sforza, *F.M. Fiorentini,* 265 n1.
66. Charas, *Histoire naturelle des animaux,* 4.
67. Charas, *Thériaque d'Andromacus,* 8, appendix.
68. On theriac ceremonies, see especially Stossl, *Lo spettacolo della triaca.* One such architecture was displayed in the Cathedral of Saint John the Divine in New York; see Renehan, "Eighteenth-Century Carved Piece."
69. McVaugh, *Medicine before the Plague,* 119–120.
70. Bosc, "Ce que fut la thériaque," 291.
71. ASV, Compilazione delle Leggi Seconda Serie, fasc. 231 n. 6. Also in Dian, *Cenni,* 39.
72. Probably after Hermann Peters, a nineteenth-century German scholar, historians interpreted this woodcut as a public production of theriac. See Peters, *Aus Pharmazeutischer Vorzeit,* 142.
73. I have not found evidence to substantiate this hypothesis, but it remains a credible possibility; see Dian, *Cenni,* 38; also Gentz, "Theriaca."
74. Alpini, *De medicina Aegyptiorum,* 133v.
75. BNM, Collegio Medico IT.VII, 2361 (= 9716), 26r.
76. Melich, *Avvertimenti nelle compositioni* (1575), 41v.
77. On charlatans' performances, see Gentilcore, *Medical Charlatanism,* chap. 9, 301–334; also Park, "Country Medicine."
78. Moryson, *Shakespeare's Europe,* 422.
79. Stossl, *Lo spettacolo della teriaca,* 15.
80. Gorman, *The Scientific Counter-Revolution,* 385.
81. Stossl, *Lo spettacolo della teriaca,* 20–21.
82. At least in 1554, 1560, and 1566, Bolognese apothecaries made theriac and mithridate with the approval of the Protomedici, but the number of substitutes they used attracted criticism and no *celebrations* were recorded; see ASB, Studio 217, 108v, 122r, 10v, 146r; Calestani, *Delle osservationi,* 250.
83. Charles V inherited the administration of this and other two religious orders. Trombelli, *Memorie istoriche,* 75.
84. BUB, Ald. Ms. 21, III, 135v; Ald. Ms. 91, 352. This is the oldest example of this kind of apothecary print I have found.
85. On Gabriele Paleotti, see Prodi, *Il cardinale Gabriele Paleotti.*

86. BUB, Ald. Ms. 21, III, 142r.
87. BUB, Ald. Ms. 21, III, 144r.
88. Masini, *Bologna perlustrata,* 267.
89. ASB, Studio 213, 27r.
90. Ferrari, "Public Anatomy Lessons," 50, 57-61. Bologna's anatomical theater was built in 1683.
91. Cardullo, *Teriaca d'Andromaco composta publicamente.*
92. Sartorio, *Discorso,* 22.
93. Grandi, "La scienza medica," 151-158.
94. Bertioli, *Breue auuiso,* 5.
95. Menegacci, *La theriaca et il mithridato,* n.p.
96. Cardullo, *Teriaca d'Andromaco,* n.p.
97. ASB, Miscellanea delle Arti, vol. 25, n9. The cost of making theriac in Bologna remains unknown because the apothecary guild's archive is lost and the documents apothecaries shared with the Collegio Medico are unreliable.
98. BNM, Collegio Medico IT.VII, 2374 (= 9694). *Compendio storico e politico dell'Italia,* 170.
99. Candrini, *Teriaca d'Andromaco,* 9.
100. Part of the discussion on theriac celebrations builds on Di Gennaro Splendore, "The Triumph of Theriac."
101. On print and festivities, see Nussdorfer, "Print and Pageantry"; Watanabe-O'Kelly, "'True and Historical Descriptions'?"
102. Catelan, *Discours et demonstration;* Guldenius et al., *Andromachi Senioris Theriaca.*
103. Menegacci, *La theriaca et il mithridato.*
104. Rossi, *Theriaca di Andromaco il Vecchio.*
105. Candrini, *Teriaca d'Andromaco.*
106. Scalcina, *Successo, giuditio, & offerta,* n.p.
107. Coltellini, *Corona d'applausi poetici.*
108. BNCF, *Facendosi la composizione di Mitridate, Teriaca, e Confezione di Giacinto nella Spezieria apostolica del Signor Camillo de Luca* (n.p., n.d.).
109. Lavoranti, *Lode della Theriaca d'Andromaco,* n.p.
110. Lavoranti, *Lode della theriaca,* n.p. Bocchi, *Descrittione del teatro teriacale,* 10.
111. ASB, Studio 251.
112. Di Gennaro Splendore, "The Triumph of Theriac," 458.
113. Bocchi, *Descrittione del teatro teriacale,* 18-19. On Simon Bocchi, see Dallasta, "Novità."
114. Candrini, *Teriaca d'Andromaco,* 9-10.
115. Candrini, *Teriaca d'Andromaco,* 14.
116. Menegacci, *La theriaca,* n.p.
117. Sartorio, *Discorso,* 60-61.
118. See, for example, ASB, Studio 196.

119. There are no specific studies on the legal value of medical or scientific *fedi*. For health documents, see Bamji, "Health Passes, Print and Public Health."

5. THERIACA MAGNA ON THE MARKETPLACE

1. Welch, "Space and Spectacle"; Wallis, "Consumption, Retailing, and Medicine."
2. On apothecary shops as centers of communication, see De Vivo, "Pharmacies as centers of communication"; De Vivo, "La farmacia"; Kostylo, "Pharmacy as a Centre"; Pugliano, "Natural History in the apothecary shop."
3. Gentilcore, *Medical Charlatanism*, 301–304; Park, "Country Medicine."
4. Strocchia, *Forgotten Healers*, chap. 3.
5. Cavallo and Storey, *Healthy Living*; Eamon, *Science and the Secrets*; Cohn, *Cultures of Plague*.
6. Guarguanti, *Della theriaca*, 6.
7. Lavoranti, *Lode della Theriaca*, 6.
8. Costa, *Discorsi sopra le compositioni*.
9. On Filippo Costa, a little-known figure, see Franchini, *La scienza a corte*, 41–51.
10. Ferdinando, *Centum historiae*, 31.
11. Melella, "La spezieria dell'Arciospedale," 2:1128, 1138.
12. Bellorini, *The World of Plants*, 213–214.
13. BUB, Ald. Ms. 21, III, 172r.
14. For the late Middle Ages, see Bénézet, and Flahaut, *Pharmacie et médicament*. For late fifteenth-century Italy, see Shaw and Welch, *Making and Marketing Medicine*. For the early modern period, see Gentilcore, *Medical Charlatanism*, esp. chap. 6; Minuzzi, *Sul filo dei segreti*; Ledermann, "Le prix des médicaments," the first attempted analysis of medicine's prices in Rome. See also Lavallée, "Appréciation de l'évolution du prix."
15. For example, during the English "kitchen physick" phase, when domestic production was primary, the market of remedies was already well developed in Italy: Curth, *From Physick to Pharmacology*; see also Jenner and Wallis, *Medicine and the Market*; Wallis, "Exotic Drugs." For the British context see also Anderson, *Making Medicines*.
16. Palmer, "Pharmacy in the Republic of Venice," 103.
17. BMC, Mariegola 209, art. 25 *Del ordine che si de tenere per gli speciali che vogliono fare Theriaca*, 30r.
18. *Libro delle teriache* was a volume kept by the Giustizia Vecchia, now lost, but a copy of theriac production from 1601 to 1618—probably made in the occasion of the honey dispute (see Chapter 6)—is in ASV, Giustizia Vecchia, 211.
19. In 1603 a light galley cost 10,000 ducats: Pullan, *Crisis and Change*, 81.
20. Official producers of theriac between 1580 and 1618 were allo Struzzo, ai Due Mori, alla Testa d'Oro, all'Aquila Negra, San Gierolamo, San Giacomo,

al Griffo, al Medico, alla Campana, alla Madonna, San Zuanne, al Paradiso, San Salvatore, al Basilisco, della Pigna, and della Cavaliera: ASV, Giustizia Vecchia 211, BMC, Mariegola 209, 145r, 168v.
21. ASV, Giustizia Vecchia, 211.
22. Wallis, "Exotic Drugs," 31.
23. King, *The British Merchant,* 122.
24. Wallis, "Exotic Drugs," 31.
25. I would like to thank Patrick Wallis for sharing his raw data on English imports taken from the English port books, and the annual ledgers of the Inspector General of Customs. On these sources, see Wallis, "Exotic Drugs," 22. Duty-free products and drugs smuggled to avoid tax were not recorded.
26. Schumpeter and Ashton, *English Overseas Trade Statistics,* 6.
27. For the production of theriac by English apothecaries, see Bayley, *A Discourse.*
28. Woodall, *The Surgions Mate,* 95.
29. Dingwall, *Physicians, Surgeons,* 187.
30. Evelyn, *Diary,* 329.
31. Woodall, *The Surgions Mate,* 95.
32. Lassels, *The Voyage of Italy,* 424–425.
33. Evelyn, *Diary,* 215.
34. Woodall, *The Surgions Mate,* 95. See also Druett, *Rough Medicine,* esp. chap. 1.
35. Raj et al., "The Real Theriac," 4.
36. Dian, "Memoria," 30n1; BMC, Mariegola 209, 33v; BUB, Ald. Ms. 21, IV, *Tassa delli pretii delle robbe medicinali.*
37. Gentilcore, *Medical Charlatanism,* 238.
38. Ledermann, "Les taxes de médicaments," 54; Dian, "Memoria," 30.
39. ASB, Collegio dei medici di Bologna, *Tassa de' medicinali* (1637), 28.
40. Trivellato, "The Moral Economies," 196. Trivellato has spoken of "moral economies" rather than relying on a single Thompsonian "moral economy."
41. Gentilcore, *Medical Charlatanism,* 236 n9.
42. Colapinto and Maviglia, "Esame analitico comparativo."
43. ASB, Studio 318, 45r–46v.
44. ASB, Studio 318, 45r–46v; 53v–54r.
45. See Ulvioni, *Il Gran Castigo di Dio,* 32.
46. Trivellato, *Fondamenta dei vetrai,* 57–67.
47. Pullan, "Wage-Earners."
48. Scalone, "Sulle relazioni tra variabili demografiche," 77.
49. Guenzi, *Pane e Fornai,* 144; Vigo, "Real Wages," 389.
50. On this debate, see Hatcher and Stephenson, *Seven Centuries of Unreal Wages.* For a different view, see de Vries, "Between Purchasing Power," and van Zanden, "Wages."
51. Viale et al., "Decomposing Economic Inequality."
52. Gentilcore, *Medical Charlatanism,* 249.

53. Collegio dei medici di Bologna, *Notificazione;* Ledermann, "Les taxes de médicaments."
54. Dian, "Memoria," 30.
55. Gentilcore, *Medical Charlatanism,* 238; Show and Welch, *Marketing Medicines,* 123–129.
56. Arte degli Speziali di Bologna, *Riforma de' statuti,* 17.
57. Collegio dei medici di Bologna, *Tassa de' medicinali ultimamente;* Rotelli, "Exotic Plants," 857–858.
58. ASB, Collegio dei medici di Bologna, *Tassa de' medicinali ultimamente.*
59. Gentilcore, *Medical Charlatanism,* 236–237, 248.
60. Gentilcore, *Medical Charlatanism,* 238. (A teaspoon is 1 gram more than a drachm.)
61. ASF, Mediceo del Principato 2944, fol. 371r, October 1607, Francesco Ormanni to unidentified addressee (MAP Doc ID# 5078).
62. ASF, Mediceo del Principato 1584, fol. nn, 9 July 1677, Andrea Galleni to unidentified addressee (MAP Doc ID# 24399).
63. BNCF, Galileiana ms. 276, 209r–209v, Giovanni Filippo Marucelli to Leopoldo II de' Medici, July 13, 1663. Theriac was sent as a gift to Prague through Vienna; see ASF, Mediceo del Principato 4339, fol. 66r, 9 May 1581, Giovanni Alberti to Francesco I de' Medici (MAP Doc ID#13537).
64. Grendler, *The University of Mantua,* 176–177.
65. ASF, Mediceo del Principato 2955, fol. nn, 29 January 1621, Ferdinando Gonzaga to Cosimo II de' Medici (MAP Doc ID#5143).
66. BCAB, *Bandi et Provisioni,* 1617, 2.
67. ASB, Studio 213.
68. ASV, Giustizia Vecchia, 98.
69. Fantasti, *Vero modo di comporre,* 56–58.
70. ASV, Studio 340; also in Pomata, *Contracting a Cure,* 178.
71. ASB, Studio 251, *Indice delle Robbe da tenersi nelle botteghe de' semplici Droghieri,* July 24, 1737.
72. ASV, Studio 340.
73. ASB, Studio 322, July 31, 1744.
74. Gentilcore, *Medical Charlatanism,* 240.
75. Elici, *Delle virtù del mithridate minore,* 14.
76. De Sgobbis, *Nuovo et universale theatro,* 449–463.
77. De Sgobbis, *Nuovo et universale theatro,* 355–356; Pancotto, *Le mirabili virtù.*
78. Mancini, *L'Officina profumo-farmaceutica,* 196.
79. Du Chesne, *La reformation des theriaques.* There are two different editions of this book with the same frontispiece; I used the online copy from the Universitad Complutense de Madrid, accessed July 8, 2020.
80. Du Chesne, *La reformation des theriaques,* 133–135.
81. Du Chesne, *La reformation des theriaques,* 143.

82. Greiff celebrated his productions in Tübingen with *Decas Nobilissimorum Medicamentorum, Galeno-Chymico modo compositorum* (1641) and *Kurtze Beschreibung Deß Chymischen oder Himm]elischen Theriacs* (1652). Wickersheimer, "La thériaque céleste,"
83. Wickersheimer, "La thériaque céleste," 155.
84. Carlo Maria Cipolla estimated that, between 1610 and 1780, the poor were 11 to 15 percent of the total population; see Cipolla, *Storia economica*, 29. According to more recent estimates, the percentage of the poor was generally higher during the early modern period; see Ammannati et al., "Poverty."
85. Bumaldi, *Formolario economico cibario*, 13.
86. ASB, Studio 354; also in Pomata, *Contracting a Cure*, 90–91.
87. On theriacs in charitable books, see also Lafont, "Les thériaques."
88. Rubbi, *Dizionario di antichità*, I, 49.
89. Galasso, *Recetario di nouo raccolto*, 4–6.
90. Elici, *Delle virtù del mithridate*; Lémery, *Farmacopea universale*, 329. Furetière, *Dictionnaire Universel*, ad vocem. On diatesseron, see Flahaut, "La thériaque diatessaron"; Flahaut, "La thériaque Diatessaron: Oligopharmacie."
91. Collegio dei medici di Bologna, *Tassa de' medicinali semplici*, 39.
92. Faber, *Rerum medicarum*, 778; also in Gentilcore, *Medical Charlatanism*, 139.
93. On Orviétan, see Gentilcore, *Healers and Healing*, 96–124.
94. Faber, *Rerum medicarum*, 778.
95. Gentilcore, *Medical Charlatanism*, 245. The term *populuxe* was coined for the twentieth century in Hine, *Populuxe*, then applied to the early modern period in Fairchilds, "Production and Marketing of Populuxe Goods." See also Berg, "New Commodities, Luxuries"; Jones and Sprang, "Sans-Culottes, Sans Café."
96. The discussion about *theriac virtues* builds on Di Gennaro Splendore, "The Triumph of Theriac."
97. De Vos, *Compound Remedies*, 8, 30, 69.
98. Butner, *De theriaca et mitridato Graecorum*, 343.
99. Gentilcore, *Medical Charlatanism*, 234.
100. De Sgobbis, *Nuovo et universale theatro*, 455.
101. Minuzzi, *Sul filo dei segreti*, 222.
102. Minuzzi, *Sul filo dei segreti*, 222–224.
103. Guarguanti, *Tria opuscula*.
104. Croce, *Triaca musicale*.
105. Melich, *Avertimenti nelle compositioni* (1596), republished in at least 1605, 1627, 1648, 1660, 1670, 1678, 1688, and 1720.
106. On early modern printed medical knowledge and its readership, see Minuzzi, "Printing Medical Knowledge."
107. Rutta, *Trionfi contro la morte*, 11–12.

108. Rutta, *Trionfi*, 18–19.
109. BUB, *Le virtù e facoltà della theriaca*.
110. See Sensi, "Cerretani e ciarlatani," document 5, 84–85; also in Gentilcore, *Medical Charlatanism*, 340n25. See also Salzberg, *Ephemeral City*, esp. chap. 4.
111. Gentilcore, *Medical Charlatanism*, 340.
112. Minuzzi, *Sul filo dei segreti*, 224.
113. See also Berveglieri, *Tutela e brevettazione*, 19. Similarly in Bologna, see Collegio dei medici di Bologna, *Conventioni*; Arte degli Speziali di Bologna, *Riforma de' statuti*.
114. Gentilcore, *Medical Charlatanism*, 353–355, n68.
115. ASB, Studio 251, *Le virtù e facoltà principali della Triaca* (1663).
116. BUB, *Le virtù e facoltà della theriaca* (1574).
117. ASB, Studio 251, *Le virtù e facoltà principali della triaca* (1730).
118. Wellcome Collection, Ms. 8687, *Of the Use, Virtues, et Doze of the Treacle*.

6. A PRESERVATIVE OF THE SOCIAL ORDER

1. Among others, see Cook, *The Decline*; Pelling and White, *Medical Conflicts*; Brockliss and Jones, *The Medical World*; Pomata, *Contracting a Cure*; Murphy, *A New Order of Medicine*.
2. BCAB, Raccolta Bandi Merlani, March 22, 1688.
3. Pomata, *Contracting a Cure*, 91.
4. BMC, Mariegola 209, I, 117v, July 30, 1621.
5. Busti, *De mellis*.
6. On Busti, see see Cicogna, *Delle iscrizioni veneziane*, v. 1, 337; Ogilvie, *The Science of Describing*, 25–27.
7. See Chapter 5, Figure 5.1.
8. Busti, *De Mellis*, 8. For a comparison, see Aldrovandi and Collegio dei medici di Bologna, *Antidotarii Bononiensis*, 99; Collegio dei medici di Roma, *Antidotario Romano* (1612), 41.
9. Ricordel and Bonmatin, "Les vertus du miel."
10. Albala, *Eating Right in the Renaissance*, 86.
11. Olmo, *De mellis opportuna*, 15.
12. Busti, *De mellis*, 32
13. ASV, Provveditori e Sopraprovveditori alla Sanità, Capitolare II 1574–1689, 61v.
14. For the institutional setup of theriac production in Venice, see Chapter 1; on the Venetian Health Office, see Vanzan Marchin, *I mali e i rimedi*, 65–102.
15. BNM, Collegio Medico IT.VII, 2329 (= 9723), Libro D 1549–1628, 131v.
16. BNM, Collegio Medico IT.VII, 2340 (= 9724), 13r; also in Dian, *Cenni*, 46.
17. For Martinelli, see Palmer, "Pharmacy," 107.
18. Martinelli, *Ragionamenti sopra l'amomo*, n.p.

19. Anonymus [Bertioli], *Giudicio sopra i raggionamenti*.
20. Bertioli, *Giudicio sopra i raggionamenti*, 24.
21. Galangal is an unidentified species of the genera *Alpinia* or *Kaempferia*. BNM, Collegio Medico IT.VII, 2340 (= 9672), 13; also in Dian, *Cenni*, 46.
22. Storax is the refined oil produced from the sap of the bark of oriental sweetgum or Turkish sweetgum (*Liquidambar orientalis*).
23. Dian, *Cenni*, 47; BMC, Mariegola 209, I 68v.
24. BMC, Mariegola 209, I 69v–70r.
25. BMC, Mariegola 209, I 69v–70r.
26. BMC, Mariegola 209, I 70r.
27. BMC, Mariegola 209, I 69v–70r, petition October 19, 1613.
28. BNM, Collegio Medico, IT.VII, 2340 (= 9672), 179r, 179v.
29. BNM, Collegio Medico, IT.VII, 2340 (= 9672), 179v.
30. BNM, Collegio Medico, IT.VII, 2340 (= 9672), 179v–180r.
31. Olmo, *De mellis*.
32. Rankin, *The Poison Trials*; Strocchia, *Forgotten Healers*, chap. 2; Leong, *Recipes and Everyday Knowledge*.
33. Universitätsbibliothek Hauptbibliothek, Basel, Frey-Gryn Mscr I 15: No. 463, Brief an Jacob Zwinger, 1597 https://www.e-manuscripta.ch/bau/849155; Campi, *Spicilegio botanico*, 92; Pona, *Monte Baldo descritto*, 234.
34. Sprechi, *Antabsinthium Clauenae*.
35. Busti, *Aduersus ea*, 16-18.
36. BNM, Collegio Medico IT.VII, 2340 (= 9672), 180r.
37. Campolongo, *Considerationi intorno alla Theriaca*.
38. The book was printed by a relative of the Martinellis in Ravenna. Mostravero, *Risposte*.
39. Mostravero, *Risposte*, 17.
40. BNM, Collegio Medico, IT.VII, 2340 (= 9672), 15r, 102r–102v, 179rv.
41. Marinelli, *Pharmacopaea*; Busti, *Adversus ea quae disputationi*.
42. BMC, Mariegola 209, I, 107r–109v. On the vicissitudes of the 1617 Venetian pharmacopoeia, see Minuzzi, *Sul filo dei segreti*, 48–53.
43. Minuzzi, *Sul filo dei segreti*, 53.
44. Busti, *Adversus ea quae disputationi*, 89.
45. ASV, Giustizia Vecchia 211, fasc. *Speziali*.
46. On the 1790 Venetian pharmacopoeia, see Giormani, "La farmacopea ufficiale."
47. ASV, Giustizia Vecchia 211, n.p.
48. ASV, Giustizia Vecchia 211, n.p.
49. ASV, Giustizia Vecchia 211, n.p.; also in Palmer, "Pharmacy," n77, 307.
50. ASV, Giustizia Vecchia 211, n.p. Also in Palmer, "Pharmacy," n77, 307.
51. ASV, Compilazione delle Leggi, Prima serie 277, c. 925. Also in BMC, Mariegola 209, 1, 117v–118v.
52. BMC, Mariegola 209, I, 117v July 30, 1621.

53. Certainly in 1600, 1606, 1610, 1655, 1663, 1665, 1667, 1675, and 1683. ASB, Studio 258; 251.
54. For Venetian production, see Chapter 5, Figure 5.1.
55. BCAB, Raccolta Bandi Merlani, 1683, 1688.
56. Pomata, *Contracting a Cure*, 10-1; 56-62.
57. The college had only fifteen full members, affiliated under three conditions: citizenship, degree from the University of Bologna, and at least one year of lectureship. More physicians could be affiliated as supernumeraries, but could obtain full membership only if a full member died. Pomata, *Contracting a Cure*, 16.
58. On Bologna apothecaries, see Baldi, *Notizie storiche;* Baldi, *Gli statuti;* Pomata, *Contracting a Cure*, 67-69; Pancino, "Malati, medici, mammane"; Piccinno, "Speziali"; Oszajca and Bela, "Granting a Licence"; Di Gennaro Splendore, "Craft, Money and Mercy"; Farolfi, "Società commerciale e società civile in una città di antico regime," 605.
59. Pomata, *Contracting a Cure*, 66.
60. For example, in 1671 and 1672 the medical college approved new restrictions to enter the apothecary professions, and in 1678, 1682, and 1683 closed several apothecary shops. ASB, Studio 258.
61. See Farolfi, "Società commerciale e società civile," 597-598.
62. ASB, Studio 258.
63. ASB, Studio 217, *Officiales aromatarios subjucunt se colegio*, 99v. Mention of the 1550 publication of the statutes, today lost, is in Arte degli speziali di Bologna, *Riforma de' statuti*, 9.
64. BUB, Ald. Ms. 21, IV, *Tassa delli pretii delle robbe medicinali semplici e composte.*
65. Collegio dei medici di Bologna, *Nuova Riforma.*
66. Pomata, *Contractig a Cure*, 67.
67. Aldrovandi and Collegio dei medici di Bologna, *Antidotarii Bononiensis.*
68. Olmi, "Farmacopea antica," 205.
69. On the theriac dispute, see Fantuzzi, *Memorie della vita*, 39-47; Benedicenti, *Malati, medici e farmacisti*, ii, 1022-1023; Zaccagnini, *Storia dello studio*, 239-240; Andreoli, "Ulisse Aldrovandi," 11-19; Olmi, "Farmacopea antica"; Di Gennaro Splendore, "Craft, Money and Mercy"; Cevolani and Buscaroli, "Dispute sulla teriaca." For theriac disputes in the creation of naturalistic collections, see Findlen, *Possessing Nature*, 241-287.
70. Calestani, *Delle osservationi*, 250.
71. Pastarino, *Ragionamento;* Di Gennaro Splendore, "Craft, Money and Mercy."
72. BUB, *Nuova riforma* (1585), 2-3.
73. Gardi, "Lineamenti della storia politica," 25, 27.
74. ASB, Studio 197, September 14, 1604.
75. Collegio dei medici di Bologna, *Conventioni*, chap. 1. Alessandro de Sangro was cardinal legate of Bologna in 1605. Between 1600 and 1610, Bologna had four different cardinal legates. Italics are mine.

76. ASB, Studio 213.
77. Collegio dei medici di Bologna, *Antidotarium*.
78. Gardi, "Lineamenti della storia politica," 26–27.
79. BCAB, *Avviso* 1617, 2.
80. ASB, Studio 319; also in Pomata, *Contracting a Cure*, 146.
81. Pomata, *Contracting a Cure*, 21.
82. Pomata, *Contracting a Cure*.
83. ASB, Studio 195, 116r.
84. ASB, Studio 195, 114r, 115r, 116r, 121r.
85. Sartorio, *Discorso*.
86. ASB, Studio 233.
87. Medici, *Le accademie scientifiche*, 12; also in Pomata, *Contracting a Cure*, 68.
88. Bartoli, *Notizie istoriche*, 136.
89. Riccardi, *Istruttione*.
90. Riccardi, *Venticinque discorsi*.
91. Montalbani, *Gl'indirizzi dell'arte*. The name of the author does not appear on the frontispiece, but the text is part of a work certainly written by Montalbani: *L'Honore de i collegi dell'arti della città*, 15–33.
92. Montalbani, *Antineotiologia*.
93. Montalbani, *Gl'indirizzi dell'arte*.
94. On measures against poverty used for social stability, see, among others, Gavitt, *Gender, Honor, and Charity;* Terpstra, *Cultures of Charity*. For poor relief and charity in early modern Bologna, see Terpstra, *Cultures of Charity*.
95. Collegio dei medici di Bologna, *Bandi et Provisioni*, 2.
96. Di Gennaro Splendore, "Craft, Money and Mercy," 104–106.
97. Strocchia, *Nuns and Nunneries;* Strocchia, "The Nun Apothecaries"; Strocchia *Forgotten Healers,* esp. chap. 3.
98. Di Gennaro Splendore, "Craft, Money and Mercy," 104–106.
99. ASB, Assunteria d'Arti. Notizie sopra il sollievo delle Arti, b. 1.
100. Collegio Medico di Bologna, *Conventioni*. This rule had already been stated in 1594; ASB, Studio 233 *Bando et Provisione*.
101. ASB, Studio 248, n.d.
102. ASB, Studio 338.
103. ASB, Studio 258.
104. ASB, Studio 318.
105. See Chapter 5, Figure 5.3.
106. ASB, Studio 237.
107. "Deve riuscire il composto per quanto si crede libbre 1.235, quali vogliamo solo libbre 1.200; dalle quali si levano libbre 50 che viene donata; resta libbre 1.150 e queste pure si vogliono credere libbre 1.100. Se libbre 1.100 costano lire 2.263, ogni libbra adunque costerà Lire 2:1/2. A considerarla solo libbre 1.000, costa ogni libbra lire 2:5:4. Il tutto è un cibaldone da non farne alcun conto e se la teriaca fosse solo libbre 900, costerebbe cinquanta bajocchi la

libbra." Producing theriac most likely cost 50-70 bajocchi or 5-7 paoli per pound. See ASB, Studio 250; also in Rosa, "La panacea dell'antichità," 335; De Tata, *All'insegna della fenice,* 230; BUB, Ms. 3938.

108. ASB, Studio 258, 248.
109. ASB, Studio 251.
110. Collegio dei medici di Bologna, *Riforma de' statuti,* 1.
111. Terpstra, *Lay Confraternities,* esp. 139-144.
112. Compared to previous statutes from 1377, this was a notable restriction, although also in the fourteenth century relatives by agnate line enjoyed a privileged entry into the guild. See Colapinto, "Gli statuti."
113. Collegio dei medici di Bologna, *Riforma de' statuti,* 25-29.
114. Collegio dei medici di Bologna, *Riforma de' statuti,* 35-36.
115. BUB, Ms. 3938, 22 *Iurate conventiones nonnullorum obedentium professorum artis aromatoriorum bononiae;* also in De Tata, *All'insegna della Fenice,* 228.
116. ASB, Studio 250.
117. BNM, IT VII 2361 (9717), fasc. H, 129r.

7. FROM "ANTIDOTE OF ALL ANTIDOTES" TO PHARMACEUTICAL MONSTER

1. Heberden, *Antitheriaka,* 11-15.
2. Cowen, "Expunctum est Mithridatium."
3. Lindemann, *Medicine and Society,* 264; Berman, "Persistence of Theriac."
4. Berman, "Persistence of Theriac," 11.
5. Berman, "Persistence of Theriac," 7.
6. Foucault, *Power/Knowledge,* 114, 131.
7. Urdang, "The Development of Pharmacopoeias."
8. Berman, "Persistence of Theriac," 10.
9. On the anti-marvelous in the Enlightenment, see Daston and Park, *Wonders,* 329-363. On the changing medical attitudes of Italian higher classes, see Brambilla, "La medicina del Settecento," 29; Cosmacini, *Storia della medicina,* 287.
10. On Galenic pharmacy in colonial context, see, among others, Newson, *Making Medicine;* De Vos, *Compounding Remedies.*
11. De Paul, *Correspondance,* 293.
12. Salle, *A New Discovery,* 102.
13. Salle, *A New Discovery,* 74, 78.
14. For a rich bibliography on Jesuit pharmacy in South America, see Boumediene, "Jesuit Recipes, Jesuit Receipts," 229-254.
15. Caminha, "Emplastros: os medicamentos," 303-304; Leite, *Artes e Ofícios,* 2:583.
16. Leite, *Artes e Ofícios,* 1:87-88, 298; 2:584. On the recipe of Triaga brasilica, see Dos Santos, *As plantas brasileiras,* 75-167, 219-225, 229-232. See also Pereira et al., "Triaga Brasilica."

17. Leite, *Artes e Ofícios*, 2:584.
18. Dos Santos, *As plantas brasileiras*, 63.
19. Dos Santos, *As plantas brasileiras*, 236–237.
20. Leite, *Artes e Ofícios*, 1:87.
21. Boumediene, "Jesuit Recipes, Jesuit Receipts," 234–235.
22. Pereira et al., "Triaga Brasilica," 312. In Europe many new products derived from theriac, such as orviétan, were secret and protected by a privilege, similarly to Triaga brasilica.
23. Leite, *Artes e Ofícios*, 1:88.
24. Semedo, *Polyanthea Medicinal*.
25. Semedo, *Polyanthea Medicinal*, 1–35, after the final index; 17–18. I was not able to consult the 1727 edition.
26. ARSI, NN 17, 400–421 also in Leite, *Artes e Ofícios*, 2:583–584.
27. Uragoda and Paranavitana, "Dutch Pharmacopoeia of 1757," 1.
28. Bruijn, *Ship's Surgeons*, 85–86.
29. Cook, *Matters of Exchange*, 305, 308–309.
30. Thunberg, *Voyages de C. P. Thunberg*, 2:9.
31. Grimm, *Insulae Ceyloniae thesaurus medicus*, 39–40.
32. Uragoda and Paranavitana, "Dutch Pharmacopoeia of 1757," 17.
33. Uragoda and Paranavitana, "Dutch Pharmacopoeia of 1757," 13–14.
34. For theriac in North America, see Eggleston, "Some Curious Colonial Remedies," 204; Sonnedecker, "Harward's 'Electuarium.'"
35. Roberts, "To Heal and to Harm," 352–353.
36. Roberts, "To Heal and to Harm," 350.
37. Boyle, *Of the reconcileableness of specific medicines*.
38. Roberts, "To Heal and to Harm," 83; Roberts, personal communication.
39. Schafer, *Golden Peaches of Samarkand*, 184.
40. Puente-Ballestreros, "Antoine Thomas Si," 237.
41. Nappi, "Bolatu's Pharmacy Theriac," 752, 753n41.
42. Nappi, "Bolatu's Pharmacy Theriac," 753.
43. Beckwith, "Tibetan Treacle."
44. Puente-Ballestreros, "Antoine Thomas Si," 237–243.
45. Waldack, "Le Père Philippe Couplet," 17.
46. Puente-Ballestreros, "Antoine Thomas Si," 230.
47. Griffin, *Mixing Medicines*, chap. 4.
48. McGowan, "The Age of Ayans," 725–727, 736.
49. Tekiner and Mat, "Les thériaques"; Leiser and Dols, "Evliyā Chelebi's Description . . . Part I"; Leiser and Dols, "Evliyā Chelebi's Description . . . Part II," 67–68.
50. Tavernier, *Nouvelle relation*, 189.
51. Küçük, *Science Without Leisure*, 161–166.
52. Tavernier, *Parte prima*, 165–166.
53. Ghobrial, *The Whispers of Cities*, 69.
54. Shay, *The Ottoman Empire*, 45, 48, 51, 52, 54.

55. Lane, *Venice*, 416–417.
56. Foscari, *Dispacci da Costantinopoli*, 27–28, 48.
57. Marin, *Storia civile e politica*, 343, 347; Ianiro, *Levante*, 321.
58. I thank Erica Ianiro for sharing this data. Venetian sources do not specify how much theriac was in a trunk. The 1750 and the 1784 tariff imposed a tariff of 1,60 and 4,60 kuruş per *occa* (a measure of weight approximately equal to 1.282 kilograms or 2.8 pounds) respectively. ASV, Cinque Savi alla Mercanzia, 605, 650, 652, 743, 749, 750.
59. BMC, Codice Cicogna 3382, 16.
60. Brugnera, "Frammenti," 88.
61. ASV, Cinque Savi alla Mercanzia, 743.
62. Brugnera, "Frammenti," 92.
63. Maehle, *Drugs on Trial*.
64. Hoffmann and Descazals, *Dissertatio inauguralis medica*, in Maehle, *Drugs on Trial*, 144.
65. Oddi, *De componendis medicamentis*, 39–40.
66. Charas, *Thériaque*.
67. Capron, *Correspondance complète* (1648): XI.
68. Capron, *Correspondance complète*, Heinrich Meibomius, July 24, 1664. It is not clear whether this is the treatise mentioned above.
69. Boyle, *Works*, 2:270.
70. Boyle, *Of the Reconcileableness*, 170.
71. Lémery, *Pharmacopée Universelle*, 602.
72. Bordeu, *Recherches*, 52–54.
73. On Venel, see Kafker and Kafker, *The Encyclopedists as Individuals*.
74. "Thériaque," in Diderot and d'Alembert, *Encyclopédie*.
75. Landouzy, preface to *Codex medicamentarius gallicus*, xvii–xviii. See also Bonnemain, "La thériaque," 309.
76. Sforza, *F.M. Fiorentini*, 265n1.
77. Gassel, *Lettere famigliari*. For the attribution to Gassel, see Melzi, *Dizionario di opere anonime*, 2, 118.
78. Gassel, *Lettere famigliari*, 227.
79. Gentilcore, *Charlatanism*, 126–127.
80. Brambilla, "La medicina del Settecento," 31–34.
81. Jarcho, *Clinical Consultations*, 91, 96, 150.
82. BCAB, Consulti Azzoguidi, Cart. 3, fasc. XXIV, XXV, XXVI, XXVII, XVIII, also in Grandi Venturi, "I consulti di Giuseppe Azzoguidi."
83. Ramazzini, *De morbis artificum diatriba*, 72, 247.
84. Azzoguidi, *La spezieria domestica*, n.p., preface. *La spezieria domestica* was republished in 1784, 1790, and 1799.
85. Azzoguidi, *La spezieria domestica*, 20.
86. Störck, *Istruzione a prevenire*.
87. ASB, Studio 248.

88. ASB, Studio 248.
89. For example, see French, *Medicine Before Science*.
90. Wellcome Collection, London, no. 816084i.
91. Goldoni, *Le donne di buon umore* (1758), 6:44, in Goldoni, *Commedie*.
92. Goldoni, *Lo spirito di contraddizione* (1758), 6:12, in Goldoni, *Commedie*. A similar image is also in *La putta onorata* (1748).
93. Infelise, "L'utile e il piacevole."
94. Piazza, *Gazzetta Urbana Veneta* (1787), 19.
95. Piazza, *Gazzetta Urbana Veneta* (1788), 54.
96. Gozzi, *La Gazzetta Veneta*, 84.
97. Mercurio, *De gli errori popolari*, 172.
98. ASB, Studio 213.
99. ASB, Studio 213, inspections dated 1640, 1657, 1658.
100. ASB, Studio 233, *Notificazione alli speciali, et altri per li medicamenti clandestinamente fatti o adulterati e specialmente la triaca*, February 27, 1717.
101. ASB, Studio 250; also in Rosa, "Medicina e salute pubblica," 33. Official quantities of theriac produced and quantities distributed do not match up, and nowhere is a reason for such a difference specified; a part of production certainly was donated to physicians and authorities.
102. BNM, Collegio Medico IT.VII, 2342 (= 9695), 121r. Document partly cited in Dian, *Cenni*, 42.
103. BNM, Collegio Medico IT.VII, 2361 (= 9716), 78r.
104. BNM, Collegio Medico IT.VII, 2374 (= 9694), published in Spada, *Una mostra di triaca*.
105. BNM, Collegio Medico IT.VII, 2374 (= 9694).
106. BNM, Collegio Medico IT.VII, 2361 (= 9716), 26r–27r.
107. VBA, O 46 inf.
108. Brugnera, "Frammenti," 88.
109. Rubbi, *L'epistolario*, 143.
110. BNM, Collegio Medico IT.VII, 2366 (= 9736).
111. Stossl, "Lo spettacolo della teriaca," 110.
112. Dian, *Cenni*, 104 n4.
113. *Pharmacopoea Austriaco-Provincialis Emendata*, 62.
114. For theriac in the Kingdom of Naples, see Gentilcore, *Healers and Healing*, 113–116; Mastroianni, *Il Reale Istituto d'incoraggiamento*; Mongelli, "Diffusione di un medicamento popolare."
115. Beltrani, *La R. Accademia di scienze*, 10.
116. ASN, Badia di Mileto, 266, 267–268, 270–272, 274–276, 279–283, 285.
117. ASN, Ministero delle Finanze 1343, April 29, 177,9 Mihar de la Sambuca to Marquis de Goyzueta; ASAN, XX B7 1.2. In 2018, during a research trip to Naples, I discovered that theriac was made in the backyard of the Museo Archeologico, right in front of the apartment where my family lived until I was eleven years old.

118. ASN, Badia di Mileto, 274, letter October 29, 1790; Badia di Mileto 266, letter April 30, 1785.
119. ASN, Badia di Mileto, 266, letter April 21, 1785.
120. ASN, Badia di Mileto, 266, letter July 18, 1785.
121. ASN, Badia di Mileto, 275, letter March 18, 1791.
122. ASN, Badia di Mileto, 275, letter March 18, 1791.

CONCLUSION

1. Defendente Sacchi, "La Teriaca di Venezia," n21, 167–168.
2. Pazzini, *La triaca in Roma,* 34–35.
3. Watson, *Theriac and Mithridatium,* 105.
4. Ackerknecht, *Therapeutics from the Primitives,* 37.
5. Bernard Palissy, *Discours admirables,* 148–156.

BIBLIOGRAPHY

PRIMARY SOURCES

MANUSCRIPTS

BASEL

Universitätsbibliothek Hauptbibliothek
Frey-Gryn Mscr I 15: Nr. 463 https://www.e-manuscripta.ch/bau/849155

BOLOGNA

Archivio di Stato di Bologna
Statuto dell'Arte degli speziali, 1303
Assunteria di Studio 87
Studio 195, 196, 197, 213, 217, 233, 237, 248, 250, 251, 258, 318, 319, 322, 338, 340, 354
Assunteria d'Arti. Notizie sopra il sollievo delle Arti, b. 1

Biblioteca Comunale dell'Archiginnasio
Ms. B2468
Raccolta Bandi Merlani
Consulti Azzoguidi, Cart. 3, fasc. XXIV, XXV, XXVI, XXVII, XVIII

Biblioteca Universitaria
Ms. 408, 3938
Ald. Ms. 21, III; 21, IV; 38, II, 69, I; 70; 79; 91; 100; 136, XI; 136, XXVI; 382, III
Giornale di Hercole Dal Buono

FLORENCE

Archivio dell'Ospedale degli Innocenti
Filza di ricevute riguardanti la spezieria del conservadorio 1705–1743
Giornale della spezieria dal 1729 al 1767

Archivio di Stato di Firenze

Arte Medici e Speziali, 269 Registro di Provvisioni e Ricordi detto C
Mediceo del Principato 241, 649, 1584, 2944, 2955, 4339

Biblioteca Nazionale Centrale di Firenze

Galileiana ms. 276

NAPLES

Archivio di Stato di Napoli

Badia di Mileto 266, 267, 268, 270, 271, 272, 274, 275, 276, 279, 280, 281, 282, 283, 285
Ministero delle Finanze 1343, 1380
Sommaria Arrendamenti Protomedicati 1071, 1119, 1157, 1217

Archivio Storico della Sovrintendenza di Napoli

XX B7

LONDON

Wellcome Collection

no. 816084i, https://wellcomecollection.org/search?query=816084i
MS. 8687

MILAN

Veneranda Biblioteca Ambrosiana

D198 inf
O 46 inf.

PARMA

Archivio di Stato di Parma

Racc. Mss. B. 33

UDINE

Archivi Storici Diocesani di Udine, Archivio dell'Ospedale S. Maria Della Misericordia

Busta 1064, *Index pretia continens omnium rerum medicinalium simplicium* (1636)

VENICE

Archivio di Stato di Venezia

Compilazione delle Leggi Prima serie, 277
Compilazione delle Leggi Seconda Serie, fasc. 231 n. 6
Giustizia Vecchia 98, 211
Provveditori e Sopraprovveditori alla Sanità, Capitolare II 1574–1689
Cinque Savi alla Mercanzia, 605, 650, 652, 743, 749, 750

Biblioteca Nazionale Marciana

Collegio Medico, IT.VII, 2329 (=9723); 2340 (=9672); 2342 (=9695); 2361 (=9716); 2366 (=9736–9737); 2374 (=9694)

Biblioteca del Museo Correr

Mariegola 209 I–IV
Codice Cicogna 3382

PRINTED PRIMARY SOURCES

Abati, Carlo Angelo. *De admirabili viperae nature, et de mirificis ejusdem facultatibus liber.* Urbino: B. Ragusium, 1589.

Adorno, Anselme. *Itineraire d'Anselme Adorno en Terre Sainte (1470–1471).* Edited by J. Heers, translated by G. de Groer. Paris: Éditions du Centre National de la Recherche Scientifique, 1978.

Aldrovandi, Ulisse, and Collegio dei medici di Bologna. *Antidotarii Bononiensis, siue de vsitata ratione componendorum, miscendorumque medicamentorum, epitome.* Bologna: Rossi, Giovanni, 1574.

Alessandrini, Giulio. *In Galeni praecipua scripta annotationes, quae commentariorum loco esse possunt: Accessit trita illa de theriaca quaestio.* Basel: apud Petrum Pernam, 1581.

Alpini, Prospero. *De medicina Aegyptiorum: Libri qvatvor.* Venice: Franciscum de Franciscis Senensem, 1591.

Arduino, Sante. *Santis Ardoyni . . . Opus de venenis . . .* Venice: per Henricum Petri et Petrum Pernam, 1562.

Arte de' medici e speziali di Firenze. *Il ricettario medicinale necessario a tutti i medici e speziali.* Florence: eredi Bernardo Giunti, 1574.

Arte de' medici e speziali di Firenze. *Ricettario utilissimo et molto necessario à tutti gli spetiali.* Venice: Vincenzo Valgrisi, 1556.

Arte degli speziali di Bologna. *Le virtù e facoltà principali della Triaca di Andromaco Seniore, Archiatro di Nerone Imperatore, fatta in Bologna l'anno 1663, dalla Honoranda Compagnia de gli Speciali Medicinalisti.* Bologna: Giacomo Monti, 1663.

Arte degli speziali di Bologna. *Riforma de' statuti dell'onoranda Compagnia de' Speziali di Bologna.* Bologna: per Giuseppe Longhi, 1690.

Arte degli speziali di Pisa. *Statuto inedito dell'Arte degli speziali di Pisa nel secolo XV.* Edited by Pietro Vigo. Bologna: G. Romagnoli, 1885.

Avicenna, Giovanni Paolo Mongiò, Giovanni Casteo, and Gherardo Andrea Alpago, eds. *Libri in re medica omnes, qui hactenus ad nos pervenere: Id est: Libri Canonis quinque.* Venice: Valgrisi, 1564.

Azzi, Francesco, and Stefano di Silvestri. *Le virtù e facoltà della theriaca di Andromaco protomedico di Claudio Nerone imperatore.* Bologna: Alessandro Benacci, 1574.

Azzoguidi, Germano. *La spezieria domestica.* Venice: stamperia Graziosi, 1782.

B.D.B. *Theriaque et anthidot prepare, pour chasser le venin, poison, ou Peste, des Heretiques, Nauarrois, et Athees Politiques de la France . . . Dedie a . . . Cardinal Caietan, Legat en France: Par le Seigneur B.* Paris: H. Duglar, 1590.

Baldi, Baldo. *Del vero opobalsamo orientale discorso apologetico.* Rome: Mascardi, 1646.

Baley, Walter. *A discourse of the medicine called mithridatium: Declaring the firste beginninge, the temperament, the noble vertues, and the true vse of the same: Compiled rather for those which are to vse it, then for the learned.* London: H. Marsh, 1585.

Bartoli, Francesco. *Notizie istoriche de' comici italiani.* Padua: Conzatti a S. Lorenzo, 1782.

Bartoli, Giorgio. *Lettere a Lorenzo Giacomini.* Edited by Anna Siekiera. Florence: Accademia della Crusca, 1997.

Bartolomeo da Orvieto, and Angelo Paglia. *In antidotarium Joannis filii Mesue cum declaratione simplicium medicinarum, & solutione multorum dubiorum, ac difficilium terminorum.* Venice: per Bartholomaeum de Zannettis, 1543.

Beauvais, Vincent de. *Speculum naturale.* Venice: Hermannus Liechtenstein, 1494.

Bernardi, Francesco. *Prospetto storico-critico dell'origine: Facoltà, diversi stati, progressi, e vicende del collegio medico-chirurgico e dell'arte chirurgica in Venezia.* Venice: Dalle stampe di D. Contantini, 1797.

Bertioli, Antonio. *Breue avviso del vero balsamo, theriaca, et mithridato: Ultimamente composti a commune beneficio: Per li fratelli Berthioli spetiali del serenissimo di Mantova.* Mantua: Francesco Osanna, 1596.

[Bertioli, Antonio.] *Giudicio sopra i raggionamenti di Cechino Martinelli sopra il nuovo Amomo e Calamo aromatico, alli speziali della città di Mantova.* Mantua: Francesco Osanna, 1605.

Blainville, J. de. *Travels Through Holland, Germany, Switzerland, but Especially Italy.* London: John Noon, 1757.

Bocchi, Simone. *Descrittione del teatro teriacale rappresentato nella pubblica piazza della nobil città di Parma l'anno 1632: Con l'autorità, e l'intervento dell'Eccellentissimo Collegio de' Signori Medici da Simon Bocchi: In fine della quale si pongono le virtuose qualità d'essa teriaca et del mitridato.* Modena: Iuliano Cassani, 1632.

Bordeu, Théophile. *Recherches sur quelques points d'histoire de la médecine, concernant l'inoculation, et qui paroissent favorable à la tolerance de cette operation.* Paris: chez Rémont 1764.

Borgarucci, Prospero. *La fabrica degli spetiali*. Venice: Vincenzo Valgrisio, 1566.

Boyle, Robert. *Of the reconcileableness of specific medicines to the corpuscular philosophy to which is annexed a discourse about the advantages of the use of simple medicines*. London: Sam. Smith, 1685. https://quod.lib.umich.edu/e/eebo/A29016.0001.001.

Boyle, Robert. *The Works of the Honourable Robert Boyle: In Six Volumes*. London: Printed for J. and F. Rivington, 1772.

Bruno, Giordano. *De la causa principio et uno*. Edited by Giovanni Aquilecchia. Turin: Einaudi, 1973.

Brunschwig, Hieronymus. *Liber de arte distilandi de compositis*. Strasbourg: 1512.

Bumaldi, Giovanni Antonio. *Formolario economico cibario, e medicinale di materie più facili, e di minor costo altretanto buone, e valeuoli, quanto le più pretiose*. Bologna: per Giacomo Monti, 1654.

Busti, Angelo. *Adversus ea quae disputationi suae De mellis convenienti atque legitimae quantitate ad theriacam componendam objecta fuere, defensio, praeclarissimo Philosophorum ac Medicorum Venetorum Collegio dicata*. Venice: ex typographia A. Muschij, 1617.

Busti, Angelo. *De mellis convenienti atque legitima quantitate ad theriacam componendam*. Venice: 1613.

Butner, Andreas. *De theriaca et mitridato Graecorum: De usu et virtutibus veræ Theriacæ et Mithridati*. Venice: Girolamo Scoto, 1546.

Calestani, Girolamo. *Delle osservationi . . . nel comporre gli antidoti, & medicamenti, che più si costumano in Italia all'uso della medicina, secondo il parere de medici antichi & moderni, esaminate: Con l'ordine di comporre, et fare diversi conditi, & col modo di conservarli*. Venice: Francesco Senese, 1568.

Calestani, Girolamo, and Giovanni Battista Bertucci. *Osservationi . . . nel comporre gli antidoti*. Venice: Francesco de Franceschi Senese, 1570.

Calogera, Angelo. *Nuova Raccolta d'opuscoli scientifici e filologici (cominciata da Angelo Calogera e continuata da Fortunata Mandelli)*. Venice: Occhi, 1771.

Calvin, John. *Commentaries on John*. Edited by Christian Classics Ethereal Library. https://ccel.org/ccel/calvin/commentaries/commentaries.i.html

Calzaveglia, Vincenzo. *De theriacae abusu in febribus pestilentibus*. Brescia: apud Vincentium Sabiensem, 1570.

Calzolari, Francesco. *Lettera di m. Francesco Calceolari spetiale al segno della campana d'oro in Verona, intorno ad alcune menzogne & calonnie date alla sua Theriaca da certo Scalcina Perugino*. Cremona: Vincenzo Conti, 1566.

Camerarius, Joachim. *De theriacis et methridateis commentariolus: Ad Pamphylianum de theriaca libellus antidotus: Item ad Parmphylianum de Theriacâ libel Galeni item Galène antidota Andromachi: Theriaca Andromachi. Antodotus Phiioni conversa in lat. adjectis his et aliis quibusdam Graecis diligenter emendates*. Nuremberg: Johann Petreius, [1533?].

Campi, Baldassarre. *Spicilegio botanico*. Lucca: Francesco Marescandoli, 1654.

Campolongo, Ottavio. *Considerationi di Ottavio Campolongo parmegiano, spetiale in Vinegia . . . intorno alla Theriaca, ove si scoprono secondo l'opinione di Galeno, et altri celebri scrittori, molti gravissimi errori fin'hora commessi da coloro che la compongono.* Venice: Gio. Battista Bertoni, 1614.

Candrini, Giuseppe. *Teriaca d'Andromaco e Mitridato di Democrate, composta da me Gioseppe Candrini.* Modena: Viviano Soliani, 1677.

Cantini, Lorenzo. *Legislazione toscana raccolta e illustrata dal dottore.* Florence: Stamp. Albizziniana da S. Maria in Campo, 1805.

Capello, Giovanni Battista, and Lorenzo Capello. *Lessico Farmaceutico-Chimico.* Venice: Antonio Graziosi, 1775.

Capron, Loïc, ed. *Correspondance complète et autres écrits de Guy Patin.* Paris: Bibliothèque interuniversitaire de santé, 2018. https://www.biusante.paris descartes.fr/patin/.

Cardullo, Domenico G. *Teriaca d'Andromaco composta publicamente in Messina.* Messina: Bianco, 1637.

Castiglione, Giovanni. *Prospectus pharmaceutici, seu Antidotarii Mediolanensis: Pars Tertia.* Milan: Carlo Giuseppe Galli, 1729.

Catelan, Laurens. *Discours et demonstration des ingrediens de la theriaque.* Lyon: par Jacques Mallet, 1614.

Ceruti, Benedetto. *Musaeum Francisci Calceolari iunioris Veronensis.* Verona: apud Angelum Tamum, 1622.

Champier, Symphorien. *Appothiquaires et Pharmacopoles par Symphorien Champier.* Edited by Paul Dorveaux. Paris: H. Welter, 1894.

Charas, Moyse. *Histoire naturelle des animaux, des plantes, et des minéraux qui entrent dans la composition de la Theriaque d'Andromachus.* Paris: Olivier de Varennes, 1668.

Charas, Moyse. *Thériaque d'Andromacus: Avec une description particulière des plantes, des animaux et des minéraux employez à cette grande composition.* Paris: D'Houry, 1685.

Cicogna, Antonio. *Delle iscrizioni veneziane raccolte et illustrate da Antonio Cicogna.* Venice: Giuseppe Orlandelli, 1824.

Cinelli Calvoli, Giovanni. *Biblioteca volante.* Edited by Dionigi Sancassani. Vol. 1. Venice: G. Albrizzi, 1735.

Colapinto, Leonardo, ed. "Gli statuti della compagnia degli speziali di Bologna (1377–1557)." In *Pagine di storia della scienza e della tecnica, allegato agli Annali di Medicina Navale*, vol. 1, nos. 24, 22. Rome: Ministero della difesa, 1966.

Collegio degli speziali di Napoli, Francesco Greco, and Giuseppe Donzelli, eds. *Antidotario napolitano di nuouo riformato, e corretto.* Naples: per Francesco Savio, 1642.

Collegio dei medici di Bologna. *Antidotarium a Bononiense medicinae collegio ampliatum ad ill.mum Senatum Bonon. cum dupl. tab. vna praesidiorum altera morborum.* Bologna: Vittorio Benacci, 1606.

Collegio dei medici di Bologna. *Avvertimenti, & prouisione intorno li Speciali, & quelli, che essercitano la medicina*. Bologna: Vittorio Benacci, 1600.

Collegio dei medici di Bologna. *Bandi et Provisioni sopra quelli che senza autorità . . . essercitano alcuna parte di Medicina*. Bologna: Vittorio Benacci, 1617.

Collegio dei medici di Bologna. *Bando et Provisione sopra quelli che senza autorità & licenza dell'Ecc. Collegio di Medicina danno, ordinano, vendono & applicano medicamenti in alcun modo*. Bologna: Vittorio Benacci, 1594.

Collegio dei medici di Bologna. *Conventioni fra l'ecc.mo Collegio de' medici, et la honorabile Compagnia delli speciali medicinalisti di Bologna*. Bologna: Vittorio Benacci, 1606.

Collegio dei medici di Bologna. *Notificazione sopra l'osservanza della tariffa de medicinali semplici, composti, e spagirici*. Bologna: 1765.

Collegio dei medici di Bologna. *Nuova Riforma et ordini aggionti alla moderatione altre volte fatta sopra li Speciali, & altri*. Bologna: Alessandro Benaccio, 1581.

Collegio dei medici di Bologna. *Tassa de' medicinali semplici, composti e spagirici*. Bologna: Barbiroli, 1711.

Collegio dei medici di Bologna. *Tassa de' medicinali ultimamente stabilita dall'eccellentissimo Collegio di Medicina, et honoranda Compagnia de' Speciali della citta di Bologna*. Bologna: eredi Benacci, 1637.

Collegio dei medici di Roma. *Antidotario romano*. Rome: Bartolomeo Zanetti, 1612.

Collegio dei medici di Roma. *Antidotario romano latino e volgare*. Rome: Ruffinelli, 1624.

Collegio dei medici di Roma. *Antidotarium Romanum, seu Modus componendi medicamenta, quae sunt in vsu*. Venice: apud Marinellus, 1585.

Coltellini, Agostino. *Corona d'applausi poetici in occasione di esporsi al pubblico la preparazione della triaca nella spezieria del convento della santissima Nunziata di Firenze dell'ordine de' Servi di M. V. dal di' 21. di luglio 1748. fino al di' 28. dello stesso mese dedicata a gl'illustrissimi signori socii della Facoltà Botanica di Firenze*. Florence: Bonducci, 1748.

Compendio storico e politico dell'Italia. Naples: G. P. Meranda, 1793–1794.

Cordus, Euricius. *Von Der Vielfaltigen Tugent Unnd Waren Bereitung Deß Rechten Edlen Theriacs Und Wie Er Lang Zeit Groblich Verfelscht Auch Noch Nit Wie Sichs Geburt Gemacht Wird Wider Die Losen Landleuffer Und Etliche Untrewe Apotecker*. Marburg: Franz Rhode, 1532.

Costa, Filippo. *Discorsi di Filippo Costa mantouano sopra le compositioni de gli antidoti & medicamenti, che più si costumano di dar per bocca*. Mantua: Giacomo Ruffinelli, 1576.

Crasso, Giunio Paolo, Bernardino Turrisani, and Marco degli Oddi. *Meditationes doctissimae in theriacam & mithridaticam antidotum*. Venice: Paulum, & Antonium Meietos fratres, 1576.

Croce, Giovanni. *Triaca musicale di Giovanni Croce chiozzotto nella quale vi sono diversi caprici a 4, 5, 6 et 7 voci*. Venice: Giacomo Vincenzi, 1595.

De Gasparis, Stefano. *Liquoris artificialis pro opobalsamo Orientali in conficienda theriaca Romae adhibiti physica oppugnatio*. Rome: ex tipographia Antonii Landini, 1640.

De Paul, Vincent. *Correspondance, entretiens, documents*. Edited by Pierre Coste. Paris: Librarie LeCoffre, 1922.

De Sgobbis, Antonio. *Nuovo et universale theatro farmaceutico*. Venice: Stamperia Iuliana, 1667.

Diderot, Denis, and Jean le Rond d'Alembert, eds. *Encyclopédie, ou dictionnaire raisonné des sciences, des arts et des métiers, etc.* University of Chicago: ARTFL Encyclopédie Project (Autumn 2022 edition). Edited by Robert Morrissey and Glenn Roe. http://encyclopedie.uchicago.edu/.

Donzelli, Giuseppe. *Additio apologetica ad suam de opobalsamo orientali synopsim*. Naples: Ottavio Beltrani, 1640.

Donzellini, Girolamo. *De natura, causis, et legitima curatione febris pestilentis: Ad Josephum Valdanium . . . epistola*. Venice: apud Camillum, & Ruttilium Borgominerios, 1570.

Donzellini, Girolamo. *Discorso nobilissimo e dottissimo preservativo et curativo della peste*. Venice: Horatio dei Gobi da Salò, 1577.

Draconi, Christophoro, and Barucino Zanni. *Theriaca fina contra il pestifero veleno delle comedie mercenarie lascive e impudiche de' nostri tempi composta da cari ingredienti di trattati di eccellenti autori secondo le regole del Gran Mitridate del Cielo.* Cremona: Christophoro Draconi e Barucino Zanni, 1614.

Du Chesne, Joseph. *La reformation des thériaques et antidotes opiatiques*. Paris: Claude Morel, 1608.

Elici, Frediano. *Delle virtù del mithridate minore contro la peste*. Pisa: per Francesco Tanagli, 1630.

Erculiani, Camilla. *Letters on Natural Philosophy: The Scientific Correspondence of a Sixteenth-Century Pharmacist, with Related Texts*. Edited by Eleonora Carinci, translated by Hannah Marcus, with a foreword by Paula Findlen. New York: Iter Press, 2021.

Evelyn, John. *The Diary of John Evelyn*. Edited by William Bray. New York: M. W. Dunne, ca. 1901.

Faber, Johannes. *Rerum medicarum Novae Hispaniae thesaurus, seu, plantarum animalium mineralium Mexicanorum historia*. Rome: Deversinus & Masotti, 1651.

Fantasti, Giovanni. *Vero modo di comporre la theriaca giusta l'intentione di Andromaco vecchio secondo Galeno*. Verona: Il Merlo, 1667.

Ferdinando, Epifanio. *Centum historiae, seu, Observationes et casus medici*. Venice: 1621. Reprint Mesagne: Biblioteca comunale "U. Granafei," 2001.

Ficino, Marsilio. *Consiglio contro la pestilenza*. Florence: Giunta, 1522.

Ficino, Marsilio. *De vita libri tres*. Basel: apud Io. Beb[elium], 1529.

Fioravanti, Leonardo. *Del reggimento della peste*. Venice: Andrea Revenoldo, 1565.

Foscari, Francesco. *Dispacci da Costantinopoli, 1757–1762*. Edited by Filippo Maria Paladini. Venice: La Malcontenta, 2007.

Fracastoro, Girolamo. *Hieronymi Fracastorii Veronensis Adami Fumani . . . et Nicolai Archii Comitis Carminum editio II.* Padua: J. Cominus, 1739.

Furetière, Antoine. *Dictionnaire Universel: Contenant généralement tous les Mots François tant vieux que modernes, & les Termes des Sciences et des Arts.* Rotterdam: 1708.

Galasso, Mario di Marino. *Recetario di nouo raccolto per l'esperto, & perito m. Mario di Marino Galasso napolitano diuiso in due parti, nella prima si contiene il regimento della sanità, & prouisione fatta l'anno 1576 . . . nella seconda il modo, che si deue tener per adoperare la gratia di san Paolo.* Milan: per Gio. Battista Bidelli, 1630.

Galasso, Mario di Marino. *Trattato molto vtile, qui dicitur flagellum Dei.* Bologna: per Alessandro Benacci, 1575.

Galenus, Claudius. *De anatomicis administrationibus libri novem: De constitutione artis medicae liber; De Theriaca, ad Pisonem commentariolus; De pulsibus, ad medicinae candidatos liber.* Translated by Johannes Guenther. Basel: apud And. Cratandrum, 1531.

Galenus, Claudius. *De theriaca ad Pisonem liber.* Translated by Johann Guenther. Paris: apud Simonem Colinaeum, 1531.

Galenus, Claudius. *Galeni librorum pars prima-quinta.* Venice: in aedibus Aldi et Andrea soceri, 1525.

Galenus, Claudius. *L'antidotario di Claudio Galeno Pergameno interpretato da Michelangelo Angelico.* Translated by Michelangelo Angelico. Vicenza: Amadio, 1613.

Garzoni, Tommaso. *La piazza universale di tutte le professioni del mondo.* Venice: Michiel Miloco, 1665.

Gasparis, Stefano de. *Liquoris artificialis pro opobalsamo orientali in conficienda theriaca Romae adhibiti physica oppugnatio.* Rome: ex tipographia Antonii Landini, 1640.

Gassel, Johan. *Lettere famigliari sopra le novelle letterarie oltramontane.* Venice: appresso Gio. Battista Recurti, 1749–1751.

Goldoni, Carlo. *Commedie del sig. Carlo Goldoni.* Venice: Antonio Zatta e figli, 1789.

Gozzi, Gasparo. *La Gazzetta Veneta.* Venice: 1760.

Greiff, Frederich. *Decas nobilissimorum medicamentorum, Galeno-Chymico modo compositoru.* Tübingen: Brunn, 1641.

Greiff, Frederich. *Kurtze Beschreibung Deß Chymischen oder Himmelischen Theriacs.* Tübingen: 1652.

Grimm, Hermanus Nicolaas. *Insulae Ceyloniae thesaurus medicus laboratorim.* Amsterdam: Henricum & Theodorum, 1679.

Guarguanti, Orazio. *Della theriaca, et sue mirabili virtù: Operetta d'Horatio Guarguanti da Soncino, medico et philosopho.* Venice: Giacomo Vincenti, 1596.

Guarguanti, Orazio. *Tria opuscula: Hoc est De theriacæ virtutibus paraphrasis; De mechioacani radice opusculum; Ac de ouo gallinarum, & eius vsu in febribus.* Venice: apud Battistam Ciottum, 1595.

Guldenius, Paulus, Franciszek Schnellboltz, and Jakub Gerhardi. *Andromachi Senioris Theriaca in usum et commodum Reipublicæ Thoruniensis.* Torún: typis Francisci Schnellboltzii, 1630.

Heberden, William. *Antitheriaka: An Essay on Mithridatium and Theriaca*. [n.p.]: 1745.
Hoffmann, Friederich, and Jaques Descazals. *Dissertatio inauguralis medica de opiatorum nova eaque mechanica operandi ratione*. Halle (Saale): literis Chr. Henckelii, 1700.
Hoffmann, Moritz. *Botanotheca Lauremergiana*. Altdorf: Georgi Hagen, 1662.
Houel, Nicolas. *Traité de la thériaque et mithridat*. Paris: Jean de Bordeaux, 1573.
Il giornale dei letterati d'Italia. Venice: Hertz, 1720.
King, Charles. *The British Merchant, or, Commerce Preserv'd: In Answer to The Mercator, or Commerce Retriev'd*. London: A. Baldwin, 1713.
Lassels, Richard. *The Voyage of Italy or a Complete Journey through Italy*. Paris: 1670.
Lavoranti, Lauro de'. *Lode della Theriaca d'Andromaco fatta in casa del Mag. M. Giulio Affaruosi spetiale in Reggio*. Reggio: appresso Hercoliano Bartoli, 1578.
Lebrija, Marcelo de. *La Triaca del alma: La triaca de amor: La triaca de tristes*. Granada, 1542.
Lémery, Nicolas. *Farmacopea universale che contiene tutte le composizioni di farmacia le quali sono in uso nella medicina, tanto in Francia, quanto per tutta l'Europa*. Venice: Gio. Gabriel Hertz, 1720.
Lémery, Nicolas. *Pharmacopée Universelle*. Paris: Laurent D'Houry, 1697.
Leoniceno, Niccolò. *Opuscula*. Basel: apud And. Cratandrum, et Io. Bebelium, 1532.
Lettere edificanti, e curiose scritte da alcuni religiosi della Compagnia di Gesù. Venice: Piotto and Valvasense, 1757.
Lettres édifiantes et curieuses, écrites des missions étrangères: Mémoires de la Chine. Paris: J. G. Merigot, 1781.
Machiavelli, Niccolò. *The Prince: A Revised Translation, Backgrounds, Interpretations*. Edited by Wayne A. Rebhorn. New York: W. W. Norton, 2020.
Manliis, Joannes Jacobus de, et al. *Luminare maggiore*. Venice: Bariletto, 1559.
Maranta, Bartolomeo. *De theriaca et mithridatio*. Translated by Joachim Camerarius. Frankfurt: Egenolph, 1576.
Maranta, Bartolomeo. *Della theriaca et del mithridato libri due ne quali s'insegna il vero modo di comporre i sudetti antidoti, et s'esaminano con diligenza tutti i medicamenti, che v'entrano*. Venice: Marcantonio Olmo, 1572.
Marin, Carlo Antonio. *Storia civile e politica del commercio de' Veneziani*. Venice: Coleti, 1808.
Marinelli, Curzio. *Pharmacopea, sive de vera pharmaca conficiendi et preparandi methodo*. Venice: Roberto Meietti, 1617.
Martinelli, Cechino. *Ragionamenti sopra l'amomo et calamo aromatico nuovamente l'anno 1604 havuto di Malaca città d'India dall'eccell. sig. Cechino Martinello suo zio*. Venice: Gratioso Perchacino, 1604.
Masini, Antonio di Paolo. *Bologna perlustrata, in cui si fa mentione ogni giorno in perpetua delle fontioni sacre profane di tutto l'anno*. Bologna, 1650.
Massa Ducale, Giuseppe di. *Dilucidazione fitologica di quelle piante specialmente italiche delle quali è necessaria la cognizione agli studenti di farmacia*. Rome: Generoso Salomoni, 1763.

Massaria, Alessandro. *De abusu medicamentorum vesicantium et theriacae in febribus pestilentibus disputatio.* Padua: Paulum Meiettum, 1591.

Mather, Cotton. *A Treacle Fetch'd Out of a Viper: A Brief Essay upon Falls into Sins.* Boston: B. Green, for Benj. Eliot, 1707.

Mattioli, Pier Andrea. *Di Pedacio Dioscoride Anazarbeo libri cinque della historia, et materia medicinale tradotti in lingua volgare italiana da M. Pietro Andrea Matthiolo Sanese medico, con amplissimi discorsi, et comenti, et dottissime annotationi, et censure del medesimo interprete, detti Discorsi.* Venice: Niccolò Bascarini, 1544.

Mattioli, Pier Andrea. *Il Dioscoride dell'eccellente dottor medico m. P. Andrea Matthioli da Siena, co i suoi discorsi, da esso la seconda uolta illustrati, & diligentemente ampliati; con l'aggiunta del sesto libro di i rimedi di tutti i ueleni da lui nuouamente tradotto, & con dottissimi discorsi per tutto commentato.* Venice: Vincenzo Valgrisi, 1548.

Mattioli, Pier Andrea. *I discorsi di M. Pietro Andrea Matthioli . . . nei sei libri di Pedacio Dioscoride Anazarbeo della materia medicinale.* Venice: Vincenzo Valgrisi, 1563.

Mattioli, Pier Andrea. *I Discorsi di M. Pietro Andrea Matthioli . . . nelli sei libri di Pedacio Dioscoride Anazarbeo della materia Medicinale.* Venice: Vincenzo Valgrisi, 1573.

Melich, Georg. *Auertimenti nelle compositioni de' medicamenti per vso della spetiaria: Con vna diligente esaminatione di molti simplici, tratta da piu degni auttori antichi & moderni.* Venice: Giovanni e Andrea Zenaro, 1575.

Melich, Georg. *Avertimenti nelle compositioni per uso della Spetiaria . . . Di nuouo aggiontoui vn bellissimo Trattato delle mirabili virtù della theriaca dell'eccellentissimo sig. Oratio Guarguanti.* Edited by Giacomo Vincenti. Venice: Niccolo Poli, 1596.

Melich, Georg. *De recta medicamentorum, quorum hodie usus est, parandorum ratione commentarij.* Translated by Samuel Keller. Wittenberg: Johannes Crato, 1586.

Melzi, Gaetano. *Dizionario di opere anonime e pseudonime di scrittori italiani.* Milan: Luigi di Giacomo Pirola, 1852.

Menegacci, Vendramino. *La theriaca et il mithridato.* Vicenza: Perin, 1587.

Mercuriale, Geronimo, ed. *Hippocratis COI. Opera quae extant graece et latine.* Venice: Giunta, 1588.

Mercurio, Scipione. *De gli errori popolari d'Italia.* Venice: G. B. Ciotti, 1603.

Metastasio, Pietro. *Lettere.* Vol. 5. Nice: Soc. Tipografica, 1787.

Montalbani, Ovidio. *Antineotiologia cioé discorso contro le nouità co gli astrologici presagij dell'anno 1662.* Bologna: per Giacomo Monti, 1661.

Montalbani, Ovidio. *Gl'indirizzi dell'arte dello spetiale medicinalista.* Bologna: per l'herede di Vittorio Benacci, 1658.

Montalbani, Ovidio. *L'Honore de i collegi dell'arti della città di Bologna: Brieve trattato fisico politico e legale.* Bologna: per l'herede del Benacci, 1670.

Monticolo, Giovanni, ed. *I capitolari delle arti veneziane: Sottoposte alla giustizia e poi alla giustizia vecchia dalle origini al MCCCXXX.* Rome: Forzani e C. tipografi del Senato, 1896-1914.

Moratti, Pietro. *Racconto de gli ordini e prouisioni fatte ne' lazaretti in Bologna, e suo contado in tempo del contagio dell'anno 1630.* Bologna: Clemente Ferroni, 1631.

Moryson, Fynes. *Shakespeare's Europe; Unpublished Chapters of Fynes Moryson's Itinerary, Being a Survey of the Condition of Europe at the End of the 16th Century; with an Introd. and an Account of Fynes Moryson's Career by Charles Hughes.* Edited by Charles Hughes. London: Sherratt and Hughes, 1903.

Mostravero, Asdrubale. *Risposte alle considerazioni d'Ottavio Campolongo Parmegiano, speciale in Venetia all'insegna del Forno, intorno alla compositione della teriaca, dove si mostra come quella è stata sempre legalissimamente composta, & si scopre la vanità de'pretesi & annoverati errori da lui, composta per mano di Asdrubale Mostravero, già speciale in Milano & hora publico professore di matematica.* Ravenna: Domenico Martinelli, 1614.

Neckam, Alexander. *De Naturis Rerum Libri Duo, with the Poem of the Same Author, De Laudibus.* Edited by Thomas Wright. London: Longman, Roberts, and Green, 1863.

Oddi, Marco. *De componendis medicamentis et aliorum diiudicandis methodus exactissima.* Padua: apud Paulum Meietum, 1583.

Olivi, Giovan Battista. *De reconditis et praecipuis collectaneis ab honestissimo, et solertiss. mo Francisco Calceolari Veronensi in musaeo adservaatis.* Venice, 1584.

Olmo, Fabio. *De mellis opportuna decentiue quantitate pro theriaca, mithridatoque componendis Fabii Vlmi philosophi ac medici Veneti responsio ad praeclarissimum philosophorum ac medicorum Venetorum collegium.* Venice: apud Petrum Dusinellum, 1614.

Palissy, Bernard. *Discours admirables de la nature des eaux et fontaines, tant naturelles qu'artificielles, des métaux, des sels et salines, des pierres, des terres, du feu et des émaux . . .* Paris: chez Martin le Iune, 1580.

Panciroli, Guido. *Rerum memorabilium iam olim deperditarum.* Amberg: Forster, 1602.

Pancotto, Michele. *Le mirabili virtù del sale dell'assenzo, del theriacale, e del perfetto elettuario contra veleni.* Bologna: Bellagamba, 1612.

Panicelli, Carlo. *Trattato de gl'effetti marauigliosi delle carni di vipere, per conseruare il corpo sano, e sicuro da veleni, prolongar la gioventù, ritardar la vecchiezza, liberare da molti mali incurabili, con altri mirabili effetti.* Florence: nella Stamperia di Simone Ciotti, 1630.

Pascual, Manuel. *Sueños ay, que verdad son, y punto en contra de los astrologos: triaca magna contra el veleno de la astrologia judiciaria.* [n.p.] 1739.

Pastarino, Filippo. *Ragionamento di Pastarino sopra l'arte della speciaria.* Bologna: Giovanni Rossi, 1575.

Patrizio, Francesco. *La città felice.* Venice: Giovan Griffio,1553.

Pharmacopoea Austriaco-Provincialis Emendata. Milan: Joseph Galeatium, 1794.

Piazza, Antonio. *Gazzetta Urbana Veneta.* Venice: 1787, 1788.

Picinelli, Filippo. *Mondo simbolico formato d'imprese scelte, spiegate, ed illustrate con sentenze, ed eruditioni, sacre, e profane.* Venice: Francesco Vigone, 1669.

Pisanelli, Baldassare. *Discorso sopra la peste diviso in due parti*. Rome: Heredi di Antonio Baldo, 1577.

Pliny the Elder. *Naturalis Historia*. Edited by Karl Friedrich and Theodor Mayhoff. Leipzig: Teubner, 1906.

Pona, Giovanni. *Monte Baldo descritto da Giouanni Pona veronese*. Venice: Roberto Meietti, 1617.

Prévost, Nicolaus. *Dispensarium Magistri Nicolai Prepositi Ad Aromatarios*. Lyon: Jacobo Huguetan, 1505.

Pulci, Luigi. *Morgante: The Epic Adventures of Orlando and His Giant Friend Morgante*. Translated by Joseph Tusiani. Bloomington: Indiana University Press, 1998.

Quattrami, Evangelista. *Tractatus perutilis atque necessarius ad theriacam, mitridaticumque antidotum*. Ferrara: Victorius Baldinus, 1597.

Rabelais, François. *Gargantua and Pantagruel: Translated and Edited with an Introduction and Notes by M.A. Screech*. Translated by Michael A. Screech. London: Penguin Classics, 2006.

Ramazzini, Bernardino. *De morbis artificum diatriba*. Utrecht: van de Water, 1703.

Ramusio, Giovan Battista. *Navigazioni e Viaggi*. Edited by Marica Milanesi. Turin: Einaudi, 1978–1988.

Redi, Francesco. *Consulti medici di Francesco Redi*. Edited by Lorenzo Martini. Capolago: Tipografia Elvetica, 1831.

Redi, Francesco. *Lettera sopra alcune opposizioni fatte alle sue osservazioni intorno alle vipere*. Florence: Pietro Matini, 1685.

Redi, Francesco. *Osservazioni intorno alle vipere*. Florence: all'insegna della Stella, 1664.

Riccardi, Adriano. *Istruttione intorno al comporre la Theriaca d'Andromaco*. Bologna: Vittorio Benacci, 1606.

Riccardi, Adriano. *Venticinque discorsi del modo di preparare i semplici medicinali*. Bologna: Bartolomeo Cocchi, 1613.

Rossi, Girolamo. *Theriaca di Andromaco il Vecchio*. Cesena: stamperia del Neri, 1643.

Rubbi, Andrea. *Dizionario di antichità sacre e profane, pubbliche e private, civili e militari comuni ai greci ed ai romani giusta il metodo di Samuele Pitisco*. Venice: Nuova Stamperia, 1793.

Rubbi, Andrea, ed. *L'epistolario ossia scelta di lettere inedite famigliari curiose erudite storiche galanti ec. ec. di donne e d'uomini celebri morti o viventi nel secolo 18° o nel 1700*. Venice: Graziosi, 1796.

Rutta, Clemente. *Trionfi contro la morte overo le rare prerogative e virtù singolari della teriaca*. Piacenza: Giovanni Bazachi, 1655.

Sacchi, Defendente. "La Teriaca di Venezia." In *Cosmorama Pittorico*, no. 21. Milan: dalla tipografia del Cosmorama, 1835.

Saggi scientifici e letterari dell'Accademia di Padova. Vol. 1. Padua: a spese dell'Accademia, 1789.

Salle, Robert de la. *A New Discovery of a Vast Country in America, extending above four thousand miles, between New France & New Mexico.* London: Henry Bonwicke, 1699.

Sanudo, Marin. *I Diarii.* Edited by Deputazione Veneta di Storia Patria. Venice: Fratelli Visentini, 1886.

Sanudo, Marin. *Le vite dei Dogi.* Edited by Angela Caracciolo Aricò. Venice: La Malcontenta, 1999.

Sartorio, Francesco. *Discorso di Francesco Sartorio speciale sopra la compositione della triaca da lui composta secondo la ricetta d'Andromaco il vecchio nell'Hospitale di S. Maria della Morte di Bologna à 15. d'Agosto 1612.* Bologna: Vittorio Benacci, 1613.

Sassetti, Filippo. *Lettere edite e inedite di Filippo Sassetti.* Edited by Ettore Marcucci. Florence: Le Monnier, 1855.

Sassonia, Ercole. *Disputatio de phoenigmorum, quae vulgo vesicantia appellantur, et de theriacae usu in febribus pestilentibus: In qua etiam de natura pestis et pestilentium febrium nonnulla tractantur.* Padua: Paulus Meiettus, 1591.

Scalcina, Hercolano. *Successo, giuditio, & offerta, circa la theriaca de Francesco de Calzolari spiciale alla Campana indorata in Verona, scritto per Herculano Scalcina Perugino.* [n. p.] post 1566.

Schott, Franz. *Italy in its Original Glory Ruine and Revival.* London: Griffin, 1660.

Semedo, João Curvo. *Polyanthea Medicinal: Noticias Galenicas e Chymicas.* Lisbon: Miguel Deslandes, 1697.

Settala, Lodovico. *Breve compendio delle virtù della Teriaca di Andromaco il Vecchio e del Mitridate di Damocrate.* Milan: Rolla, 1633.

Settala, Lodovico. *Preservatione dalla peste.* Brescia: Bartholomeo Fontana, 1630.

Severino, Marco Aurelio. *Vipera Pythia: Id est, De viperæ natura, veneno, medicina, demonstrationes, & experimenta noua.* Padua: Paolo Frambotti, 1651.

Sprechi, Pompeo. *Antabsinthium Clauenae idest quod absinthium vmbelliferum in Monte Seruae Belluni et alijs Italiae montibus ortum sit idem cum absinthio alpino vmbellifero Carolj Clusij.* Venice: apud Antonium Turinum, 1611.

Sterlich, Romualdo de. *Lettere a G. Bianchi (1754–1775).* Edited by Giuseppe F. de Tiberis. Naples: Arte tipografica, 2006.

Stigliola, Nicola Antonio. *Theriace, et mithridatia Nicolai Stelliolae Nolani libellus, in quo harum antidotorum apparatus, atque vsus monstratur.* Naples: Marinum de Alexandro, 1577.

Störck, Anton von. *Istruzione a prevenire, ed a guarire i morsi de' cani rabbiosi.* Translated by Giulio Zandt. Rome: per Luigi Perego Salvioni, 1784.

Tasso, Torquato. *Lettere.* Edited by Cesare Guasti. Florence: Le Monnier, 1854.

Tavernier, Jean-Baptiste. *Nouvelle relation de l'intérieur du serrail du Grand Seigneur.* Paris: Varennes, 1675.

Tavernier, Jean-Baptiste. *Parte prima de' viaggi nella Turchia, Persia et India.* Rome: Giuseppe Corvo, 1632.

Teodosio, Giovan Battista. *Medicinales epistolae LXVIII.* Basel: apud Nicolaus Episcopius, 1553.

Theriaca Andromachi senioris ex Gal. Cum succedaneis ab Excell. Coll. Medicorum Venet. electis. Venice: Joanne Baptista Albricci, 1756.

Thunberg, Carl Peter. *Voyages de C. P. Thunberg au Japon par le Cap de Bonne-Espérance.* Paris: Dandré, 1796.

Tiraboschi, Girolamo, Antonio Lombardi, and Tommaso Maria Mamachi. *Storia della letteratura italiana: Dall'anno MD fino all'anno MDC.* Venice: 1796.

Trombelli, Giovanni Crisostomo. *Memorie istoriche concernenti le due canoniche di S. Maria di Reno e di San Salvatore.* Bologna: per G. Corciolani ed eredi Colli, 1752.

Turner, William. *A Perservative, or Triacle, Agaynst the Poyson of Pelagius Lately Renued, by the Furious Secte of the Annabaptistes.* London: Steven Mierdman for Andrew Hester, 1551.

Valdagni, Giuseppe. *De theriacae usu in febribus pestilentibus.* Brescia: apud Vincentium Sabiensem, 1570.

Villanova, Arnaldus de. *Arnaldi de Villanova Opera Medica Omnia. Tractatus de Amore Heroico: Epistola de Dosi Tyriacalium Medicinarum.* Edited by Michael R. McVaugh. Barcelona: Seminarium Historiae Medicae Granatensis, 1985.

Voiture, Vincent de. *Les oeuvres de Monsieur de Voiture.* Paris: A. Courbé, 1650.

Woodall, John. *The Surgions Mate: The First Compendium on Naval Medicine, Surgery and Drug Therapy (London 1617).* Edited by Irmgard Müller. Cham: Springer International, 2016.

Zanella, Girolamo. *Della triaca e sue meravigliose virtù con il modo e regola d'usarla breve et utile discorso.* Padua: Stampator Camerale, 1650.

Zevi, Shlomo Zalman. *Theriaca Judaica.* Hanau: 1615.

SECONDARY SOURCES

Ackerknecht, Erwin. *Therapeutics from the Primitives to the 20th Century.* New York: Hafner Press, 1973.

Ahnfelt, Nils-Otto, and Hjalmar Fors. "Making Early Modern Medicine: Reproducing Swedish Bitters." *Ambix* 63, no. 2 (2016): 162–183.

Ahnfelt, Nils-Otto, Hjalmar Fors, and Karin Wendin. "Making and Taking Theriac: An Experimental and Sensory Approach to the History of Medicine." *British Journal for the History of Science Themes* 7 (2022): 39–62.

Ait, Ivana. *Tra scienza e mercato: Gli speziali a Roma nel tardo Medioevo.* Rome: Istituto nazionale di studi romani, 1996.

Albala, Ken. *Eating Right in the Renaissance.* Berkeley: University of California Press, 2002.

Alberi, Eugenio, ed. *Relazioni degli ambasciatori veneti al Senato.* Florence: Clio, 1839.

Alfani, Guido. *Il grand tour dei cavalieri dell'Apocalisse: L'Italia del "lungo Cinquecento," 1494–1629.* Venice: Marsilio, 2010.

Ammannati, Francesco, Guido Alfani, and Wouter Ryckbosch. "Poverty in Early Modern Europe: New Approaches to Old Problems," ESEH Working Paper 222 (2022): 1–60.

Anagnostou, Sabine, Florike Egmond, and Christoph Friedrich, eds. *A Passion for Plants: Materia Medica and Botany in Scientific Networks from the 16th to the 18th Centuries.* Stuttgart: Wissenschaftliche, 2011.

Anderson, Stuart. *Making Medicines: A Brief History of Pharmacy and Pharmaceuticals.* Grayslake, UK: Pharmaceutical Press, 2005.

Andretta, Elisa. *Roma Medica: Anatomie d'un système médical au XVIe siècle.* Rome: École française de Rome, 2011.

Anonye, Blessing, Valentina Nweke, Jessica Furner-Pardoe, et al. "The Safety Profile of Bald's Eyesalve for the Treatment of Bacterial Infections." *Scientific Reports* 10, report 1753 (2020). https://www.nature.com/articles/s41598-020-74242-2.

Baldi, Giovanni. *Gli statuti dell'Arte degli speziali in Bologna.* Pisa: Pacini Mariotti, 1958.

Baldi, Giovanni. *Notizie storiche sulla farmacia bolognese.* Bologna: Società Tipografica Mareggiani, 1955.

Bamji, Alexandra. "Health Passes, Print and Public Health in Early Modern Europe." *Social History of Medicine* 32, no. 3 (2019): 441–464.

Beckwith, Christopher. "Tibetan Treacle: A Note on Theriac in Tibet." *Tibet Society Bulletin* 15 (1980): 49–51.

Beecher, Donald. "Ficino, Theriaca and the Stars." In *Marsilio Ficino: His Theology, His Philosophy, His Legacy,* edited by Michael J. B. Allen, Valery Rees, and Martin Davies. Leiden: Brill, 2002.

Bellorini, Cristina. *The World of Plants in Renaissance Tuscany: Medicine and Botany.* Burlington, VT: Ashgate, 2016.

Beloch, Karl Julius. *Storia della popolazione d'Italia.* Florence: Le lettere, 1994.

Beltrani, Giovanni. *La Real Accademia di scienze e belle lettere fondata in Napoli nel 1778: Memoria letta all'Accademia Pontaniana nelle tornate del 20 maggio e 1 luglio 1900 dal socio corrispondente Giovanni Beltrani.* Naples: Stabilimento tipografico nella R. Università di Alfonso Tessitore e Figlio, 1900.

Benedicenti, Alberico. *Malati, medici e farmacisti: Storia dei rimedi traverso i secoli e delle teorie che ne spiegano l'azione sull'organismo.* Milan: Hoepli, 1924–1925.

Bénézet, Jean-Pierre, and Jean Flahaut. *Pharmacie et médicament en Méditerranée occidentale (XIIIe–XVIe siècles).* Paris: H. Champion; Geneva: Slatkine, 1999.

Benzi, Gaia. *Tra prìncipi e saltimbanchi: Medicina e letteratura nel tardo Rinascimento.* Rome: Sapienza Università Editrice, 2020.

Berg, Maxine. "New Commodities, Luxuries and Their Consumers in Eighteenth-Century England." In *Consumers and Luxury: Consumer Culture in Europe, 1650–1850,* edited by Maxine Berg and Helen Clifford. New York: Manchester University Press, 1999.

Berman, Alex. "The Persistence of Theriac in France." *Pharmacy in History* 1, no. 12 (1970): 5–12.

Bernhard, Joseph. *Les médicaments oubliés: La Thériaque, étude historique et pharmaceutique*. Paris: J. B. Baillière et fils, 1893.

Bertucci, Paola. *Artisanal Enlightenment: Science and the Mechanical Arts in Old Regime France*. New Haven, CT: Yale University Press, 2017.

Berveglieri, Roberto. *Tutela e brevettazione in campo medico farmaceutico*. Cavriana: Tecnologos, 2006.

Biagioli, Mario. *Galileo, Courtier: The Practice of Science in the Culture of Absolutism*. Chicago: University of Chicago Press, 1993.

Biagioli, Mario. "Galileo's System of Patronage." *History of Science* 28, no. 79 (1990): 1-62.

Biller, Peter, and Joseph Ziegler, eds. *Religion and Medicine in the Middle Ages*. Woodbridge: York Medieval Press, 2001.

Blair, Ann M. *Too Much to Know: Managing Scholarly Information Before the Modern Age*. New Haven, CT: Yale University Press, 2010.

Bloch, Marc. *The Royal Touch: Sacred Monarchy and Scrofula in England and France*. London: Routledge and Kegan Paul, 1973.

Blockmans, Willem Pieter, André Holenstein, and Jon Mathieu, eds. *Empowering Interactions: Political Cultures and the Emergence of the State in Europe, 1300–1900*. Burlington, VT: Ashgate, 2009.

Bonnemain, Bruno. "La thériaque à l'époque moderne (XVIIe au XXe siècle)." In *Revue d'histoire de la pharmacie* 97, no. 367 (2010): 301–310.

Bosc, Jean-Louis. "Ce que fut la thériaque de Montpellier." *Revue d'histoire de la pharmacie* 97, no. 367 (2010): 285–294.

Boudon-Millot, Véronique. "Anecdote et antidote: Fonction du récit anecdotique dans le discours galénique sur la thériaque." In *Antike Medizin im Schnittpunkt von Geistes- und Naturwissenschaften: Internationale Fachtagung aus Anlass des 100-jährigen Bestehens des Akademievorhabens "Corpus Medicorum Graecorum / Latinorum."* Edited by Christian Brockmann, Wolfram Brunschön, and Oliver Overwien. Berlin: De Gruyter, 2009.

Boudon-Millot, Véronique, ed. and trans. *Claudius Galenus, Œuvres*. Vol. 6, *Thériaque à Pison*. Paris: Les Belles Lettres, 2016.

Boudon-Millot, Véronique, and Françoise Micheau, eds. *La Thériaque: Histoire d'un remède millénaire*. Paris: Les Belles Lettres, 2020.

Boumediene, Samir. "Jesuit Recipes, Jesuit Receipts: The Society of Jesus and the Introduction of Exotic Materia Medica into Europe." In *Cultural Worlds of the Jesuits in Colonial Latin America*, edited by Linda A. Newson. London: Institute of Latin American Studies, 2020.

Boumediene, Samir, and Valentina Pugliano. "La route des succédanés: Les remèdes exotiques, l'innovation médicale et le marché des substituts au XVIe siècle." *Revue d'histoire moderne contemporaine* 66, no. 3 (2019): 24–54.

Brambilla, Elena. "Dagli antidoti contro la peste alle Farmacopee per i poveri: Farmacia, alchimia e chimica a Milano 1600-1800." In *Studi in onore di Franco della Peruta,* vol. 2, edited by Maria Luisa Betri and Duccio Bigazzi. Milan: Angeli, 1996.

Brambilla, Elena. "La medicina del Settecento: Dal monopolio dogmatico alla professione scientifica." In *Storia d'Italia 7: Malattia e medicina,* edited by Franco Della Peruta. Turin: Einaudi, 1984.

Breen, Benjamin. *The Age of Intoxication: Origins of the Global Drug Trade.* Philadelphia: University of Pennsylvania Press, 2019.

Bremer-David, Charissa, with Peggy Fogelman, Peter Fusco, and Catherine Hess. *Decorative Arts: An Illustrated Summary Catalogue of the Collections of the J. Paul Getty Museum.* Malibu: J. Paul Getty Museum, 1993.

Brighetti, Antonio. *Bologna e la peste del 1630: Con documenti inediti dell'Archivio segreto Vaticano.* Bologna: Antonio Gaggi, 1968.

Brockliss, Lawrence, and Colin Jones. *The Medical World of Early Modern France.* Oxford: Oxford University Press, 1997.

Brugnera, Mariano. "Frammenti di un processo per la falsificazione della Teriaca veneta." *Atti e Memorie Rivista di storia della farmacia* 8, no. 2 (1991): 87–93.

Bruijn, Iris. *Ship's Surgeons of the Dutch East India Company: Commerce and the Progress of Medicine in the Eighteenth Century.* Leiden: Leiden University Press, 2009.

Bynum, W. F., and Roy Porter, eds. *Medicine and the Five Senses.* Cambridge: Cambridge University Press, 1993.

Calvet, Antoine. "À la recherche de la médecine universelle: Questions sur l'élixir et la thériaque au 14e siècle." In *Alchimia e medicina nel Medioevo,* edited by Chiara Crisciani and Agostino Paravicini Bagliani. Tavarnuzze: SISMEL edizioni del Galluzzo, 2003.

Calvi, Giulia. *Histories of a Plague Year: The Social and the Imaginary in Baroque Florence.* Berkeley: University of California Press, 1989.

Caminha, Viviane Machado São Bento. "Emplastros: Os medicamentos das boticas jesuítas no auxílio do cotidiano na América Portuguesa." *Revista História e Cultura* 3, no. 2 (2014): 299–315.

Carinci, Eleonora. "Una 'speziala' padovana: Lettere di philosophia naturale di Camilla Erculiani (1584)." *Italian Studies* 68, no. 2 (2013): 202–229.

Carmichael, Ann G. "Contagion Theory and Contagion Practice in Fifteenth-Century Milan." *Renaissance Quarterly* 44, no. 2 (1991): 213–256.

Catellani Patrizia, and Renzo Console. "Moyse Charas, Francesco Redi, the Viper and the Royal Society of London." *Pharmaceutical Historian: Newsletter of the British Society for the History of Pharmacy* (2004): 2–10.

Cavallo, Sandra. "Secrets to Healthy Living: The Revival of the Preventive Paradigm in Late Renaissance Italy." In *Secrets and Knowledge in Medicine and Science, 1500–1800,* edited by Elaine Leong and Alisha Rankin. Burlington, VT: Ashgate, 2011.

Cavallo, Sandra, and Tessa Storey. *Healthy Living in Late Renaissance Italy.* Oxford: Oxford University Press, 2013.

Cevolani, Enrico, and Carla Buscaroli. "Dispute sulla teriaca tra gli speziali e Ulisse Aldrovandi nella Bologna del XVI secolo." *Atti e Memorie: Accademia Italiana di Storia della Farmacia* 35, no. 1 (2018): 39–50.

Charlesworth, James H. *The Good and Evil Serpent: How a Universal Symbol Became Christianized.* New Haven, CT: Yale University Press, 2010.

Chase, Melissa P. "Fevers, Poisons and Apostemes: Authority and Experience in Montpellier Plague Treatises." In *Science and Technology in Medieval Society,* edited by Pamela O. Long. New York: New York Academy of Sciences, 1985.

Chittolini, Giorgio, Anthony Molho, and Pierangelo Schiera, eds. *Origini dello stato: Processi di formazione statale in Italia fra medioevo ed età moderna.* Bologna: Il Mulino, 1994.

Cipolla, Carlo M. *Miasmas and Disease: Public Health and the Environment in the Pre-Industrial Age.* New Haven, CT: Yale University Press, 1992.

Cipolla, Carlo M. "Origine e sviluppo degli Uffici di Sanità in Italia." *Annales cisalpines d'Histoire sociale* 1, no. 4 (1973): 89–90.

Cipolla, Carlo M. *Public Health and the Medical Profession in the Renaissance.* Cambridge: Cambridge University Press, 1976.

Cipolla, Carlo M. *Storia economica dell'Europa preindustriale.* Bologna: Il Mulino, 1974; 2nd ed., 1990.

Ciuti, Francesco. "Il Collegio dei fisici e l'arte dei medici e speziali di Firenze: Dalla Repubblica allo Stato mediceo (XIV–XVI Secolo)." *Archivio Storico Italiano* 170, no. 1631 (2012): 3–28.

Clericuzio, Antonio. "Chemical Medicine and Paracelsianism in Italy, 1550–1650." In *The Practice of Reform in Health, Medicine, and Science, 1500–2000,* edited by Margaret Pelling and Scott Mandelbrote. London: Routledge, 2017.

Cohn, Samuel K. *Cultures of Plague: Medical Thinking at the End of the Renaissance.* Oxford: Oxford University Press, 2010.

Colapinto, Leonardo, and Alessandro Maviglia. "Esame analitico comparativo di tre tariffe di medicinali contemporaneamente vigenti nel 1689 in Roma e suo distretto, Marche e Romagna, e Stato Ecclesiastico." *Rivista di Storia della Medicina* 14 (1970): 180–94.

Collard, Franck. *The Crime of Poison in the Middle Ages.* Westport, CT: Praeger, 2008.

Collard, Franck. *Pouvoir et poison: Histoire d'un crime politique de l'antiquité à nos jours.* Paris: Seuil, 2007.

Collard, Franck, and Evelyne Samama, eds. *Pharmacopoles et apothicaires: Les pharmaciens de l'antiquité au Grand siècle.* Paris: L'Harmattan, 2006.

Cook, Harold J. *The Decline of the Old Medical Regime in Stuart London.* Ithaca, NY: Cornell University Press, 1986.

Cook, Harold J. "Markets and Cultures: Medical Specifics and the Reconfiguration of the Body in Early Modern Europe." *Transactions of the Royal Historical Society* 21 (2011): 123–45.

Cook, Harold J. *Matters of Exchange: Commerce, Medicine, and Science in the Dutch Golden Age*. New Haven, CT: Yale University Press, 2007.

Cooper, Alix. *Inventing the Indigenous: Local Knowledge and Natural History in Early Modern Europe*. Cambridge: Cambridge University Press, 2007.

Corradi, Alfonso. *Annali delle epidemie occorse in Italia dalle prime memorie fino al 1850*. Bologna: Gamberini e Parmeggiani, 1865.

Corradi, Alfonso. "Degli esperimenti tossicologici in anima nobili nel Cinquecento." *Annali universali di medicina e chirurgica* 277 (1886): 73–100.

Corradi, Alfonso. "Gli antichi statuti degli speziali." *Annali universali di medicina e chirurgia* 1, no. 277, f. 834 (1886): 153–213.

Cosmacini, Giorgio. *Storia della medicina e della sanità in Italia*. Rome: Laterza, 2010.

Coturri, Enrico. "Perché il 'De usu Theriacae ad Pamphilianum' non è da ritenersi opera di Galeno." *Galeno* 4 (1959).

Cowen, David L. "Expunctum est Mithridatium." *Pharmaceutical Historian* 15, no. 3 (1985): 2–3.

Crawshaw, Jane L. Stevens. *Plague Hospitals: Public Health for the City in Early Modern Venice*. Burlington, VT: Ashgate, 2012.

Cuna, Andrea. "Editoria e testi 'de re medica.'" In *Nicola Stigliola: Enciclopedista e linceo*, edited by Saverio Ricci. Rome: Atti della Accademia Nazionale dei Lincei, 1996.

Curth, Louise, ed. *From Physick to Pharmacology: Five Hundred Years of British Drug Retailing*. Burlington, VT: Ashgate, 2006.

Dallasta, Federica. "Novità sul semplicista Evangelista Quattrami (1527–1608) e sul suo collaboratore Simon Bocchi." In *Ulisse Aldrovandi: Libri e immagini di Storia naturale nella prima Età moderna*, edited by Giuseppe Olmi and Fulvio Simoni. Bologna: Bononia University Press, 2018.

Daston, Lorraine, and Katharine Park. *Wonders and the Order of Nature, 1150–1750*. New York: Zone Books, 1998.

Davis, Norman, ed. *Paston Letters and Papers of the Fifteenth Century*. Oxford: Early English Text Society, 2004.

De Ninno, Giuseppe. *Memorie storiche degli uomini illustri della città di Giovinazzo*. Bari: Pansini 1890.

De Tata, Rita. *All'insegna della Fenice: Vita di Ubaldo Zanetti speziale e antiquario bolognese (1698–1769)*. Bologna: Comune di Bologna, 2007.

De Toni, Giovan Battista. "Notizie bio-bibliografiche intorno Evangelista Quattrami semplicista degli Estensi." *Atti del reale Istituto Veneto di Scienze, Lettere ed Arti* 77 (1917–1918): 373–396.

De Vivo, Filippo. "La farmacia come luogo di cultura: Le spezierie di medicine in Italia." In *Interpretare e curare: Medicina e salute nel Rinascimento*, edited by Maria Conforti, Andrea Carlino, and Antonio Clericuzio. Rome: Carocci, 2013.

De Vivo, Filippo. "Pharmacies as Centres of Communication in Early Modern Venice." In *Spaces, Objects and Identities in Early Modern Italian Medicine*, edited by Sandra Cavallo and David Gentilcore. Oxford: Blackwell, 2008.

De Vos, Paula. *Compound Remedies: Galenic Pharmacy from the Ancient Mediterranean to New Spain*. Pittsburgh: University of Pittsburgh Press, 2020.

De Vos, Paula. "The 'Prince of Medicine': Yūḥannā Ibn Māsawayh and the Foundations of the Western Pharmaceutical Tradition." *Isis* 104, no. 4 (2013): 667–712.

De Vries, Jan. "Between Purchasing Power and the World of Goods: Understanding the Household Economy in Early Modern Europe." In *Consumption and the World of Goods*, edited by John Brewer and Roy Porter. London: Routledge, 1993.

Debru, Armelle, ed. *Galen on Pharmacology: Philosophy, History, and Medicine: Proceedings of the Vth International Galen Colloquium, Lille, 16–18 March 1995*. Leiden: Brill, 1997.

Debus, Allen G. *The French Paracelsians: The Chemical Challenge to Medical and Scientific Tradition in Early Modern France*. Cambridge: Cambridge University Press, 1991.

Del Panta, Lorenzo. *Le epidemie nella storia demografica italiana (secoli XIV–XIX)*. Turin: Loescher, revised edition 2021 (first edition 1980).

DeLancey, Julia. "Dragonblood and Ultramarine: The Apothecary and Artist Pigments in Renaissance Florence." In *The Art Market in Italy: 15th–17th Centuries*, edited by Marcello Fantoni, Louisa C. Matthew, and Sara F. Matthews Grieco. Modena: F. C. Panini, 2003.

Della Peruta, Franco, "Infanzia e famiglia nella prima metà dell'Ottocento." *Studi Storici* 20, no. 3 (1979): 473–491.

Delumeau, Jean. *La peur en Occident, XIVe–XVIIIe siècles: Une cité assiégée*. Paris: Fayard, 1978.

Deputazione Veneta di Storia Patria. *L'Ufficio della Giustizia Vecchia a Venezia dalle origini sino al 1330*. Venice: A spese della Società, 1892.

Di Gennaro Splendore, Barbara. "Aldrovandi's *Farmaceptica*: Global Knowledge, Local Remedies." In *Global Aldrovandi: Exchanging Nature in the Early Modern World*, edited by Lia Markey and Davide Domenici. Leiden: Brill, forthcoming.

Di Gennaro Splendore, Barbara. "Craft, Money and Mercy: An Apothecary's Self-Portrait in Sixteenth-Century Bologna." *Annals of Science* 74, no. 2 (2017): 91–107.

Di Gennaro Splendore, Barbara. "Mediterranean Botany: Making Cross-Cultural Knowledge About Materia Medica in the Sixteenth Century." In *Plants in 16th and 17th Century: Botany between Medicine and Science*, edited by Fabrizio Baldassarri. Berlin: De Gruyter, 2023.

Di Gennaro Splendore, Barbara. "The Triumph of Theriac: Print, Apothecary Publications, and the Commodification of Ancient Antidotes (1497–1800)." *Nuncius* 36, no. 2 (2021): 431–470.

Dian, Girolamo. *Cenni storici sulla farmacia veneta al tempo della Repubblica*. Venice: Tip. Societa m. s. fra compositori tipografi, 1900–1908.

Dian, Girolamo. "Memoria sulle condizioni sugli statuti e sugli ordinamenti dei farmacisti sotto la repubblica Veneta." In *Atti del terzo congresso nazionale chimico-farmaceutico tenuto in Venezia dal 2 al 7 agosto 1891*. Rome: Tipografia M. Armanni, 1892.

Dingwall, Helen M. *Physicians, Surgeons and Apothecaries: Medicine in Seventeenth-Century Edinburgh*. East Linton: Tuckwell Press, 1995.

Dorner, Zachary. *Merchants of Medicines: The Commerce and Coercion of Health in Britain's Long Eighteenth Century*. Chicago: University of Chicago Press, 2020.

Dos Santos, Fernando Santiago. *As plantas brasileiras, os jesuítas e os indígenas do Brasil: História e ciência na Triaga Brasílica (séc. XVII–XVIII)*. São Paulo: Casa do Novo Autor, 2009.

Druett, Joan. *Rough Medicine: Surgeons at Sea in the Age of Sail*. New York: Routledge, 2000.

Eamon, William. *The Professor of Secrets: Mystery, Medicine and Alchemy in Renaissance Italy*. Washington, DC: National Geographic Society, 2010.

Eamon, William. *Science and the Secrets of Nature: Books of Secrets in Medieval and Early Modern Culture*. Princeton, NJ: Princeton University Press, 1994.

Eggleston, Edward. "Some Curious Colonial Remedies." *American Historical Review* 5, no. 2 (1899): 199–206.

Egmond, Florike. "Apothecaries as Experts and Brokers in the Sixteenth-Century Network of the Naturalist Carolus Clusius." *History of Universities* 23 (2008): 59–91.

Fairchilds, Cissie. "The Production and Marketing of Populuxe Goods in Eighteenth-Century Paris." In *Consumption and the World of Goods*, edited by John Brewer, Roy Porter, and William Andrews Clark Memorial Library. New York: Routledge, 1993.

Farolfi, Bernardino. "Società commerciale e società civile in una città di antico regime." In *Storia di Bologna*, vol. 3, edited by Adriano Prosperi. Bologna: Bononia University Press, 2005.

Fausti, Daniela. "Su alcune traduzioni cinquecentesche di Dioscoride: Da Ermolao Barbaro a Pietro Andrea Mattioli." In *Sulla tradizione indiretta dei testi medici greci: Le traduzioni: Atti del III seminario internazionale di Siena, Certosa di Pontignano, 2009*, edited by Ivan Garofalo, Alessandro Lami, and Amneris Roselli. Pisa: Serra Editore, 2010.

Favaro, Antonio. *Galileo Galilei e lo Studio di Padova*. Florence: Succ. Le Monnier, 1883.

Ferrari, Giovanna. "Public Anatomy Lessons and the Carnival: The Anatomy Theatre of Bologna." *Past & Present*, no. 117 (1987): 50–106.

Findlen, Paula. "Controlling the Experiment: Rhetoric, Court Patronage and the Experimental Method of Francesco Redi." *History of Science: An Annual Review of Literature, Research and Teaching* 31, no. 91 (1993): 35–64.

Findlen, Paula. "The Death of a Naturalist: Knowledge and Community in Late Renaissance Italy." In *Professors, Physicians and Practices in the History of Medicine: Essays in Honor of Nancy Siraisi, edited by Cynthia Klestinec and Gideon Manning. Cham: Springer, 2017.

Findlen, Paula. "Foreward: Aristotle in the Pharmacy: The Ambitions of Camilla Erculiani in Sixteenth-Century Padua." In Camilla Erculiani *Letters on Natural Philosophy: The Scientific Correspondence of a Sixteenth-Century Pharmacist, with Related Texts*, edited by Eleonora Carinci, translated by Hannah Marcus, with a foreword by Paula Findlen. New York: Iter Press, 2021.

Findlen, Paula. *Possessing Nature: Museums, Collecting, and Scientific Culture in Early Modern Italy*. Berkeley: University of California Press, 1994.

Findlen, Paula. "Why Put a Museum in a Book? Ferrante Imperato and the Image of Natural History in Sixteenth-Century Naples." *Journal of the History of Collections* 33, no. 3 (2021): 419–433.

First Historical Archive, ed. *Complete Translation of Imperially Rescripted Manchu Palace Memorials of the Kangxi Period*. Beijing: Zhongguo shehui kexue chubanshe, 1996.

Flahaut, Jean. "La thériaque Diatessaron: Oligopharmacie contre polypharmacie." *Revue d'histoire de la pharmacie* 97, no. 367 (2010): 295–300.

Flahaut, Jean. "La thériaque diatessaron ou thériaque des pauvres." *Revue d'histoire de la pharmacie* 86, no. 318 (1998): 173–182.

Foucault, Michel. *Power/Knowledge: Selected Interviews and Other Writings, 1972–1977*. Brighton, UK: Harvester Press, 1980.

Franchini, Dario A., ed. *La scienza a corte: Collezionismo eclettico, natura e immagine a Mantova fra Rinascimento e Manierismo*. Rome: Bulzoni, 1979.

French, Roger. *Medicine Before Science: The Rational and Learned Doctor from the Middle Ages to the Enlightenment*. Cambridge: Cambridge University Press, 2003.

Furner-Pardoe, Jessica, Blessing Anonye, Ricky Cain, John Moat, Catherine Otori, Christina Lee, et al. "Anti-Biofilm Efficacy of a Medieval Treatment for Bacterial Infection Requires the Combination of Multiple Ingredients." *Scientific Reports* 10, no. 12687. https://www.nature.com/articles/s41598-020-69273-8.

Gabriel, Joseph M. *Medical Monopoly: Intellectual Property Rights and the Origins of the Modern Pharmaceutical Industry*. Chicago: University of Chicago Press, 2014.

Galassi, Adriano. "Antonio Bertioli aromatario e speziale." *Civiltà Mantovana* 6 (1985): 53–57.

Galluzzi, Paolo. "Motivi paracelsiani nella Toscana di Cosimo II e di Don Antonio dei Medici: alchimia, medicina, 'chimica' e riforma del sapere." In *Scienze, credenze occulte, livelli di cultura*, edited by Giancarlo Garfagnini. Florence: Olschki, 1982.

García Ballester, Luis. *Galen and Galenism: Theory and Medical Practice from Antiquity to the European Renaissance*. Burlington, VT: Ashgate, 2002.

Gardi, Andrea. "Lineamenti della storia politica di Bologna." In *Storia di Bologna*, vol. 3.1, edited by Adriano Prosperi. Bologna: Bononia University Press, 2005.

Garello Alberto. "Sopra un vecchio campione di triaca conservato nell'ospedale Pammatone di Genova." *Atti Società Ligustica di Scienze e Lettere* 7 (1928): 283–294.

Gavitt, Philip. *Gender, Honor, and Charity in Late Renaissance Florence.* Cambridge: Cambridge University Press, 2011.

Gentilcore, David. "'All That Pertains to Medicine': Protomedici and Protomedicati in Early Modern Italy." *Medical History* 38, no. 2 (1994): 121–142.

Gentilcore, David. *Healers and Healing in Early Modern Italy: Social and Cultural Values in Early Modern Europe.* Manchester: Manchester University Press, 1998.

Gentilcore, David. "Il Regio Protomedicato nella Napoli Spagnola." *DYNAMIS Acta Hispanica ad Medicinae Scientiarumque Historiam Illustrandam* 16 (1996): 219–236.

Gentilcore, David. *Medical Charlatanism in Early Modern Italy.* Oxford: Oxford University Press, 2006.

Gentilcore, David, ed. "The World of the Italian Apothecary, 1400–1750." Special issue, *Pharmacy in History* 45, no. 3 (2003).

Gentz, Lauritz. "Theriaca." In *Festschrift zum 73 Geburtstag von E. Urban,* edited by G. E. Dann. Stuttgart: Verlag Dr. Roland Schmiedel, 1949.

Gestrich, Andreas. "The Social Order." In *The Oxford Handbook of Early Modern European History, 1350–1750,* vol. 1, *Peoples and Places,* edited by H. M. Scott. Oxford: Oxford University Press, 2015.

Ghobrial, John-Paul A. *The Whispers of Cities: Information Flows in Istanbul, London, and Paris in the Age of William Trumbull.* Oxford: Oxford University Press, 2013.

Gibbs, Frederick W. *Poison, Medicine, and Disease in Late Medieval and Early Modern Europe.* New York: Routledge, 2019.

Gibbs, Frederick W. "Specific Form and Poisonous Properties: Understanding Poison in the Fifteenth Century." *Preternature: Critical and Historical Studies on the Preternatural* 2, no. 1 (2013): 19–46.

Gillispie, Charles C. ed. *Complete Dictionary of Scientific Biography.* Detroit: Scribner's, 2008.

Ginzburg, Carlo. *Paura Reverenza Terrore.* Milan: Adelphi, 2015.

Giormani, Virgilio. "La farmacopea ufficiale della Serenissima nel 1790: Un libro sfortunato." *Atti e memorie dell'Accademia patavina di scienze lettere ed arti* 52, no. 2 (1989–1990): 95–119.

Gorman, Michael J. *The Scientific Counter-Revolution: The Jesuits and the Invention of Modern Science.* London: Bloomsbury Academic, 2020.

Grafton, Anthony, with April Shelford and Nancy Siraisi. *New World, Ancient Texts: The Power of Tradition and the Shock of Discovery.* Cambridge, MA: Belknap Press of Harvard University Press, 1995.

Grandi, Claudio. "La scienza medica e farmaceutica in accademia e a Mantova nel XVI secolo: Marcello Donati, Antonio Bertioli e i loro 'colleghi.'" In *Il mecenatismo accademico dei Gonzaga e la loro cultura antiquaria e umanistica nel Cinquecento,* edited by Paola Tosetti. Mantua: Accademia nazionale virgiliana di scienze, lettere e arti, 2016.

Grandi Venturi, Graziella. "I consulti di Giuseppe Azzoguidi e la medicina a Bologna nella prima metà del XVII secolo." *L'Archiginnasio* 82 (1987): 93–137.

Granel, François. "La thériaque de Montpellier." *Revue d'histoire de la pharmacie* 64, no. 229 (1976): 75–83.

Greene, Jeremy A. *Generic: The Unbranding of Modern Medicine*. Baltimore: Johns Hopkins University Press, 2014.

Grell, Ole Peter, Andrew Cunningham, and Jon Arrizabalaga, eds. *"It All Depends on the Dose": Poisons and Medicines in European History*. New York: Routledge, 2018.

Grendler, Paul F. *The University of Mantua, the Gonzaga and the Jesuits, 1584–1630*. Baltimore: Johns Hopkins University Press, 2009.

Griffin, Claire. *Mixing Medicines: The Global Drug Trade and Early Modern Russia*. Montreal: McGill-Queen's University Press; 2022.

Griffin, J. P. "Venetian Treacle and the Foundation of Medicines Regulations." *British Journal of Clinical Pharmacology* 58, no. 3 (2004): 317–325.

Guenzi, Alberto. *Pane e Fornai a Bologna in età moderna*. Venice: Marsilio Editori, 1982.

Halikowski-Smith, Stefan. "'The Physician's Hand': Trends in the Evolution of the Apothecary and His Art Across Europe over the Early Modem Period." *Nuncius* (2009): 101–125.

Hankinson, R. J., ed. *The Cambridge Companion to Galen*. Cambridge: Cambridge University Press, 2008.

Harkness, Deborah E. *The Jewel House: Elizabethan London and the Scientific Revolution*. New Haven, CT: Yale University Press, 2007.

Harley, David. "Medical Metaphors in English Moral Theology, 1560–1660." *Journal of the History of Medicine and Allied Sciences* 48 (1993): 396–435.

Hatcher, John, and Judy Z. Stephenson, eds. *Seven Centuries of Unreal Wages: The Unreliable Data, Sources and Methods That Have Been Used for Measuring Standards of Living in the Past*. New York: Palgrave Macmillan, 2018.

Hein, Wolfgang-Hagen. *Christus als Apotheker*. Frankfurt am Main: Govi, 1974.

Henderson, John. *Florence Under Siege: Surviving Plague in an Early Modern City*. New Haven, CT: Yale University Press, 2019.

Herlihy, David, and Christiane Klapisch-Zuber. *Les toscans et leurs familles: Une étude du catasto florentin de 1427*. Paris: Presses de la Fondation Nationale des Sciences Politiques, 1978.

Hine, Thomas. *Populuxe*. New York: Knopf, 1986.

Hobsbawm, Eric J., and T. O. Ranger, eds. *The Invention of Tradition*. Cambridge: Cambridge University Press, 1983.

Holste, Thomas. *Der Theriakkrämer: E. Beitr. zur Frühgeschichte D. Arzneimittelwerbung*. Pattensen: Wellm, 1976.

Holzmair, Eduard. *Katalog der Sammlung Dr. Josef Brettauer "Medicina in Nummis."* Vienna: 1937. Reprint, Vienna: Verlag der Österr. Akademie der Wissenschaften, 1989.

Ianiro, Erica. *Levante. Veneti e Ottomani nel XVIII secolo*. Venice: Marsilio, 2014.

Infelise, Mario. "L'utile e il piacevole: Alla ricerca dei lettori italiani del Secondo Settecento." In *Lo spazio del libro nell'Europa del XVIII secolo: Atti del Convegno di Ravenna 15–16 dicembre 1995,* edited by Maria Gioia Tavoni and Françoise Waquet. Bologna: Patron, 1997.

Jacquart, Danielle. "La thériaque dans l'Occident medieval latin." In *La Thériaque: Histoire d'un remède millénaire,* edited by Véronique Boudon-Millot and Françoise Micheau. Paris: Les Belles Lettres, 2020.

Jarcho, Saul ed. *Clinical Consultations and Letters by Ippolito Francesco Albertini, Francesco Torti and Other Physicians.* Boston: Countway Library, 1989.

Jardine Nicholas, James A. Secord, and Emma C. Spary, eds. *Cultures of Natural History.* Cambridge: Cambridge University Press, 1996.

Jenner, Mark S. R., and Patrick Wallis, eds. *Medicine and the Market in England and Its Colonies, c.1450–c.1850.* Basingstoke: Palgrave Macmillan, 2007.

Jones, Colin. "Plague and Its Metaphors in Early Modern France." *Representations,* no. 53 (1996): 97–127.

Jones, Colin, and Rebecca Sprang. "Sans-Culottes, sans Café, sans Tabac: Shifting Realms of Necessity and Luxury in Eighteenth-Century France." In *Consumers and Luxury: Consumer Culture in Europe, 1650–1850,* edited by Maxine Berg and Helen Clifford. New York: Manchester University Press, 1999.

Kadam, Snehal, with Vandana Madhusoodhanan, Anuradha Bandgar, and Karishma S. Kaushik. "From Treatise to Test: Evaluating Traditional Remedies for Anti-Biofilm Potential." *Frontiers in Pharmacology* 11 (2020).

Kafker, Frank A., and Serena L. Kafker. *The Encyclopedists as Individuals: A Biographical Dictionary of the Authors of the Encyclopédie.* Oxford: Voltaire Foundation, 1988.

Keller, Vera. "Accounting for Invention: Guido Pancirolli's Lost and Found Things and the Development of Desiderata." *Journal of the History of Ideas* 73, no. 2 (2012): 223–245.

Keller, Vera. "Storied Objects, Scientific Objects, and Renaissance Experiment: The Case of Malleable Glass." *Renaissance Quarterly* 70, no. 2 (2017): 594–632.

Kertzer, David I. *Ritual, Politics, and Power.* New Haven, CT: Yale University Press, 1988.

Kluge, Martin. "Das Theriak-Experiment." In *Materialwissen: Experimentelle Geschichte im Pharmaziemuseum,* edited by Barbara Orland and Byron Cole Dowse. Zurich: Intercom, 2022.

Knoefel, Peter K. "Abati's Work on the Amazing Nature of the Viper and Its Miraculous Powers." *Toxicon* 29, no. 3 (1991): 301–309.

Knoefel, Peter K. *Francesco Redi on Vipers.* Leiden, 1988.

Knoefel, Peter K., and Madeline C. Covi. *A Hellenistic Treatise on Poisonous Animals (the "Theriaca" of Nicander of Colophon): A Contribution to the History of Toxicology.* Lewiston: E. Mellen Press, 1991.

Kostylo, Joanna. "Pharmacy as a Centre for Protestant Reform in Renaissance Venice." *Renaissance Studies* 30, no. 2 (2016): 236–253.

Krafft, Fritz, and Beiträgen von Christa. *Christus ruft in die Himmelsapotheke: Die Verbildlichung des Heilandsrufs durch Christus als Apotheker: Begleitbuch und Katalog zur Ausstellung im Museum Altomunster.* Stuttgart: Wissenschaftliche, 2002.

Krumholz McDonald, Diana. "The Serpent as Healer: Theriac and the Ancient near Eastern Pottery." *Notes in the History of Art* 13, no. 4 (1994): 21–27.

Küçük, Harun K. *Science Without Leisure: Practical Naturalism in Istanbul, 1660–1732.* Pittsburgh: University of Pittsburgh Press, 2019.

Lafont, Olivier. "Les thériaques dans les ouvrages charitables aux XVIIe et XVIIIe siècles." *Revue d'histoire de la pharmacie* 97, no. 367 (2010): 311–318.

Landouzy, Louis. "Préface." In *Codex medicamentarius gallicus: Pharmacopée française, rédigée par ordre du Gouvernement.* Paris, 1908.

Lane, Frederic. *Venice: A Maritime Republic.* Baltimore: Johns Hopkins University Press, 1973.

Laughran, Michelle A. "Medicating With or Without 'Scruples': The Professionalization of the Apothecary in Sixteenth-Century Venice." *Pharmacy in History* 45, no. 3 (2003): 95–107.

Lavallée, Hue Lafont. "Appréciation de l'évolution du prix des médicaments à Rouen de 1640 à 1788." *Annales pharmaceutiques françaises* 51, no. 1 (1993): 1–7.

Ledermann, Francois. "Le prix des médicaments à Rome: Économie et pharmacie de 1700 à 1870." *Medicina nei secoli* (1999): 117–133.

Ledermann, Francois. "Les taxes de médicaments de Rome et de l'État Pontifical: Une histoire complexe et presque immobile." *Bulletin Cercle Benelux d'Histoire de la Pharmacie*, no. 98 (2000): 52–61.

Leigh, Robert. *On Theriac to Piso, Attributed to Galen: A Critical Edition with Translation and Commentary.* Leiden: Brill, 2015.

Leiser, Gary, and Michael Dols. "Evliyā Chelebi's Description of Medicine in Seventeenth-Century Egypt: Part I: Introduction." *Sudhoffs Archiv* 71, no. 2 (1987): 197–216.

Leiser, Gary, and Michael Dols. "Evliyā Chelebi's Description of Medicine in Seventeenth-Century Egypt: Part II: Text." *Sudhoffs Archiv* 72, no. 1 (1988): 49–68.

Leite, Serafim. *Artes e ofícios dos Jesuítas no Brasil, 1549–1760.* Lisbon: Edições Brotéria, 1953.

Leong, Elaine. *Recipes and Everyday Knowledge: Medicine, Science, and the Household in Early Modern England.* Chicago: University of Chicago Press, 2019.

Leong, Elaine, and Alisha Rankin, eds. *Secrets and Knowledge in Medicine and Science, 1500–1800.* Burlington, VT: Ashgate, 2011.

Lindemann, Mary. *Medicine and Society in Early Modern Europe.* 2nd ed. Cambridge: Cambridge University Press, 2010.

"Literary Notes." *British Medical Journal* 2, no. 2120 (1901).

Maehle, Andreas-Holger. *Drugs on Trial: Experimental Pharmacology and Therapeutic Innovation in the Eighteenth Century.* Amsterdam: Rodopi, 1999.

Maggioni, Giuseppe. "La teriaca 'farmaco di Stato' e le sue forme di pubblicità presso i farmacisti veneti." *Estratto da Atti e memorie dell'Accademia italiana di storia della farmacia: La Farmacia Nuova* 36, no. 1 (1980).

Mancini, Gabriella, ed. *L'Officina profumo-farmaceutica di Santa Maria Novella in Firenze*. Florence: Chitarrini, 1994.

Mani, Nikolaus. "Die griechischte Editio princeps des Galenos (1525), ihre Entstehung und ihre Wirkung." *Gesnerus: Swiss Journal of the History of Medicines and Sciences* 13 (1956): 29–52.

Manzi, Leonello. "Un maestro dello studio bolognese tra umanesimo e rinascimento: G. B. Teodosio." *Bullettino delle scienze mediche, organo della Società medica chirurgica di Bologna* (1965): 144–170.

Martelli, Matteo, Caroline Petit, and Lucia Raggetti, eds. "Galen's Treatise on Simple Drugs: Interpretation and Transmission." *Archives internationales d'histoire des sciences* 70, no. 184–185 (2020): 1–328.

Martin, Colin. "De theriaca." *Nouvelles pages d'histoire Vaudoise* 15 (1967): 117–129.

Mastroianni, Emanuele O. *Il Reale Istituto d'incoraggiamento di Napoli, MDCCCVI–MCMVI*. Naples: L. Pierro, 1907.

Mattoli, Luisa, Anna Gaetano, Michela Burico, et al. "Mass Spectrometry Studies of an Ancient Sample of Theriac from the Spezieria di Santa Maria della Scala in Rome." In *Drugs, Colors and Aromatics: Tradition and Innovation in the Materia Medica of Italian Baroque: Studies from the Spezieria of Santa Maria della Scala*, edited by Vázquez de Ágredos-Pascual, María Luisa, Cavallo Giovanni, and Rita Pagiotti. Sansepolcro: Aboca Museum, 2021.

Mayor, Adrienne. *The Poison King: The Life and Legend of Mithradates the Great, Rome's Deadliest Enemy*. Princeton, NJ: Princeton University Press, 2010.

McGowan, Bruce. "The Age of Ayans, 1699–1812." In *An Economic and Social History of the Ottoman Empire*, edited by Halil İnalcık and Donald Quataert. Cambridge: Cambridge University Press, 1994.

McVaugh, Michael R. "Chemical Medicine in the Medical Writings of Arnau de Vilanova." In *Actes de la "Il Trobada Internacional d'Estudis sobre Arnau de Vilanova,"* edited by Josep Perarnau. Barcelona: Institut d'Estudis Catalans, 2005.

McVaugh, Michael R. *Medicine Before the Plague: Practitioners and Their Patients in the Crown of Aragon, 1285–1345*. Cambridge: Cambridge University Press, 1993.

McVaugh, Michael R. "Theriac at Montpellier." *Sudhoffs Archiv* 56 (1972): 113–144.

Medici, Michele. *Le accademie scientifiche e letterarie della città di Bologna*. Bologna: Sassi nelle Spaderie, 1852.

Melella, Patrizia. "La spezieria dell'Arciospedale di S. Spirito in Sassia di Roma nei secoli XVI e XVII." In *Gli archivi per la storia della scienza e della tecnica: Atti del Convegno internazionale Desenzano del Garda, 4–8 giugno 1991*, edited by G. Paoloni. Rome: Ministero per i beni culturali e ambientali, 1995.

Mendelsohn, J. Andrew, Annemarie Kinzelbach, and Ruth Schilling, eds. *Civic Medicine: Physician, Polity, and Pen in Early Modern Europe*. New York: Routledge, 2020.
Meneghini, Gino. *La farmacia attraverso i secoli e gli speziali di Venezia e Padova*. Padua: Istituto veneto di arti grafiche, 1946.
Micca, G. "The 'De Theriaca e del Mithridato' of Bartolomeo Maranta." *Minerva Medica* 61, no. 15 (1970): 705-715.
Milwright, Marcus. "Balsam in the Mediaeval Mediterranean: A Case Study of Information and Commodity Exchange." *Journal of Mediterranean Archaeology* 14, no. 1 (2001): 3-23.
Milwright, Marcus. "The Balsam of Matariyya: An Exploration of a Medieval Panacea." *Bulletin of the School of Oriental and African Studies* 66, no. 2 (2003): 193-209.
Minard, Philippe. *La fortune du colbertisme: État et industrie dans la France des Lumières*. Paris: Fayard, 1998.
Minuzzi, Sabrina, ed. "Printing Medical Knowledge: Vernacular Genres, Reception and Dissemination." Special issue, *Nuncius* 36, no. 2 (2021).
Minuzzi, Sabrina. *Sul filo dei segreti: Farmacopea, libri e pratiche terapeutiche a Venezia in età moderna*. Milan: Unicopli, 2016.
Mongelli, Nicola. "Diffusione di un medicamento popolare nel Regno di Napoli: La teriaca di Andromaco." *Lares* 42, no. 3-4 (1976): 308-344.
Moran, Bruce T. *Chemical Pharmacy Enters the University: Johannes Hartmann and the Didactic Care of Chymiatria in the Early Seventeenth Century*. Madison, WI: American Institute for the History of Pharmacy, 1991.
Moran, Bruce T. "A Survey of Chemical Medicine in the 17th Century: Spanning Court, Classroom, and Cultures." *Pharmacy in History* 38, no. 3 (1996): 121-133.
Mozzato, Andrea. "Oppio, triaca e altre spezie officinali a Venezia nella seconda metà del Quattrocento." In *Venice and the Veneto During the Renaissance: The Legacy of Benjamin Kohl*, edited by Michael Knapton, John E. Law, and Alison A. Smith. Florence: Firenze University Press, 2014.
Mozzato, Andrea. "Uno speziale aretino a Venezia nel secondo Quattrocento." *Annali Aretini* 15/16 (2009): 117-148.
Murphy, Hannah. *A New Order of Medicine: The Rise of Physicians in Reformation Nuremberg*. Pittsburgh: University of Pittsburgh Press, 2019.
Musatti, Cesare. *La teriaca e il mitridato nel 1532 in Venezia*. Venice: Stab. tip. lit. M. Fontana, 1836.
Musi, Aurelio. "Medicina e sapere medico a Salerno in età moderna." In *Salerno e la sua Scuola Medica*, edited by Italo Gallo. Naples: Guida, 1994.
Naphy, William G. *Plagues, Poisons, and Potions: Plague-Spreading Conspiracies in the Western Alps, c. 1530-1640*. Manchester: Manchester University Press, 2002.
Naphy, William G., and Penny Roberts, eds. *Fear in Early Modern Society*. Manchester: Manchester University Press, 1997.

Nappi, Carla. "Bolatu's Pharmacy Theriac in Early Modern China." *Early Science and Medicine* 14 (2009): 737–764.

Newson, Linda A. *Making Medicines in Early Colonial Lima, Peru: Apothecaries, Science and Society*. Leiden: Brill, 2017.

Nockels Fabbri, Christiane. "Treating Medieval Plague: The Wonderful Virtues of Theriac." *Early Science and Medicine* 12 (2007): 247–283.

Nussdorfer, Laurie. "Print and Pageantry in Baroque Rome." *Sixteenth Century Journal* 29, no. 2 (1998): 439–464.

Nutton, Vivian. "Greek Science in Sixteenth-Century Renaissance." In *Renaissance and Revolution: Humanists, Scholars, Craftsmen and Natural Philosophers in Early Modern Europe* edited by Judith V. Fields and Frank A. J. L. James. Cambridge: Cambridge University Press, 1993.

Ogilvie, Brian W. *The Science of Describing: Natural History in Renaissance Europe*. Chicago: University of Chicago Press, 2006.

Olmi, Giuseppe. "Farmacopea antica e medicina moderna." *Physis* 19 (1977): 197–246.

Olshin, Benjamin B. *Lost Knowledge: The Concept of Vanished Technologies and Other Human Histories*. Leiden: Brill, 2019.

Ongaro, Giuseppe, and Elda Martellozzo Fiorin. "Girolamo Mercuriale e lo studio di Padova." In *Girolamo Mercuriale: Medicina e cultura nell'Europa del Cinquecento: Atti del convegno "Girolamo Mercuriale e lo spazio scientifico e culturale del Cinquecento Forlì, 8–11 Novembre 2006*, edited by Alessandro Arcangeli and Vivian Nutton. Florence: Olschki, 2008.

Oszajca, Paulina. "Trocisci viperini nelle preparazioni teriacali." *Rivista di storia della farmacia atti e memorie* 10 (2018): 111–120.

Oszajca, Paulina, and Zbigniew Bela. "Granting a Licence for Opening a Pharmacy in Bologna During Activity of the Bolognese Arte de' speziali (13th–18th Century)." *Medicina nei secoli* 27, no. 1 (2015): 215–240.

Overduin, Floris. "The Anti-Bucolic World of Nicander's *Theriaca*." *Classical Quarterly* 64, no. 2 (2014): 623–641.

Pagano, Matheo, and Guillaume Postel. *The True Description of Cairo: A Sixteenth-Century Venetian View*. Edited and translated by Nicholas Warner. Oxford: New York: Oxford University Press, 2006.

Palmer, Richard. "Girolamo Mercuriale and the Plague of Venice." In *Girolamo Mercuriale: Medicina e cultura nell'Europa del Cinquecento: Atti del convegno "Girolamo Mercuriale e lo spazio scientifico e culturale del Cinquecento Forlì, 8–11 Novembre 2006*, edited by Alessandro Arcangeli and Vivian Nutton. Florence: Olschki, 2008.

Palmer, Richard. "In Bad Odour: Smell and Its Significance in Medicine from the Antiquity to the Seventeenth Century." In *Medicine and the Five Senses*, edited by W. F. Bynum and Roy Porter. Cambridge: Cambridge University Press, 1993.

Palmer, Richard. "La Gran Moría." *Kos* 2, no. 18 (1985): 17–48.

Palmer, Richard. "Medical Botany in Northern Italy in the Renaissance." *Journal of the Royal Society of Medicine* 78, no. 2 (1985): 149–157.

Palmer, Richard. "Pharmacy in the Republic of Venice in the Sixteenth century." In *The Medical Renaissance of the Sixteenth Century*, edited by Andrew Wear, R. K. French, and Iain M. Lonie. Cambridge: Cambridge University Press, 1985.

Palmer, Richard. "Physicians and the State in Post Medieval Italy." In *The Town and State Physician in Europe from the Middle Ages to the Enlightenment*, edited by Andrew Wear and Society for the Social History of Medicine. Wolfenbüttel: Herzog August Bibliothek, 1981.

Palmer, Richard. *The Studio of Venice and Its Graduates in the Sixteenth Century*. Trieste: Lint, 1983.

Pancino, Claudia. "Malati, medici, mammane, saltimbanchi. Malattia e cura nella Bologna d'età moderna." In *Storia di Bologna*, vol. 3.2, edited by Adriano Prosperi. Bologna: Bononia University Press, 2005.

Paracelsus. *Paracelsus (Theophrastus Bombastus von Hohenheim, 1493–1541): Essential Theoretical Writings*. Edited and translated by Andrew Weeks. Leiden: Brill, 2008.

Park, Katharine. "Country Medicine in the City Marketplace: Snakehandlers as Itinerant Healers." *Renaissance Studies* 15 (2001): 104–120.

Park, Katharine. *Doctors and Medicine in Early Renaissance Florence*. Princeton, NJ: Princeton University Press, 1985.

Pastore, Alessandro. "Poisoning as Politics." In *"It All Depends on the Dose": Poisons and Medicines in European History*, edited by Ole Peter Grell, Andrew Cunningham, and Jon Arrizabalaga. New York: Routledge, 2018.

Pastore, Alessandro. *Veleno: Credenze, crimini, saperi nell'Italia moderna*. Bologna: Il Mulino, 2010.

Pazzini, Adalberto. *La triaca in Roma: Brevi notizie sulla vita della farmacia romana*. Rome: Tip. del Senato, G. Bardi, 1933.

Pellegrini, Paolo. "Lonigo, Niccolò da" DBI 78 (2013): 409–414. https://www.treccani.it/enciclopedia/niccolo-da-lonigo_%28Dizionario-Biografico%29/.

Pelling, Margaret, and Frances White. *Medical Conflicts in Early Modern London: Patronage, Physicians, and Irregular Practitioners, 1550–1640*. Oxford: Oxford University Press, 2003.

Pereira, N. A., R. J. Jaccoud, and W. B. Mors. "Triaga Brasilica: Renewed Interest in a Seventeenth-Century Panacea." *Toxicon: Official Journal of the International Society on Toxinology* 34, no. 5 (1996): 311–316.

Peters, Hermann. *Aus Pharmazeutischer Vorzeit in Bild und Wort*. Berlin: J. Springer, 1886.

Pezzolo, Luciano. "The Venetian Economy." In *Companion to Venetian History, 1400–1797*, edited by Eric R. Dursteler. Leiden: Brill 2013.

Piccinini, Guido Maria, Ludovico Sorrentino, and Massimo Di Rosa. *Una ulteriore luce, storica e sperimentale, su la Teriaca: Con 41 figure di documentazione storica e sperimentale.* Naples: Genovese, 1962.

Piccinno, Lucia. "Speziali." In *Atlante delle Professioni,* edited by Maria Malatesta. Bologna: Bononia University Press, 2009.

Pomata, Gianna. *Contracting a Cure: Patients, Healers, and the Law in Early Modern Bologna.* Baltimore: Johns Hopkins University Press, 1998.

Pomata, Gianna. "Malpighi and the Holy Body: Medical Experts and Miraculous Evidence in Seventeenth-Century Italy." *Renaissance Studies* 21, no. 4 (2007): 568–586.

Pomata, Gianna. "Practicing Between Heaven and Earth: Women Healers in Seventeenth-Century Bologna." *Dynamis* 19 (1999), 119–143.

Pomata, Gianna. "The Recipe and the Case: Epistemic Genres and the Dynamics of Cognitive Practices." In *Wissenschaftsgeschichte und Geschichte des Wissens im Dialog/Connecting Science and Knowledge,* edited by Kaspar von Greyerz, Silvia Flubacher, and Philipp Senn. Göttingen: Vanderhoeck und Ruprecht, 2013.

Preto, Paolo. *Peste e società a Venezia.* Vicenza: Neri Pozza, 1978.

Prodi, Paolo. *Il cardinale Gabriele Paleotti (1522–1597).* Rome: Edizioni di storia e letteratura, 1959.

Puente-Ballestreros, Beatriz. "Antoine Thomas Si as a 'Patient' of the Kangxi Emperor (r. 1662–1722): A Case Study on the Appropriation of Theriac at the Imperial Court." *Asclepio* 64, no. 1 (2012): 213–250.

Pugliano, Valentina. "Botanical Artisans: Apothecaries and the Study of Nature in Venice and London, 1550–1610." PhD dissertation, Oxford University, 2012.

Pugliano, Valentina. "Natural History in the Apothecary Shop." In *Worlds of Natural History,* edited by Helen A. Curry, Nicholas Jardine, James A. Secord, and Emma C. Spary. Cambridge: Cambridge University Press, 2018.

Pugliano, Valentina. "Pharmacy, Testing, and the Language of Truth in Renaissance Italy." *Bulletin of the History of Medicine* 91, no. 2 (2017): 233–273.

Pullan, Brian S. *Crisis and Change in the Venetian Economy in the Sixteenth and Seventeenth Centuries.* London: Methuen, 1968.

Pullan, Brian S. "Wage-Earners and the Venetian Economy, 1530–1630." *Economic History Review* 16, no. 3 (1964): 407–426.

Radici, Livia. *Nicandro di Colofone nei secoli XVI–XVIII: Edizioni, traduzioni, commenti.* Pisa: F. Serra, 2012.

Raj, Danuta, Katarzyna Pękacka-Falkowska, Maciej Włodarczyk, and Jakub Węglorz. "The Real Theriac: Panacea, Poisonous Drug or Quackery?" *Journal of Ethnopharmacology* 281 (2021): 114535.

Rambaldi, Susanna Peyronel. *Speranze e crisi nel Cinquecento modenese: Tensioni religiose e vita cittadina ai tempi di Giovanni Morone.* Milan: F. Angeli, 1979.

Rankin, Alisha. "On Anecdote and Antidotes: Poison Trials in Sixteenth-Century Europe." *Bulletin of the History of Medicine* 91, no. 2 (2017): 274–302.

Rankin, Alisha. *The Poison Trials.* Chicago: University of Chicago Press, 2020.

Redmond, Linda Colleen. "Girolamo Donzellino, Medical Science and Protestantism in the Veneto." PhD dissertation, Stanford University, 1984.

Reeds, Karen. *Botany in Medieval and Renaissance Universities.* New York: Garland, 1991.

Reinhard, Wolfgang, and European Science Foundation, eds. *Power Elites and State Building.* Oxford; Oxford University Press, 1996.

Renehan, Robert. "An Eighteenth-Century Carved Piece with Medical Associations." *Journal of the Warburg and Courtauld Institutes* 26, no. 3-4 (1963): 361-363.

Renzi, Salvatore de. *Storia della medicina in Italia.* Naples: Filiatre-Sebezio, 1845.

Ricordel, Joëlle. "Ibn Djuljul: Propos sur la thériaque." *Revue d'histoire de la pharmacie* 88, no. 325 (2000): 157-166.

Ricordel, Joëlle. "Le traité sur la thériaque d'Ibn Rushd (Averroes)." *Revue d'histoire de la pharmacie* 88, no. 325 (2000): 81-90.

Ricordel, Joëlle. "Variations sur le thème de la Grande thériaque dans la tradition arabe." In *La Thériaque: Histoire d'un remède millénaire,* edited by Véronique Boudon-Millot and Françoise Micheau. Paris: Les Belles Lettres, 2020.

Ricordel, Joëlle, and Jean-Marc Bonmatin. "Les vertus du miel dans les thériaques selon les médecins arabo-musulmans (IXe-XIIIe s.)." *Revue d'histoire de la pharmacie* 91, no. 337 (2003): 21-28.

Roberts, Carolyn. "To Heal and to Harm: Medicine, Knowledge, and Power in the Atlantic Slave Trade." PhD diss. Harvard University, 2017.

Roberts, Lissa. "The Death of the Sensuous Chemist: The 'New' Chemistry and the Transformation of the Sensuous Technology." In *Empire of the Senses: The Sensual Culture Reader,* edited by David Howe. Oxford: Berg, 2005.

Rosa, Edoardo. "La panacea dell'antichità approda all'Archiginnasio." In *L'Archiginnasio: Il Palazzo, l'Università, la Biblioteca,* vol. 1, edited by Giovanni Roversi. Bologna: Credito Romagnolo, 1987.

Rosa, Edoardo. "La teriaca a Bologna fra scienza e incredulità secoli XVI-XVIII." *Il Carrobbio* 10 (1984): 257-273.

Rosa, Edoardo. "Medicina e salute pubblica a Bologna nel Sei e Settecento." *Quaderni Culturali Bolognesi* 2, no. 8 (1978): 1-49.

Rosenberg, Charles E. "The Therapeutic Revolution: Medicine, Meaning, and Social Change in Nineteenth-Century America." In *The Therapeutic Revolution: Essays in the Social History of American Medicine,* edited by Morris J. Vogel and Charles E. Rosenberg. Philadelphia: University of Pennsylvania Press, 1979.

Rossi, Ettore. "La Sultana Nūr Bānū (Cecilia Venier-Baffo) moglie di Selīm II (1566-1574) e madre di Murād III (1574-1595)." *Oriente Moderno* 33, no. 11 (1953): 433-441.

Rota Ghibaudi, Silvia. *Ricerche su Ludovico Settala: Biografia, bibliografia, iconografia e documenti.* Florence: Sansoni, 1959.

Rousseau, Nathalie. "Des Thériaques (Θηριακά) à 'la thériaque' (θηριακή): Formation et histoire du terme." In *La Thériaque: Histoire d'un remède millénaire*, edited by Véronique Boudon-Millot and Françoise Micheau. Paris: Les Belles Lettres, 2020.

Roy, Bruno. "La trente-sixieme main: Vincent de Beauvais et Thomas de Cantimpré." In *Vincent de Beauvais: Intentions et réceptions d'une œuvre encyclopédique au Moyen-Age: Actes du XIVe colloque de l'Institut d'études médiévales*, edited by Monique Paulmier-Foucart, Serge Lusignan, and Alain Nadeau. Paris: Bellarmin, 1990.

Rubin, Jonathan. "The Use of the 'Jericho Tyrus' in Theriac: A Case Study in the History of the Exchanges of Medical Knowledge Between Western Europe and the Realm of Islam in the Middle Ages." *Medium Aevum* 2, no. 83 (2014): 234–253.

Russo, Andrea. "Contributo alla storia della farmacia attraverso l'archivio di Napoli." In *Estratto dagli Atti del IV Convegno di Studi AISF Varese 3–4 Ottobre 1959*. Pisa: Arti Grafiche Pacini Mariotti, 1961.

Russo, Andrea. *L'arte degli speziali in Napoli*. Naples: Arte Tipografica, 1969.

Sabbatani, Luigi. "Di un trattato del Maranta attribuito al Ghini." *Archeion* 6, no. 3 (1925): 235–241.

Saggi scientifici e letterari dell'Accademia di scienze, lettere ed arti di Padova. Vol. 5. Padua: a spese dell'Accademia, 1840.

Salzberg, Rosa. *Ephemeral City: Cheap Print and Urban Culture in Renaissance Venice*. Manchester: Manchester University Press, 2014.

Scalone, Francesco. "Sulle relazioni tra variabili demografiche ed economiche in Emilia Romagna durante i secoli XVII–XVIII." In *Prezzi, Redditi, popolazioni in Italia: 600 anni (dal secolo XIV al secolo XX)*, edited by Marco Breschi, Paolo Malanima, and Società italiana di demografia storica. Udine: Forum, 2002.

Scarborough, John. "Nicander's Toxicology II: Spiders, Scorpions, Insects and Myriapods." *Pharmacy in History* 21, no. 1 (1979): 3–34.

Scarborough, John. "The Opium Poppy in Hellenistic and Roman Medicine." In *Drugs and Narcotics in History*, edited by Roy Porter and Teich Mikula. Cambridge: Cambridge University Press, 1995.

Schafer, Edward H. *The Golden Peaches of Samarkand: A Study of T'ang Exotics*. Berkeley: University of California Press, 1963.

Schickore, Jutta. *About Method: Experimenters, Snake Venom, and the History of Writing Scientifically*. Chicago: University of Chicago Press, 2017.

Schickore, Jutta. "Trying Again and Again: Multiple Repetitions in Early Modern Reports of Experiments on Snake Bites." *Early Science and Medicine* 15, no. 6 (2010): 567–617.

Schiebinger, Londa. *Plants and Empire: Colonial Bioprospecting in the Atlantic World*. Cambridge, MA: Harvard University Press, 2007.

Schiebinger, Londa, and Claudia Swan, eds. *Colonial Botany: Science, Commerce, and Politics in the Early Modern World*. Philadelphia: University of Pennsylvania Press, 2005.

Schumpeter, Elizabeth Boody, and T. S. Ashton. *English Overseas Trade Statistics, 1697–1808*. London: Clarendon Press, 1960.

Sensi, Mario. "Cerretani e ciarlatani nel secolo XV: Spigolature d'archivio." *Medicina nei secoli* 15 (1978): 69-91.

Sforza, Giovanni. *F. M. Fiorentini ed i suoi contemporanei lucchesi: Saggio di storia letteraria del secolo XVII*. Florence: F. Menozzi, 1879.

Shapin, Steven. "The Sciences of Subjectivity." *Social Studies of Science* 42, no. 2 (2012): 170-184.

Shapin, Steven. "The Tastes of Wine: Towards a Cultural History." *Rivista di estetica*, no. 51 (2012): 49-94.

Shaw, James, and Evelyn Welch. *Making and Marketing Medicine in Renaissance Florence*. Amsterdam: Rodopi, 2011.

Shay, Mary Lucille. *The Ottoman Empire from 1720 to 1734 as Revealed in Despatches of the Venetian Baili*. Urbana: University of Illinois Press, 1944.

Silini, Giovanni. *Umori e farmaci: Terapia medica tardo-medievale*. Gandino: Servitium, 2001.

Siraisi, Nancy. *Avicenna in Renaissance Italy: The Canon and Medical Teaching in Italian Universities after 1500*. Princeton, NJ: Princeton University Press, 1987.

Sismondo, Sergio, and Jeremy A. Greene, eds. *The Pharmaceutical Studies Reader*. New York: Wiley, 2015.

Skinner, Quentin. *The Foundations of Modern Political Thought*. Cambridge: Cambridge University Press, 1978.

Smith, Pamela H. *The Body of the Artisan: Art and Experience in the Scientific Revolution*. Chicago: University of Chicago Press, 2004.

Smith, Pamela H. *From Lived Experience to the Written Word: Reconstructing Practical Knowledge in the Early Modern World*. Chicago: University of Chicago Press, 2022.

Smith, Pamela H., and Paula Findlen, eds. *Merchants and Marvels: Commerce, Science and Art in Early Modern Europe*. New York: Routledge, 2002.

Soll, Jacob. "Healing the Body Politic: French Royal Doctors, History, and the Birth of a Nation, 1560-1634." *Renaissance Quarterly* 55, no. 4 (2002): 1259-1286.

Sonnedecker, Glenn. "Harward's 'Electuarium...': Earliest Drug Treatise Published by an American Colonist?" *Pharmacy in History* 19, no. 1 (1977): 24-38.

Spada, Niccolò. *Una mostra di triaca a Venezia*. Rome: Istituto nazionale medico farmacologico Serono, 1934.

Stannard, Jerry, Richard Kay, and Katherine E. Stannard. *Herbs and Herbalism in the Middle Ages and Renaissance*. Aldershot: Ashgate, 1999.

Stein, Michael. "La Theriaque chez Galen: Sa préparation et son usage thérapeutique." In *Galen on Pharmacology: Philosophy, History, and Medicine: Proceedings of the 5th International Galen Colloquium, Lille, 16–18 March 1995*, edited by Armelle Debru. Leiden: Brill, 1997.

Stendardo, Enrica. *Ferrante Imperato: Collezionismo e studio della natura a Napoli tra Cinque e Seicento*. Naples: Accademia Pontaniana, 2001.

Stieb, E. W. "Drug Adulteration and Its Detection, in the Writings of Theophrastus, Dioscorides, and Pliny." *Journal mondial de pharmacie* (1938): 117–134.

Stossl, Marianne. *Lo spettacolo della triaca, produzione e promozione di una "Droga Divina" a Venezia dal Cinque al Settecento.* Venice: Centro Tedesco di Studi Veneziani, 1983.

Strocchia, Sharon T. *Forgotten Healers: Women and the Pursuit of Health in Late Renaissance Italy.* Cambridge, MA: Harvard University Press, 2019.

Strocchia, Sharon T. "The Nun Apothecaries of Renaissance Florence: Marketing Medicines in the Convent." *Renaissance Studies* 25, no. 5 (2011): 627–647.

Strocchia, Sharon T. *Nuns and Nunneries in Renaissance Florence.* Baltimore: Johns Hopkins University Press, 2009.

Tekiner, Halil, and Afife Mat. "Les thériaques dan la litterature turque." *Turkish Studies: International Periodical for the Languages, Literature and History of Turkish or Turkic* 9, no. 7 (2014): 517–524.

Temkin, Owsei. *Galenism; Rise and Decline of a Medical Philosophy.* Ithaca, NY: Cornell University Press, 1973.

Tergolina-Gislanzoni-Brasco, Umberto. "Francesco Calzolari speziale veronese." *Bollttino storico italiano dell'arte sanitaria* 33, f. 6 (1934): 3–20.

Terpstra, Nicholas. *Cultures of Charity: Women, Politics, and the Reform of Poor Relief in Renaissance Italy.* Cambridge, MA: Harvard University Press, 2013.

Terpstra, Nicholas. *Lay Confraternities and Civic Religion in Renaissance Bologna.* Cambridge: Cambridge University Press, 1995.

Terrusi, Leonardo. "Guittone, la triaca e il veneno: Per la storia di un antico tema letterario." In *Studi in onore di Michele Dell'Aquila*, vol. 1. Pisa: Istituti Editoriali e Poligrafici Internazionali, 2002.

Terrusi, Leonardo. *"Secondo che Galieno pone": Testi e temi extraletterari da Guittone a Boccaccio al Casa.* Padua: Libreriauniversitaria.it, 2019.

Tognetti, Sergio. "Prezzi e salari a Firenze nel tardo medioevo: Un profilo." *Archivio storico italiano* 153, no. 2 (1995): 263–333.

Totelin, Laurance. "Mithradates' Antidote: A Pharmacological Ghost." *Early Science and Medicine* 9, no.1 (2004): 1–19.

Totelin, Laurance. "Technologies of Knowledge." Oxford Handbooks Online, https://doi.org/10.1093/oxfordhb/9780199935390.013.94.

Touwaide, Alain. "Quid pro Quo: Revisiting the Practice of Substitution in Ancient Pharmacy." In *Herbs and Healers from the Ancient Mediterranean through the Medieval West*, edited by Anne van Arsdall and Timothy Graham. Burlington, VT: Ashgate, 2012.

Tribby, Jay. "Cooking (with) Clio and Cleo: Eloquence and Experiment in Seventeenth-Century Florence." *Journal of History of the Ideas* 52, no. 3 (1991): 417–439.

Trivellato, Francesca. *Fondamenta dei vetrai: Lavoro, tecnologia e mercato a Venezia tra sei e settecento.* Rome: Donzelli, 2000.

Trivellato, Francesca. "The Moral Economies of Early Modern Europe." *Humanity: An International Journal of Human Rights, Humanitarianism, and Development* 11, no. 2 (2020): 193–201.

Tugnoli Pattaro, Sandra. *Metodo e sistema delle scienze nel pensiero di Ulisse Aldrovandi.* Bologna: CLUEB, 1981.

Ulvioni, Paolo. *Il gran castigo di Dio: Carestia ed epidemie a Venezia e nella Terraferma, 1628–1632.* Milan: F. Angeli, 1989.

Uragoda, C. G., and K. D. Paranavitana. "Dutch Pharmacopoeia of 1757: Probably the Earliest such Document from Sri Lanka." *Journal of the Royal Asiatic Society of Sri Lanka,* n.s., vol. 51 (2005): 1–40.

Urdang, George. "The Development of Pharmacopoeias: A Review with Special Reference to the Pharmacopoea Internationalis." *Bulletin of the World Health Organization* 4, no. 4 (1951): 577–603.

Urdang, George. "How Chemicals Entered the Official Pharmacopoeias." *Archives internationales d'histoire des sciences* 28–29 (1954): 303–14.

Vallieri, Weiner. "Le 22 Lettere di Bartolomeo Maranta ad Aldrovandi." *Rivista di Storia della Medicina* 8 (1964): 197–229.

Van Zanden, Jan L. "Wages and the Standard of Living in Europe, 1500–1800." *European Review of Economic History,* no. 2 (1999): 175–197.

Vanzan Marchin, Nelli-Elena, ed. *Dalla scienza medica alla pratica dei corpi: Fonti e manoscritti marciani per la storia della sanità.* Vicenza: Neri Pozza, 1993.

Vanzan Marchin, Nelli-Elena. *I mali e i rimedi della Serenissima.* Vicenza: Neri Pozza, 1995.

Vanzan Marchin, Nelli-Elena. "Medici ebrei e assistenza cristiana nella Venezia del '500." *La rassegna mensile di Israel* 45, no. 4/5 (1979): 132–161.

Vedova, Giuseppe. *Biografia degli scrittori padovani.* Padua: Coi tipi della Minerva, 1831.

Viale, Matteo, Edoardo Demo, and Roberto Ricciuti. "Decomposing Economic Inequality in Early Modern Venice ca. 1650–1800." Historical Household Budgets Working Papers Series 12 (2018).

Vigo, Giovanni. "Real Wages of the Working Class in Italy: Building Workers' Wages (14th to 18th Century)." *Journal of European Economic History* 3 (1974): 378–399.

Vogt, Sabine. "Drugs and Pharmacology." In *The Cambridge Companion to Galen,* edited by R. J. Hankinson. Cambridge: Cambridge University Press, 2008.

Voinier, Sarah, and Guillaume Winter, eds. *Poison et antidote dans l'Europe des XVIe et XVIIe siècles.* Arras: Artois Presses Université, 2011.

Von Eschenbach, Wolfram. *Parzival.* Translated by A. S. Kline. https://www.poetryintranslation.com/eschenbachparzival.php.

Waldack, C. F. "Le Pere Philippe Couplet, Malinois, S.J., Missionnaire en Chine (1623–1694)." *Analectes pour servir à l'histoire ecclésiastique de la Belgique* 9 (1872).

Wallis, Patrick. "Consumption, Retailing, and Medicine in Early-Modern London." *Economic History Review* 61, no. 1 (2008): 26–53.

Wallis, Patrick. "Exotic Drugs and English Medicine: England's Drug Trade, c. 1550–c. 1800." *Social History of Medicine* 25, no. 1 (2012): 20–46.

Wallis, Patrick, and Catherine Wright Smith. "Evidence, Artisan Experience, and Authority in Early Modern England." In *Ways of Making and Knowing: The Material Culture of Empirical Knowledge*, edited by Pamela H. Smith, Amy R. W. Meyers, Harold J. Cook, and Peter N. Miller. Ann Arbor: University of Michigan Press, 2014.

Warner, John H. *The Therapeutic Perspective: Medical Practice, Knowledge, and Identity in America, 1820–1885.* Princeton, NJ: Princeton University Press, 1997.

Warolin, Christian. "Nicolas Houel and Michel Dusseau, Apothecaries of the XVIth Century in Paris." *Revue d'histoire de la pharmacie* 88, no. 327 (2000): 319–336.

Watanabe-O'Kelly, Helen. "'True and Historical Descriptions'? European Festivals and the Printed Record." In *The Dynastic Centre and the Provinces*, edited by Jeroen Duindam and Sabine Dabringhaus. Leiden: Brill, 2014.

Watson, Gilbert. *Theriac and Mithridatium: A Study in Therapeutics.* London: Wellcome Historical Medical Library, 1966.

Wear, Andrew. *Knowledge and Practice in English Medicine, 1550–1680.* Cambridge: Cambridge University Press, 2000.

Welch, Evelyn S. "Space and Spectacle in the Renaissance Pharmacy." *Medicina & Storia* (2011): 127–158.

Welch, Evelyn S. *Shopping in the Renaissance: Consumer Cultures in Italy, 1400–1600.* New Haven, CT: Yale University Press, 2005.

Wexler, Philip, ed. *Toxicology in the Middle Ages and Renaissance.* London: Academic Press, Elsevier, 2017.

Wheeler, Jo. *Renaissance Secrets, Recipes and Formulas.* London: Victoria and Albert Museum, 2009.

Whyte, Susan Reynolds, Sjaak van der Geest, and Anita Hardon. *Social Lives of Medicines.* New York: Cambridge University Press, 2002.

Wickersheimer, Ernest. "La thériaque céleste dite de 'Strasbourg.'" *Revue d'histoire de la pharmacie* 8, no. 25 (1920): 152–159.

Youyou, Tu. "The Discovery of Artemisinin (Qinghaosu) and Gifts from Chinese Medicine." *Nature Medicine* 17, no. 10 (2011): 1217–1220.

Zamuner, Ilaria. "Un volgarizzamento fiorentino *dell'Antidotarium Nicolai* (sec. XIII ex.)." In *L'Opera del Vocabolario Italiano per Pietro G. Beltrami*, edited by Pär Larson, Paolo Squillacioti, and Giulio Vaccar. Alessandria: Edizioni dell'Orso, 2013.

ACKNOWLEDGMENTS

I started this research during my graduate years at Yale University, under the mentorship of Paola Bertucci and Francesca Trivellato, a remarkable team of advisors, who offered insightful, rigorous, and consistent feedback, while giving me the freedom to experiment and develop my project in whatever direction I desired. I thank them together with John H. Warner, who also influenced me with his *Pharmaceutical Perspective*, his teachings, and his mentorship.

I am very thankful to Paula Findlen, whose pathbreaking *Possessing Nature* shaped my work. Without her affable, disinterested, and kind support, my early research would never have developed into this book. I am deeply grateful to Nick Terpstra, who saw the potential of my research and shared my vision for the project. I am also grateful to two anonymous reviewers for their insights, observations, and comments that helped me enrich this work. Of course, all responsibility for this volume remains my own.

Several organizations were kind enough to provide the time and support that enabled me to do the early research that eventually led to writing this book. My first archival research was funded by the John F. Enders Research Grant and the MacMillan Center Grant for International and Area Studies at Yale University. In 2020 the project was also funded by the American Institute of the History of Pharmacy (AIHP). The Research Institute of the University of Bucharest Fellowship for Young Researchers allowed me to revise the manuscript in 2022–2023, and I am grateful to Dana Jalobeanu and the wonderful community of scholars at ICUB in Bucharest. The time ICUB allowed me was crucial, and I am especially obliged for that. My confidence was boosted by the 2023 Reinerman Prize for the best unpublished manuscript, awarded by the Society for Italian Historical Studies, and the 2022 Santorio Award Honourable Mention, awarded by Centre for the Study of Medicine and the Body in the Renaissance, Pisa.

Chapters 2, 4, and 5 build on ideas first published in "The Triumph of Theriac: Print, Apothecary Publications, and the Commodification of Ancient Antidotes (1497–1800)," *Nuncius* 36, no. 2 (2021): 431–470.

At Yale I benefited from a lively academic community that offered generous feedback on some early drafts. Whether formally or informally, I could exchange ideas that helped me shape my project with mentors, friends, and colleagues. Among them—although many are no longer at Yale—I would like to thank especially Naomi Rogers, Bill Rankin, Henry M. Cowles, Melissa Grafe, Alan Mikhail, Carolyn Roberts, Catie Mas, Choon Hwee Koh, Jennifer Strtak and the Early Modern Interdisciplinary Graduate Lunch we created and ran, the Holmes Workshop, Ivano Dal Prete, Caroline Lieffers, Laurel Waycott, Alicia Peterson, Charlotte Abney, Tommaso Stefini, Sarah Pickman, Megann Licskai, and many others. I owe a lot to my friends Ian Hathaway and Justine Walden, who shared these years emotionally and intellectually.

I visited and contacted several archives and libraries in the course of my research, accruing many debts in the process. I owe thanks to Martina Caroli, Giovanna Flamma, Stefania Filippi, Elisa Pederzoli, Rita Bertani, Glenda Furini, Roberta Napoletano, and Giacomo Nerozzi at the Biblioteca Universitaria in Bologna; to Tiziana Di Zio, Massimo Giansante, Armando Antonelli, and Rita De Tata at the Archivio di Stato di Bologna; Michela Dal Pozzo at the Archivio di Stato di Venezia; Leonardo Mezzaroba, Cristina Crisafulli, and Monica Viero at Museo Correr; Orsola Braides and Elisabetta Sciarra at Biblioteca Marciana; Katja Piazza at the Archivio Diocesano of Udine; Laura Sbicego at the Civica Bertoliana of Vicenza; Maria Carmela Schisani at DISES Napoli; Giovanna Bergantino at the Biblioteca del Seminario di Padova; Emilio Lucia at the Museo Archeologico of Napoli; and Sarah Manthei at Städtische Museen Schloss Philippsruhe in Hanau.

Many thanks are due to several colleagues who helped me more than I can say. Patrick Wallis was especially generous in sharing records and offering comments on Chapter 5. Erica Ianiro, Antonio Mazzucco, Luca Massei, Noemi Di Tommaso, Sophia Spielmann, Beth Petitjean, Giovanni Mazzaferro, and Oana Baboi shared records, documents, or little trouvailles they came across during the course of their own research. Other colleagues engaged in fruitful conversations, shared information, or were especially kind during the pandemic when access to libraries was almost impossible. I am grateful to Francois Ledermann, Alisha Rankin, Paula De Vos, Nükhet Varlik, Sharon Strocchia, Frederick Gibbs, Lawrence Principe, Hjialmar Fors, Giovanni Bazzana, Maria Conforti, Maria Teresa Guerrini, Tillman Taape, Sandra Cavallo, Justin Rivest, Maria Fusaro, Umberto Signori, Barbara Orland, Andrea Mozzato, Francesca Rotelli, Nichola Harris, Katarzyna Pe̦kacka-Falkowska, Leonardo Terrusi, and the Associazione di storia della Farmacia Italiana. For Chapter 5, I also owe thanks to Matteo Viale, Alberto Guenzi, and Francesco Scalone. I also thank Giampiero Bettinetti, Michael Beckers at Dorotheum, Alex Helmstaedtern, Daniele Di Rosa, president of the APAE (Associazione Padovana Acquatologica Erpetologica), and Matteo di Nicola.

The support and friendship of my friend Sabrina Minuzzi, as well as my colleagues Danuta Raj, Jakub We̦glorz, and Fabrizio Baldassarri, have been invaluable over the last few years. I am deeply grateful to them. The Centro Prospero Alpini and the late Giuseppe Ongaro were particularly generous to me, and I wish to remember Professor Ongaro here with special affection.

Language issues and barriers required a lot of attention. Learning to write academically in a foreign language was a challenge for me. For support in this area, I thank James Tierney and all the writing partners at the Center for Teaching and Learning at Yale, especially Ila Tyagi, Marco Ladd, Joshua Metanko, and Breeanna Elliot. Joseph Bennet, Wendy Nelson, and Sherry Gerstein helped me with editing and copyediting, and I am also thankful to my friend Illisa Kellman. I am indebted to Paolo Pirini, Alberto Taccucci, and my dearest friend Giuliana Gambari for difficult passages translated from Latin. I thank Frank Griffel and Constantin Cless, as well as my affectionate friends Claudia Mazzocchi, Niamh Warde, and Franziska Ellinger, who helped me with German, Andrea van Leerdam, who helped with Dutch, and Justin Stearne and Anass Benmokhtar Razik for their help with Arabic. For digital elaboration of quantitative information, I thank Catherine De Rose and Damon Crockett from the Digital Humanities Lab at Yale, Christian Biasco and Luca Di Gennaro Splendore for Excel, and Russ Gasdia for helping me "scrape" book titles. At Harvard University Press, I thank Emily Silk, Stephanie Vyce, Sana Mohtadi, and Jillian Quigley for their work.

My dear aunt Paola Splendore has supported both me and my work in numerous ways, and I am deeply grateful for her generosity. During these years, Antonio Barocci has shown an inexhaustible sense of humor, supply of patience, and faith in life, which is the main reason this book could be achieved, and he remains my beloved husband. Mira Aurora and Neri had to grow up with theriac—I'll leave it to them to say whether it was harmful or beneficial. Whatever their verdict, it is about time we all take leave from it.

INDEX

Page numbers in italics refer to images.

Abanus, Peter, 167
Abati, Carlo Angelo, 75
abdominal cramps, 166
Abruzzo, 79
Academy of Science, French, 215
Academy of Science and Fine Letters, Neapolitan, 228, 229, 234
Accademia dei Lincei, 162
Accademia del Cimento, 123
Accoramboni, Francesco, 62, 105
account books, 213, 235
Ackerknecht, Erwin, 7, 232
Adrian, emperor, 96
Adriatic Sea, 213; ports, 212
Affaruosi, Giulio, 45
Agaricum albissimum, 59
Agathimero, Alessandro, 38, 42
age, aging, (of theriac), 54. *See also* fermentation
Alberghini, Antonio Maria, 134, 189–190
Albricci, Giovan Battista, 67
alchemy, 11, 34–35, 77, 94–95
Aldrovandi, Ulisse, 19, 26, 60, 78–79, 96, 98, 101, 115, 134, 147–148, 186, 221; activity to regulate apothecaries, 48, 106–110, 134, 159, 188–190; measures, 59; research on theriac, 44–45, 118
Aldrovandis, Paolo de, 196
Aleppo, 212
Alessandrini, Giulio, 119, 252n56
Aligine, Domenico, 188
alkermes, 121
Alpini, Prospero, 27, 130
Alps, 99, 216

Altucci, Agostino, 24
Al Zahrawi (Abulcasis), 32
Amfortas, knight, 53
amomum, 36, 42, 180–181
Anatolia, 211
ancien régime, 12, 16, 46, 202, 214, 230, 233, 238
ancient texts, 4, 10, 25, 186; for bioprospecting, 249n34
Ancona, 212
Andromachus the Elder, 19–20, 32, 36, 42, 43, 49, 66, 75–76, *80*, 87, *88*, 91–*92*, *126*, *129*, 130, *168*, 207, 208, 216
Andromachus the Younger, 66
An Duo. *See* Thomas, Antoine
animism (medical system), 213
Antigua, 151
Antoninus, emperor, 96
Antwerp, 151
Apennines, 79
apothecary, 250n16; Christmas gifts to, 186; Counsel of the Eight, 104; Florence guild, 263n53; guild, 14, 16, 23–24, 27, 29, 35–36, 40, 67, 69–70, 90, 99, 104, 106, 109, 111, 126, 130, 139, 159, 175–190, 194, 196–198, 224–225, 229, 233, 235, 239–240, 251, 269; inspections, 27, 67, 69, 70, 74, 104, 180, 188, 221, *224*, 229, 234, 259, 264, 281; "learned apothecaries," 14, 23, 46–49, 58, 61, 89–90, 92, 94–96, 99, 102, 105, 106, 111, 122–123, 138, 164, 176, 192, 239; statutes, 28, 67, 149, 189, 196–197, 251, 276n63, 278n112

325

apprentice. *See* apprenticeship
apprenticeship, 24, 106, 142, 171, 180
Ardoini, Sante, 34
Arezzo, 24
Arnald of Villanova, 33
arthritis, 31
Asclepius, 74-77, 260n103
Ascoli, 60
Assurbanipal, 76
asthma, 31
Atkins, John, 208
Austrian Empire. *See* Habsburg Empire
Austrian-Venetians provinces, 228
Averroes. *See* Ibn Rushd
Avicenna. *See* Ibn Sīnā
Azzoguidi, Germano, 218
Azzoguidi, Giuseppe, 217

Bacci, Andrea, 118
Baffo, Cecilia. *See* Nur Banu, sultana
Baghdad, 26
Bahia, 205-206
Bahunin, Caspar, 178
Baldi, Baldo, 122
balsam, New World, 95. *See also* opobalsamum
Barbados, 151
Barberini, Francesco, cardinal, 122, 123
Bartoli, Giorgio, 50
Bartolomeo from Orvieto, 77
Bayley, Walter, 50
bdellium resin, 53
Beaucaire fair, 24
Beauvais, Vincent de, 76, 260
beer, 55
Bellobuono, Galeno, 106
Bergamo, 52, 119
Bertioli, Antonio, 46, 47, 61, 144
Bible, Jewish, 77-78
biomedicine, 232, 242
bioprospecting, 205, 207. *See also* ancient texts
Bissingen, Ferdinand von, 228
bitter vetch, 58
bloodletting, 121
Bocchi, Simon, 143
Bolis, Giuseppe, 81, 226

Bologna, 6, 202, 218-220, 239-240; anatomical theater, 239; *Antidotarium*, 189; apothecaries and physicians, 105-111, 186-196; cardinal legate, 187; cardinal vice-legate, 190; Certosa, 194; church of San Salvatore, 134, 169, 189, 194; Collegio Medico, 57, 70, 135, 154, 176-184, 187-191, 193-197, 219, 224-225; convent of san Domenico, 194-195; convent of San Francesco, 192; cost of medicines, 162; cost of theriac, 153-158; hospital of Santa Maria della Morte, 138, 192, 195; lazaretto, 121; Opera de' Poveri Mendicanti, 162; production of theriac, 221-226; Senate, 5, 57, 187-190, 198, 218-220; theriac making ceremony, 134-139; university, 72, 99, 108, 134-135, 188, 196, 198, 214, 276n57; *virtues*, 169-171
Bontius, Jacobus, 54
Bonus, Petrus, 77
Bordeu, Théofile, 216
Borgarucci, Prospero, 105, 107, 110
botany, 97, 255
Bottoni, Albertino, 120
Boulliau, Ismael, 158
Boyle, Robert, 206, 215, 236
brand, branding (of theriac), 14, 22, 27, 29-30, 160, 233
Brazil, 205-206
Brescia, 62, 112, 119, 139, 141
British Empire, 3, 201, 208, 209
bronze serpent, 77
Broschi, Carlo, 57
Brosses, Charles de, 131
broth, 54, 170
Bruni, Domenico, 192
Bruno, Giordano, 37
Brunschwig, Hyeronimus, *127*
Bumaldi, Antonio. *See* Montalbani, Ovidio
Busti, Angelo, 178, 181-184
Butij, Michelangelo, 196
Byron, George, 25

Cairo, 26, 127, 211; Mosque called Morestan, 130
Calestani, Girolamo, 19, 20, 24, 47, 189

calumba, 208
Calvin, John, 77
Calzaveglia, Vincenzo, 119
Calzolari, Francesco, 20, 37, 38, 45–47, 96, 97, 105
Camerarius, Joachim the Elder, 44
Camerarius, Joachim the Younger, 102, 264n69
Campi, brothers, 183
Campolongo, Emilio, 120
Campolongo, Ottavio, 183
Canada, 221
Candariello, Santolillo, 79
Candrini, Gioseffo, 65, 140, 141
caper spurge, 28
Capodivacca, Girolamo, 117
Caracalla (emperor), 91
Cardullo, Gian Domenico, 135, 139
cassia (*cassia lignea*), 36, 59, 191
Castelli, Pietro, 135
cataplasm, 55, 120. See also *vescicatori*
Ceccarelli, Ippolito, 60
Çelebi, Evliya, 211
celebrations (publications), 14, 114, 134, 139–144, 237, 268
Celestial theriac, 35, 160–161, 201
Celsius, Aulus Cornelius, 30
certification(s), 61, 78, 80, 125, 126, 144, 159, 164, 227, 233, 236, 239
Cesena, 141
Champier, Symphorien, 42, 43
Charas, Moyse, 123–125, 214–215
charity, 100, 162, 163
charlatans, 11, 43, 45, 48, 67, 131, 145, 163, 169, 174, 237; counterpoison, 114; handbills, 164, 165, 172; licenses, 100, 217; prices, 153, 158; wares, 16, 25
Charles V, Habsburg emperor
Charles IX, Valois, king, 96
China, 55, 209, 217, 230; imperial court of, 1, 13, 210
China electa, 158
Choch, Pietro, 213
Christ, 51, 75–78, 83, 220, 241; *Christus medicus*, 78; as snake, 77
Christina of Sweden, queen, 131
Cinelli Calvoli, Giovanni, 122

clay, 59, 121; red clay from Armenia, *68*
Clement VIII, pope, 190
Clusius, Carolus, 107
Coch, Pietro, 213
collections, *21*, 27, 46, 135, 138, 175, 276n69
Colli Euganei, 80–83, 241
Cologne, 24
Colombo. *See* Sri Lanka
colonial empires. *See* colonization
colonization, 3, 13, 204, 211, 230, 242, 278n10; colonial subjects, 228
Commiphora opobalsamum. *See* opobalsamum
Commiphora wightii. *See* bdellium resin
contagion, 116, 118
container (of theriac), 54, 159; falsified, 227; tin, 178; unsold, 229; wrapped, 165
Conventioni, 190–191, 194, 276n75. *See also* regulation
Corcullo, 79
cordons sanitaires, 5, 113
Cordus, Euricius, 42–43
Corniani, Galeazzo, 40
Cortona, 77
Costa, Filippo, 62, 138, 147
costus (*costus odoratus*), 36, 42, 91
cough, 166
counterfeiting (of theriac), 25, 27, 28, 37, 69, 125, 146, 152, 159, 160, 172, 206, 212–213, 227, 229, 234
Couplet, Philippe, 209
Crasso, Paolo, 102–103, 105, 110
Crete, 40, 180
Croce, Giovanni, 166
crucifixion, 76, 83
cubeba, 208
Cyperus longus, 91
Cyprus, 24, 40, 180, 212
Cytinus hypocistis, 59

Dal Buono, Hercole, 72–73, 75
Dalmatian coast, 213
Damocrates, 40, 41, 65, 91, 142
Danzig, 107, 153
daryakan, 209
dead fetus, 166

deliyage, 1, 209
Della Rovere, Francesco Maria II, 120; Guidobaldo II, 105
de Luca, Gaetano, *126*
Denmark, 161
Descazals, Jacques, 214
De Sgobbis, Antonio, 59, 160, 165
Discalced Carmelites, 231
distilled waters, 11, 95, 197
Doglioni, Niccolò, 166
Dominichini brothers (trial), 69–74
Donati, Marcello, 138
Donato, Andrea, 26
Dondini, Sigismundo, 108
Donzellini, Girolamo, 117, 119
dosing, 59, 121; dose (of theriac), 25, 55, 59, 121, 153, 156, 157, 159, *173*, 195, 248n26, 257n31
Drimia maritima. *See* maritime squill
Duchesne, André, 160
Du Chesne, Joseph, 160–161
dunameis, 30. *See also* virtues

earths. *See* clay
Eastern Mediterranean, 26, 127, 211–212, 226, 233
East India Company, 152
edema, 166
effectiveness (of theriac), 25, 113, 119, 120, 122, 123, 125, 144; of medicaments, 216, 219, 238–240; social and biological, 3, 6–9, 50, 176, 238
Egypt, 20, 26–27, 127–130, 211
Egyptian theriac, 23, 26–27, 30, 106, 127–130, 211, 233
ekaweriya, 208
Eleonora di Toledo, 94–95
Emo, Angelo, 212
empirics, 67, 100, 145
Encyclopédie, 216, 266n11
England, 15, 24, 29, 100, 148–149, 151–152, 208, 216, 230, 251
environmental impact (of theriac production), 14, 52, 241
epilepsy, 31
Erculiani, Camilla, 7, 47
Eschenbach, Wolfram von, 53
Euphorbia lathyrism. *See* caper spurge

Evelyn, John, 152
exotica (materia medica from places considered "exotic"), 5, 10, 16, 61, 180–181, 214, 235; "exotic" drugs or remedies, 55, 148, 151, 152, 158, 237
experiment, 9, 15, 20, 42, 47, 94, 95, 123, 124, 158, 169, 177, 178, 183, 186, 194, 214, 217, 248n21, 249n31
exports, 28, 148; ban, 15, 117; of cheese, 139; duties, 178; of medicaments, 205; of theriac, 14, 24, 29, 149, 151, 152, 159, 167, 182, 185, 186, 201, 211–213, 242; of tyrus, 36; of vipers, 75, 79, 80
Extractum china, 158
Extractum guaiacum, 158

Faber, Johannes, 162–163, 237
Fabrici d'Acquapendente, Girolamo, 120
fake theriac. *See* counterfeiting
Falconieri, Alessio, 142
Fantasti, Giovanni, 122
Farinelli. *See* Broschi, Carlo
Farnese, Ranuccio I, 108
Farnese, Vittoria, 105
fede, 61, 78, 143
Ferdinando, Epifanio, 147
fermentation, 9, 32, 59, 65, 70, 182
Ferrara, 25, 42, 96, 105, 108, 148, 213; university, 38
fevers, 31; pestilential, 119; putrid, 120, 166
Ficino, Marsilio, 34, 53
Fioravanti, Leonardo, 55, 116, 236
Fiorentini, Francesco Maria, 121, 124, 216, 236
Florence, 6, 44, 48, 93, 95–96, 100, 120–123, 142, 148, 158, 178, 248n21, 262, 263; Collegio Medico, 59; A Giglio shop, 25, 148; monastery of Nunziatina, 55; Pharmacology Institute, 54; pharmacopoeia, 262
Fonderie, 95
Fontaney, Jean de, father, 55
Fonte, Moderata, 166
forgeries (of theriac). *See* counterfeiting
formula (list of ingredients), 140, 259n78

formulas (publications), 66, 67, *68*, 69, 164, 237
Foscari, Francesco, 212, 213
Fracastoro, Girolamo, 36
fragments of Hyacinthus prepared (remedy), 158
France, 4, 24, 42, 78, 96; king of, 110, 140, 203
Frankfurt, 161
Friuli, 62, 81
Fulginate, Pellegrino, 77

galangal (*Alpinia officinarum*), 181
Galasso, Mario di Marino, 162
Galen of Pergamon, 10, 25, 30-34, 36, 42-44, 47, 58, 66, 71, 75, 78, *80*, 83, 92-93, 95, 119, *126*, 146, 162, 165-167, 174; Galenic texts, 181, 182, 252n56. *See also* medicine
Galvani, Luigi, 218-22, 238
Galvano from Levanto, 77
Gambia, 208
Gandino, 23
Garzoni, Tommaso, 48
Gassel, Johan, 217
Geneva, 161
Genoa, 24, 28, 93, 112, 151, 250
German States (Germany), 11, 24, 42, 75, 77, 80, 94, 101, 126, 140-141, 161, 185, 266n11
Ghini, Luca, 101, 263
Gibraltar, 151
Giessen, 161
Giustizia Vecchia, 28-29, 37, 39-41, *68*, 130, 149-*150*, 157, 159, 179-180, 184-185, 197, 226, 251, 270n18
Goa, 210
Goldoni, Carlo, 220
Gonzaga (family), 107, 138; Ferdinando I, 97, 158; Francesco (duke), 97; Vespasiano, 45
Gonzaga Nevers, Ferdinando Carlo, 158
Goodwin, James, 209
Gorizia, 213
Grandi, Domenico, 159
Grand Tour, 131
Gregory XIII, pope, 95, 190

Greiff, Frederic, 161, 273n82
Grimm, Hermanus Nicolaas, 207
guaiacum wood, 10
Guarguanti, Orazio, 56, 166
Guenther, Johann, 44
Guilandino, Melchiorre (Guilandinus, Melchior Weiland), 26-27, 101
Guild. *See* apothecary

Habsburg Empire, 110, 231
Hanau, 161
Hanover, 161
headaches. *See* migraines
health, 19, 26, 46, 50, 97, 98, 143, 185, 187, 192; board, 5, 116-117, 120, 143, 179, 213, 234; business, 145, 157; care, 15, 194, 240, 242; common, 95; documents, 270n119; hazards to, 100; magistrate, 15; passport, 5; pharmacy as tool for, 109; for the poor, 193; public, 97, 112-118, 144, 233, 236-237
heating qualities (of theriac), 31, 53, 57, 83
Heberden, William, 2, 114, 201, 202
herbalist, 46, 51, 108
herbarium, 51
Hercules, 92
heresy, 4, 109
heretics. *See* heresy
Hippocrates, *80*, 92, 93, 117, *128*, 130
Hoffmann, Friedrich, 214
Hoffmann, Moritz, 56
Holy Land, 26
honey, 16, 40, 52-53, 58, 65, 73-74, 97, 152, 158-159, 176-186, 198, 252
hospital, 138, 148, 162-163, 192, 195, 207, 211, 213, 229, 237, 251n27
Houel, Nicolas, 96
hyacinthus, 121

iatrochemestry, 213
Ibn Juljul, 32
Ibn Rushd (Averroes), 33
Ibn Sīnā (Avicenna), 9, 32-33, 38, 39, 41-42, 65, *80*, 106, 167
Illinois nation, 205

Imperato, Ferrante, 45–47, 78, 101–104, 107, 147
India, 55, 91, 206, 212
inventories, 23, 147–148, 235
Istanbul, 26, 60, 211–212

Jateorhiza palmata. See calumba
Jesuits, 30, 205, 206, 208, 209, 210
juniper berries, 66

Kangxi (emperor), 1, 210, 242
Kassel, 161
kidney stones, 31
knowledge embodied, 71, 239; sensory, 69–74

labels, 19, 54, 80, 151, 213, 234
lacrima (*Liquidambar orientalis Mill.*), 181
Larnaca, 212
La Salle, Robert de, 205
Lassels, Richard, 152
Lavoranti, Lauro de', 45
Law, John, 220
lazaretto, 5, 55, 113, 116, 118, 120–121, 144, 236, 267n43
Leanciani, Domenico, 73
Leghorn, 151
Leiden, 54
Lémery, Nicolas, 215
Leoniceno, Niccolò, 38–39
levantine musk, 158
licorice, 91
Lizhong tang, 1
lower classes, 7, 44, 146, 159, 191, 204, 237; social perception of, 221
Lucca, 40, 48, 93, 121, 183, 192
Lyon, 140

Macau, 210
Machiavelli, Nicolò, 95, 96
Madagascar, 205. *See also* Port Dauphin
Magliabecchi, Antonio, 56
malabathrum, 36
Malacca, 180
Mantua, 6, 48, 97, 107, 112–113, 118, 120, 138, 148, 158, 180, 192
manual, 107; apothecary, 19, 39, 105; theriac, 101–102

Maranta, Bartolomeo, 8, 57, 61, 65, 92, 98, 101–105, 107, 110, 160
Marburg, 161
Marche, 154
Marcus Aurelius, 31, 91, 96, 204
Marinelli, Curzio, 183–184
Marini, Andrea, 106
maritime squill, 58
Marsi (people), 79
Martinelli family, 40; Cechino, 39–41; Francesco (Cechino) Jr., 180 (*see also* Mostravero); Francesco (Cechino) Sr., 180; Zuan Alberto, 41
Martin V (pope), 26
Maryland, 151
Masini, Antonio, 134–135
Masini, Margherita, 55
Massaria, Alessandro, 120
materia medica, 6, 10–12, 27, 35, 37, 40–41, 43–44, 46, 49, 60, 71, 79, 90, 94, 106, 108–110, 131, 135, 151, 177, 180, 183, 187, 201, 204–205, 207, 209, 213
Mattia, Elia, 142
Mattioli, Pier Andrea, 43–46, 74, 78, 95, 101, 112, 252, 255
Maximilian II, emperor, 102
Medici (family), 5; Cosimo I, 94; Cosimo II, 97; Cosimo III, 56; Ferdinando, 95; Francesco, 95; Leopoldo II, 158
Medici-Gonzaga, Eleonora de', 55, 158
medicine, 78; Ayurvedic, 208; Galenic, 3, 11–12, 83, 165, 172; humoral, 10, 30–31, 34, 117, 169, 172, 178, 214; magical, 78; neo-Hippocratic, 217; preventive, 51, 56, 164; rational, 32, 83, 92–93, 98, 232; religious, 76, 98, 261n11
Mediterranean Sea, countries, 11, 32, 230; cultural roots, 3; exchanges across, 27; pharmacopoeias, 107; plants, 12
Meibomius, Heinrich, 215
melancholy, 166
Melich, Georg, 46–48, 58, 105–107, 110, 130, 166
Menegacci, Vendramino, 95, 139, 140, 142–143

Mercuriale, Girolamo, 117, 120, 130, 166, 252
Mesagne, 147
Messina, 122, 135, 139
Mesue, 44, 66, 71, 106, 162, 165
Metastasio, Pietro, 57
Middle East, 1, 10, 32, 40, 76, 87
migraines, 31, 166, 218
Ming dinasty, 209
Mithradates Eupator IV, king, 4, 87, 91–92, 94, 96, *129*, 130, 143, 162, 192, 261
Modena, 118, 140–141, 143, 156, 159
Moderatione, 189. *See also* regulation
Mongio, Paolo, 106
monopoly (on theriac), 159, 197, 228, 229
Monselice castle, 80
Montagnana, Bartolomeo, 39
Montalbani, Ovidio, 162, 192, 193, 277n91
Montpellier, 33, 104, 125
mortars, 62, 77, 131–132, 220
Moseley, Joseph, 208
Moses, 77, 260
Mostravero, Asdrubale, 183. *See also* Martinelli, Francesco Jr.
Mousnier, Jean-Francois, 205
mumia, 210
musk, 26, 158

Nancy (France), 57
Naples, 6, 44–46, 48, 93, 99, 101–105, 110, 122, 192, 229, 230, 233, 264, 281; kingdom of, 202, 228, 238; king of, 222, 228
nardo indicae, 66
Nascimbeni, Baccio, 78
Neckam, Alexander, 77
Nero, emperor, 4, 20, 87, *88*, 91, 134, *170*, 204
Netherlands, 140, 151, 152, 207
Nicander of Colophon, 36, 44, 98, 263
normative model of intoxication, 6
nuns, 55, 56, 194, 257
Nur Banu, sultana, 26
Nuremberg, 12, 44, 101, 122, 127, 159, 161, 202, 215
nutmeg oil, 66, 226

Oddo, Marco, 72, 102–103, 105, 110
oil, 54, 179, 197
Olmo, Fabio, 182–184
opium, 1, 8–9, 20, 53, 58, 62, 65, 75, 97, 158, 161, 213–214, 248n21, 248n26
opobalsamum, 36, 42, 59, 60–61, 66, 74, 95, 122–123, 226
opopanax (*Opopanax chironium*), 53
Origanum dictamnus, 59
origin story (of theriac), 4, 14, 51–52, 75–78, 83, 89, 91–93, 111, 220, 235
Orimbelli, Angelo, 121
orviétan, 162–163, 205
Ottoman Empire, 27, 201, 204, 211, 213, 242; court, 212; officials, 212

Padua, 6–7, 25, 44–45, 47, 48, 78, 80–*81*, 96–97, 99, 101–106, 110–112, 117, 122, 141, 148, 161, 166, 179, 214; botanical garden, 26; Collegio Medico, 104–105; university, 74–75, 105, 120, 178, 214
Paglia, Angelo, 44
Paitoni, Giambattista, 217
Palazzi, Giuseppe, *223*
Paleotti, Camillo, 134
Paleotti, Gabriele, cardinal, 60, 134
Palissy, Bernard, 236
Palladio, 139
palsy, 31
panacea, 2, 172, 232, 266n11
Panciroli, Guido, 35
Pannei, Giuseppe, 160
Paracelsus, 11, 34
Paris, 43, 96, 104, 125, *129*, 158, 202, 258
Parma, 47, 107–108, 143, 148, 183, 189
Parzival, 53
Passarowitz, treaty of, 212
Patent, 11, 65, 140, 227, 234
Patin, Guy, 215, 236
Paul, Vincent de, 205
Paul III, pope, 44
pauliani, 77
Paul the Apostle, 77
Peretti, Felice. *See* Sixtus V, pope
Persia, 211
Perugia, 44
Peruvian bark, 208, 213
pest house. *See* lazaretto

pestles, 62, 127
Peter the Great, czar, 210
pharmacology, 11, 214, 252n57
pharmacopoeias (non-official), 9, 59, 62, 65–66, 74, 107, 205, 217, 234; *Antidotarium Nicolai*, 66, 107, 258n70; Borgarucci, 105, 107; De Sgobbis, 59, 160, 165; Melich, 166; Sumerian, 76
pharmacopoeias (official), 5, 7, 9, 59, 65–66, 100, 104, 202–203, 216; Bologna, 109, 117, 156, 187–190, 194–195; Edinburgh, 202; Florence, 262n21; French, 216; lack of, 217; London, 202, 217; Milan, 65; Parma and Piacenza, 47; Rome, 60; Sri Lanka (Dutch), 207, 209, 216; Strasbourg, 161; Venice, 7, 183–184, 228, 275n42
pharmacy, alchemical, 10–11, 35; Christian, 206; Galenic, 2, 3, 9–13, 197, 201–206, 209, 211, 214–215, 217, 219, 230, 233, 241–242; spagyric, 197
philology, 10, 36, 39, 41, 44
Piacenza, 47, 167
Piccinelli, Filippo, 78
Pisa, 27, 28, 101
Pisanelli, Baldassarre, 112
placebo effect, 218
plague, 2, 5, 8, 19, 29, 33, 42, 54–55, 113, 115, 117–120, 147, 153–154, 166–167, 236; of 1575–77, 96, 112–113, 117–118, 144, 236; of 1630, 15, 99, 113, 118, 120–122, 144, 236; Black Death, 33, 116; etiology, 117; measures against, 116–118; and poison, 34, 120
Platen Hallermünde, August von, 131
Pliny, 38, 87, 89
poison, 2, 4, 31, 33–34, 37, 45, 55, 77, 79, 87, 97–98, 112–115, 117–120, 123–124, 142, 144, 166, 208, 216, 219, 253, 262n17; powders, 94; snake venom in Western science, 75
Poitiers, 79
Poland, *81*, 140
Polani, Giovanni, 121
polypharmacy, 215, 217
Pompey (Gneus Pompeius Magnus), 4, 87, 91, 201

Pona, Giovanni, 61
populuxe, 163, 273n95
Port Dauphin, (Madagascar), 205
Portuguese Empire, 201, 204–208
Posi, Paolo, *222*
Preti, Ludovico, 227–228
price, of theriac, 15, 21, 24–25, 153–156, 158, 162–163, 172, 195, 197, 209, 229, 237; changes, 154; of drugs, 48, 158, 181; series, 157; of wheat, 156, 157
production of theriac, 24–29, 42, 45, 47, 49, 51–52, 57–65, 81–83, 90, 91, 95, 121–122, 124–139, 143, 144, 147–152, 164, 167, 172, 175–187, 194–198, 203, 204, 212–214, 221–230, 231–241
Protomedici, 69–72, 104, 120, 122, 134, 141, *170*, 180, 189, 191–192, 194–195, 217–218, 221, 225, 229, 259n82; Bologna, 268n82
Puglia, 147, 213
Pulci, Luigi, 25
purge, 55, 92

Qing dynasty, 209–210
quarantine, 5, 113, 116
Quattrami, Evangelista, 46, 47, 75, 106, 108–110
quid pro quo. See substitution

Rabelais, François, 25
Ramazzini, Bernardino, 217
Ramponi, Domenico, *136*
Ramusio, Giovan Battista, 36, 38, 40–41
Rauwolfa serpentina. See ekaweriya
reconstruction (of theriac), 9, 249n31
Redi, Francesco, 75, 79, 123, 124, 214, 216
regulation, and Aldrovandi, 265n99; consumer goods, 28; medical, 100, 111, 190, 232, 234; pharmaceutical, 27, 109, 180, 189, 251n35; theriac, 15, 23, 28–29, 41, 225, 251n42. See also *Conventioni*
Republic of Letters, 158, 187, 190
Riccardi, Adriano, 61, 192
Robustelli brothers, 212
Romagna, 154
Rome, 6, 23–24, 29, 44, 47–48, 76, 78, 93, 96–97, 101, 107, 122–123, *126*,

135, 153–154, 157, 178, 206, 229, 237, 248n21; Aracoeli monastery, 194; Collegio Medico, 122; Collegio Romano, 131; Festival of Chinea, 221; hospital of Santo Spirito, 162–163; Jesuit headquarters, 207; Santa Maria alla Scala pharmacy (Trastevere), 231; university of, 162
Rossetti, Fortunato, 158
Royal African Company, 201, 208–209
Royal Society, 217
Royal Society for the Promotion of the Natural Sciences (Istituto di Incoraggiamento). *See* Academy of Science and Fine Letters, Neapolitan
Ru Huang, 1
rum, 54
Russian Empire, 201, 204, 209–210, 242
Rutta, Clemente, 167–*168*

Sacchi, Defendente, 231
Salerno, 104, 229
San Domenico Abate, 73
Sartorio, Francesco, 138, 143, 192
Sassetti, Filippo, 55
Sassonia, Ercole, 120
Savonarola, Michele, 25
Scalcina, Herculano, 141
Scribonius Largus, 30
seals (of theriac), 28, 54, 213, 227, 229
secrets, medicines, 100, 114; books of, 145, 162
Semedo, João Curvo, 206
Septimius Severus, emperor, 91, 96
Settala, Ludovico, 99, 120, 236
Severino, Marco Aurelio, 75, 123
Sicily, 23, 112
Sixtus V, pope, 118
skink, 74
smell (of theriac), 51, 53–54, 70–71, 82, 232, 241
snakebites, 77, 123
social order, 3–5, 175, 193, 240, 242; cohesion, 144, 233–234
Societé libre de Pharmaciens de Paris, 202
Sozzi, Jacopo, 79
Spada, Bernardino, cardinal, 121

Spada, Virgilio, father, 121
spicae nardi, 66
spleen, 158
Sprechi, Pompeo, 143, 182–183
Sri Lanka, 207
state building, 15, 94, 236, 241
Stecchini, Alberto, 159
Stein, Michael, 7
Sterlich, Romualdo de, 56
Stigliola, Nicola, 103–104, 123
storax, 36, 275n22
Störck, Anton von, 218
Strasbourg, *127*, 161
substitution, 12, 61, 181
Succi, falsifier of theriac, 213
sugar, 27, 45
Sweden, 161
symbolism, religious, 14
syphilis, 10, 158
Syria, 24, 26, 38–39, 180
syrup, 121, 147, 158, 191, 217

tariffs, 154, 157, 234
Tasso, Torquato, 97
taste (of theriac), 14, 51, 53–54, 70–71, 82, 241
Tavernier, Jean-Baptiste, 211–212
tea, 54
Tempesta, Antonio, *81*
Teodosio, Giovanni Battista, 42–43
terra lemnia, 59
terra sigillata. *See* clay
Terzi, Aleardo, *136*
Teucrium scordium, 59
Theofrastus, 36
Theriaca coelestis. *See* Celestial theriac
Theseus, 92
Thessaloniki, 212, 213
thlaspi (possibly field pennycress or *Thlaspi arvense*), 53
Thomas, Antoine, 1
Thorn, 153
Thucydides, 115
Thunberg, Carl Peter, 207
Thyrrenian Sea, 79
Tomas de Cantimpré, 76
Torti, Francesco, 217
Trent, 48; council of, 134

Trevisano, Bernardino, 102, 103, 110
Treviso, 81
Triaga brasilica, 205–207, 209, 279n22
Trieste, 212, 213
trocisci, 39, 58–59; *hedicroi*, 47, 58; *scyllitici*, 59, 62; *viperini*, 39, 42, 75, 79, 80–81, 135
Trumbull, William, 212
trust, 55, 110, 235, 236, 240, 258n68
Tubingen, 161, 273n82
Tuscia, 60
tyrus snake, 26, 37–38, 76, 254

United East India Company (VOC), 207
Urbino, 44, 75, 96
urine, 54, 162

vaccines, 4, 219
Valdagni, Giuseppe, 119
Valgrisi, Vincenzo, 43, 78
Varè, Vincenzo, 139, 226
Vasi, Giuseppe, *223*
Venel, Gabriel-François, 216
Venice, 5–6, 9, 13–14, 16, 22–29, 37–42, 46, 48–49, 52, 56, 60, 122, 125, 135, 141, 148, 152, 168, 175–187, 192, 198, 206, 212, 217, 220, 221, 226–229, 231, 233, 235, 239; Austrian governor of, 7; Avogaria di Comun, 184; charlatans, 158, 169; Collegio dei Savij, 5; Collegio Medico, 29, 38–41, 81, 166, 226; commercial network, 6, 22, 28, 40, 89; Golden Head apothecary shop, *132*, 213, 232; Rialto bridge, 28, 131–*132*, 232; Signoria, 5, 185, 186; theriac ceremonies, 127–134, 146; *Treacle of*, 149–150, 151
venom. *See* poison

vermin, 166
Verona, 27, 36, 44, 45, 48, 81, 112, 141, 148; Collegio Medico, 61
vertigo, 166
vescicatori, 120, 121. *See also* cataplasm
Vicenza, 6, 81, 113, 138–141, 143; Collegio Medico, 95; Palazzo della Ragione, 139
Vicia ervilia. *See* bitter vetch
Vincenti, Giacomo, 166
viper, 1, 14, 20, 23, 26, 36–39, 51, 59, 74, 78–*80*, 82, 115, 123–124, 161–162, 166, 196, 216, 231; cost of, 261n128; symbolism, 74, 76–77
viperai, snake-catchers, 79–81, 231
Virginia (state), 151
virtues (drug's qualities), 9, 32, 73, 75, 122, 161, 165, 167, 169–172, 207, 215
virtues (publications), 15, 16, 146, 163–174, 213, 237, 273n96
vitalism (medical system), 213
Voiture, Vincent, 57

Washington, George, 54
water, 54
wax, 28, 197
wine, 54, 55, 56, 58, 62, 70, 74, 76, 81, 170, 178
Woodall, John, 152
World Health Organization (WHO), 74
Wroclaw, 53
Württemberg, 161

Yuan dinasty, 209

Zanella, Girolamo, 75, 80–81
Zilli, Derviş Mehmed, 211
Zwinger, Jacob, 183